Oral Bioscience

An Authors OnLine Book

First published by Churchill Livingstone 1999

Cover layout by James Fitt

ISBN 0 7552 0229 5

Authors OnLine Ltd
19 The Cinques
Gamlingay, Sandy
Bedfordshire SG19 3NU
England

Preface

Clinical dentistry will be able to adapt to a rapidly changing world only if it is based upon a sound understanding of the structure, metabolism and function of the oral tissues, and this understanding must itself be placed in the context of these being specific examples or specialisations of the structure, metabolism and function of the body as a whole. Such understanding should be not only of the healthy and normal but should also include a knowledge of the effects of microbiological and pathological interactions with tissues.

As new techniques become available the scientific basis of dentistry extends and our understanding becomes at once more detailed and more integrated. Whilst research journals provide the cutting edge information and specialised monographs synthesise state of the art reviews of segments within the field of study, there remains a place for books and other media which can present an integrated view across the whole scientific basis of clinical dentistry. The earliest works of this kind were almost entirely structural in their approach, reflecting the state of dental research at the time. Little change occurred up to the middle of the twentieth century. At least one textbook of 'special, or dental, anatomy, histology and embryology' in use in the 1950s had seen its first edition 50 years earlier and showed little change in approach from that first edition. Textbooks of general anatomy, biochemistry or physiology paid little attention to the special needs of dentistry.

After World War II the great extension of scientific research and knowledge in the basic dental sciences resulted in Britain in the publication of two books which changed the emphasis of dental education. One of these was a general basic science book written specifically for dentists (Anderson D J 1952 *Physiology for Dental Students* Edward Arnold, London), the other a book extending the 'special or dental' basis into the areas of biochemistry and physiology (G N Jenkins 1954 *The Physiology of the Mouth* Blackwell, Oxford). This latter which was renamed *The Physiology and Biochemistry of the Mouth*, became a classic text for research workers and students, remaining a valuable reference source even 20 years after the publication of the fourth and last edition. A massive multi-author text from Harvard (Shaw J H, Sweeney E A, Cappuccino C C, Meller S M 1978 *Textbook of Oral Biology* Saunders, Philadelphia), followed much later, but never attained the wide readership of *The Physiology and Biochemistry of the Mouth*. Since then the trend has been towards producing books covering the whole area of a basic science — particularly biochemistry — with oral biology sections (such as

Williams R A D, Elliot J C 1979 *Basic and Applied Dental Biochemistry* 1st edn. Churchill Livingstone, Edinburgh), or to extending the coverage of dental anatomy/histology texts (such as Ten Cate A R 1998 *Oral Histology* 4th edn. Mosby, St Louis or Schroeder H E 1991 *Oral Structural Biology* Thieme, Stuttgart), into the biochemical and functional fields.

There remains, however, a need for a book to integrate histological and biochemical information with our knowledge of the physiology of the oral cavity. The techniques of immunocytochemistry, of molecular biology and genetic research have transformed understanding of many biological phenomena and are likely to be the foundation of future advances in clinical dentistry. Although much of the material in this present book is informed by these advances, my original intention to devote chapters to molecular biology and genetics proved impracticable because of the patchy nature of our current knowledge.

I have tried here to put oral structure and metabolism in the context of oral function, and the arrangement of the book results from this. The first section deals with oral tissues and structures but even then must include the background of calcium metabolism and complexities of the process of calcification. The second section becomes more functional in looking at secretions, deposits on the tooth surface, their metabolism and their significance in dental disease, and then the related areas of nutrition and the effects of fluoride. The final section is structural and functional, dealing with the mechanisms of oral sensation, of the activity of the oral structures in food intake and in speech, and the effects of ageing upon oral function. Inevitably, the outline of this book has become very similar to that of *The Physiology and Biochemistry of the Mouth*. This present book does not pretend to be a successor to that work, although it does reflect the subsequent increase in knowledge; it is aimed primarily at a student audience. Thus the lists of further reading include reviews and monographs but not original papers, and I have deliberately not referenced original work. This was a difficult decision, but I believe that the average student reader finds references distracting rather than helpful. Perhaps the versatility of modern electronic media should provide a 'book' to be read at several levels. In the meantime, I hope that *Oral Bioscience* will provide today's students and practitioners with an overview of the state of our knowledge of the basis of oral function.

David B. Ferguson — Manchester 1998

Acknowledgements

I must acknowledge, firstly, the debt I owe to Dr Adrian Shuttleworth for his advice, reading of many early versions of the manuscript, and his patient correction of my idiosyncratic views on some biochemical topics, and secondly, the generosity of Dr David Whittaker in searching out and allowing me to use illustrative photomicrographs from his collection. All but a small number of the photographic illustrations come from him. Of remainder, Figures 3.4, 6.1a and b, 6.2 and 11.8 were provided by Mr M. Mahon of the School of Biological Sciences, Manchester University; Figures 4.1a and b and 5.3 were provided by Dr M. Watt of the Glasgow Dental Hospital and School and Figures 8.1, 8.2, 8.3 and 8.5 are reproduced with permission from Gibbs Oral Hygiene Service slide set, 'Plaque the Unseen Enemy'. I am deeply grateful to all of these. The originals of the line drawings were all produced by myself.

Contents

Errata and Corrigenda

p.5 *Table 1.1* Units should be mg/100 g for Ca and P and Vitamin D
p.17 *line 16* for "2% of its volume", substitute "3-5% of its volume"
p.24 for "cells from the future pulp" substitute "preodontoblasts from the future pulp"
p 21 *Table 2.1* for "1,25 DHC" read "1,25 $(OH)_2D_3$".
p.27 *Fig. 2.6b* Caption: omit "calcifying" Label: for "apatite crystals" substitute "collagen fibrils"
p.32 *Fig 2.3*: all numbers in elastic modulus column should be x 10^4.
p.34 and subsequently: for "Calcified tissues" substitute "mineralised tissues"
p.34 *line 4* in The fibres of..: for "some" substitute "some 11%."
p.36 *line 17* for "epithethial" substitute "epithelial"
p.49 *lines 7 and 10* for "tranform(s)" read "transform(s)"
p.55 insert after "insulin growth factor beta" abbreviation "(IGFβ)"
p.68 "when secretion beings" should be "when secretion begins"
p.61 *line 9* omit "as" and *line 12* omit "some writers prefer to call it the dental organ"
p.62 and 63 *Figs. 3.8 and 3.9* Labels on figure should be outer and inner enamel epithelium and not external and internal. *Caption to 3.9* for "calcification" substitute "formation"
p.63 *line 9* for "calcification" substitute "mineralisation"
p.65 Title – for "calcification" substitute "mineralisation"
p.69 *Fig 3.11b* Caption: for "wide intercellular space" substitute "narrow intercellular space"
p.70 6 lines from bottom for "Protein synthesis occurs in the RER" read "Protein synthesis occurs on the ribosomes of the RER"
4 lines from bottom "Phophorylation" should be "phosphorylation"
p.87 Neurotrophic substances *line 2* add abbreviation for nerve growth factor "(NGF)"
p.110 *Fig 5.7* "drft" should be "drift"
p.124 *line 19* "parasympathetic" should be "sympathetic" in both instances on this line
Margin note 3 for "by taste and smell" substitute "by intraoral mechanical and taste stimuli, and by smell"
p.125 *line 9* for "saliva" substitute "oral fluid". This statement may not be true of all salivary glands.
p.132 *Fig 6.10* for "Lysozome" substitute "lysozyme"
p.133 *line 7* for "intercalated duct" substitute"striated duct"
p.136-138 *Table 6.3* MG1 add "(=MUC5B)", for MG2 add "(=MUC7)"
p.143 Mucins *line 3* add "However, mucins usually contain at least 70% carbohydrate." line 11 substitute "MG2 (MUC7) has 54 potential O-glycosidic chains and 5 potential N-chains"
p.144 add at end of page "The N-part of lactoferrin is a basic protein with bacteriocidal activity." SLP1 is only one of the salivary proteins involved in HIV inactivation. Histatins are also bacteriocidal to S. Mutans.
p.146 The greater part of the bloodgroup substance in saliva is present in the oligosaccharide chains of the mucins, particularly MG1. Blood group status can therefore be determined in saliva for 80% of the population.
p.147 Margin *note 1* for "hence more calcium" substitute "hence more mucins and calcium"
p.150 In periodontal disease oral fluid contains more albumin, and cystatin and cystatin C activity is increased
p.188 Dietary modification *line12* after "involved" add " in the different groups"
p.195 The discovery of the effects of fluoride line19 "pubic" should be "public"
p.206 *lines 14-15* for "is more soluble than hydroxyapatite" substitute "is more easily lost than if it were incorporated into hydroxyapatite"

SECTION ONE

Oral hard and soft tissues

1 Calcium and phosphorus metabolism

The importance of calcium in the body

Calcium has many vital roles in the body

Calcium, in both ionised and non-ionised forms, is arguably one of the most important body components. The rigidity of the skeleton, which provides support and protection for the soft tissues of the body and enables human beings to stand, carry out movements and move from place to place by acting as a firm base for muscle contraction, depends entirely upon the aggregation of hard crystals of calcium phosphate. Teeth, essential structures for the initial processing of food, are made up of dental enamel and dentine, whose hardness and fitness for purpose is again due to the crystals of calcium phosphate of which they are composed. Even the retention of the teeth in the jaws depends upon the anchoring of periodontal fibres in the firm calcified tissues of bone and cementum. Calcium is essential for the stability of cell membranes. Its ionic concentration in cells can be an important determinant of membrane potential because the ratio of concentrations inside and outside the cell is of the order of at least 1:250 and possibly as much as 1:2000. Cell membranes are normally almost impermeable to calcium ions and the opening of calcium channels can therefore change membrane potential dramatically. The pacemaker potential of the sino-atrial node cells depends upon the opening of calcium channels, as does the plateau phase of the action potential in cardiac muscle generally. Calcium ions are necessary for synaptic and neuromuscular transmission. Inside cells calcium ions can act as second messengers and are also used in second messenger systems involving G-proteins and inositol trisphosphate. Calcium ions are needed for muscle contraction and for exocytosis in secretory cells. A number of enzyme reactions, notably several involved in the blood clotting cascade, are calcium dependent.

Calcium balance

The concentrations of calcium in cells are maintained constant by an elaborate balance of calcium-ATPase pumps in the cell membrane and in organelles, by membrane sodium–calcium exchangers, by storage in cell organelles and by calcium-binding proteins such as troponin and calmodulin. All these systems,

Table 1.1
Typical calcium balance in a young adult

Intake			
Total calcium intake	1.00 g (25 mmol)		
Amount absorbed	15.00 mmol	Unabsorbed	10.00 mmol
Output		**Faecal output**	
Gut cells/secretions	10.75	Unabsorbed	10.00
Urine	3.75	Intestines	10.75
Sweat	0.50	Total in faeces	20.75 mmol
Total	15.00 mmol		

however, depend on the constancy of the extracellular environment in relation to calcium. Although the calcium concentrations in the interstitial fluid are not the same as those in plasma because of the different degree of protein binding in the two fluids, the plasma calcium concentration is in equilibrium with that in the interstitial fluid. If the plasma calcium concentration is to be maintained constant, there must be a system of control which can adjust for varying intake and varying demands. Calcium balance indicates whether this system is operating and whether calcium is being stored or released. Table 1.1 shows typical figures for calcium balance in an adult male.

Dietary intake of calcium and its absorption

The daily requirement for calcium is about 300 mg (8 mmol), but more must be ingested because only some 60% is absorbed

Dietary intake of calcium is typically around 1.0 g/day (25 mmol/day). It is derived from milk and dairy products (excluding butter) and other sources are relatively minor (Table 1.2). It is necessary to have this much calcium in the diet because calcium readily forms insoluble salts which cannot be absorbed. Thus phosphates and oxalates in the diet reduce calcium absorption, but proteins increase it. The phytate content of wholemeal flour can reduce calcium intake markedly by forming insoluble calcium phytate in the gut. In World War II, when less wheat was imported into Britain, a higher extraction rate for flour was used and the part of the grain discarded in white flour manufacture was retained: nutritionists advised that calcium in the form of chalk should be added to the National Loaf in order to overcome the loss of calcium by precipitation of calcium phytate. As a result of the difficulties of maintaining calcium in the duodenum and jejunum in a soluble form, the overall absorption is only around 60% of the ingested amount. Calcium is secreted in the digestive secretions and lost by the shedding of mucosal cells; and this too must be reabsorbed to stay in balance, so that, in practice, some of the absorbed calcium is endogenous. Absorption takes place almost entirely in the duodenum because the alkaline conditions in the small intestine render calcium insoluble. Later parts of the small intestine are theoretically able to take up calcium by the same process as that in the duodenum: passive diffusion into the cells and then binding by a calcium-binding protein whose

Table 1.2
Calcium, phosphorus and vitamin D content of typical foodstuffs

Food		Calcium	Phosphorus	Vitamin D
RDA	(mmol/day)	17.5	17.5	None necessary
	(mg/day)	700	550	
Milk		123	112	0.001
Cream 35%		90	70	
Cheese (cheddar)		694	346	0.001
Butter		12	5	0.004
Eggs		25	96	0.0025
Beef		8	182	0
Ham		4	140	0
Cod		5	148	0
Mashed potato		7	26	0
Carrot		34	32	0
Cauliflower		33	22	0
Apple tart		9	28	0
Apple		5	10	0
Orange		40	20	0
Bread		50	200	0
Fruitcake		40	110	0
Shortbread biscuit		80	260	0
Cornflakes		0.5	50	0.028

synthesis is controlled by the active metabolite of vitamin D, 1,25-dihydroxycholecalciferol. From the binding protein calcium is passed on out of the cells by active calcium pumps in the basolateral cell membranes.

The recommended dietary allowance for calcium is 0.5–0.8 g/day, but there is evidence that people on low calcium intakes in fact absorb a higher percentage of the ingested load. The World Health Organization has progressively lowered its recommendations as this has become evident. Even the adverse effect of wholemeal flour on absorption is much less than expected because people adapt to the lower intake by more efficient absorption. A possible explanation of this is the ease with which saturation of the cell's active transport mechanism occurs as calcium intake rises. This recommended intake is that for an adult male in calcium balance but a higher intake is necessary to support bone formation and growth. In pregnancy, therefore, the recommended dietary intake is increased to around 1.5 g/day and during lactation, when calcium is being secreted into the milk for the growing infant, it is recommended that 2.0 g/day are ingested by the mother. In the first 30 years of life bone mass increases but thereafter calcium is lost from bones, most markedly in women immediately after the menopause.

Pregnancy and lactation increase the need for calcium

There has been increasing disquiet about the incidence of osteoporosis in postmenopausal women: although many women now take calcium supplements as inorganic salts, there is little evidence that this slows the process and some evidence that higher calcium intakes early in life are more important in reducing the risk. It is still unclear, therefore, what the optimal calcium intake should be.

Blood calcium concentrations

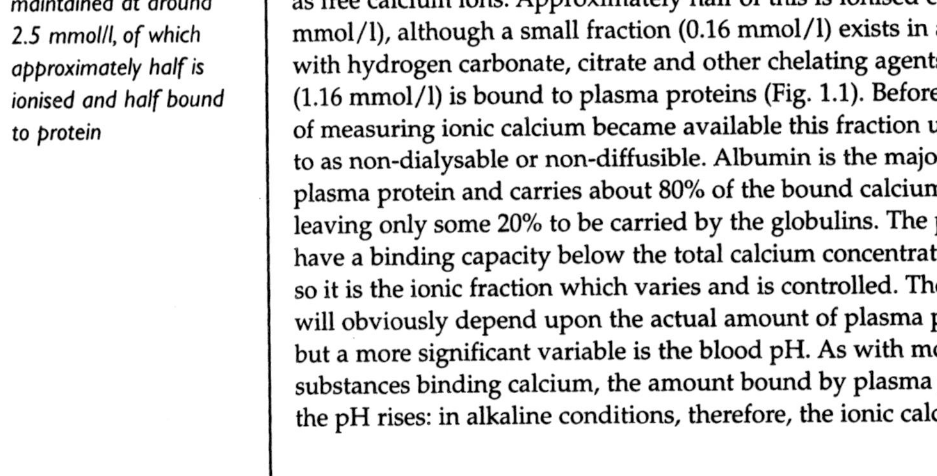

Plasma calcium concentrations are maintained at around 2.5 mmol/l, of which approximately half is ionised and half bound to protein

The calcium concentration in blood plasma is normally maintained between 2.25 and 2.75 mmol/l. This represents all forms of calcium, whether bound or as free calcium ions. Approximately half of this is ionised calcium (1.18 mmol/l), although a small fraction (0.16 mmol/l) exists in a complexed form with hydrogen carbonate, citrate and other chelating agents. The remainder (1.16 mmol/l) is bound to plasma proteins (Fig. 1.1). Before specific methods of measuring ionic calcium became available this fraction used to be referred to as non-dialysable or non-diffusible. Albumin is the major calcium-binding plasma protein and carries about 80% of the bound calcium in the blood, leaving only some 20% to be carried by the globulins. The plasma proteins have a binding capacity below the total calcium concentrations in blood and so it is the ionic fraction which varies and is controlled. The binding capacity will obviously depend upon the actual amount of plasma protein available, but a more significant variable is the blood pH. As with most organic substances binding calcium, the amount bound by plasma protein increases as the pH rises: in alkaline conditions, therefore, the ionic calcium concentrations

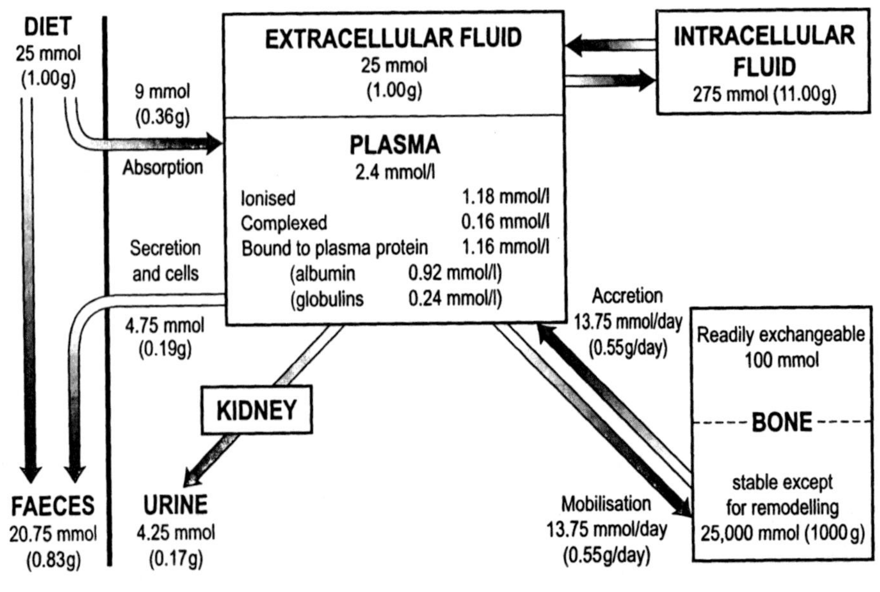

Calcium metabolism in a young adult.

decrease. This is sometimes shown rather dramatically by nervous patients as one of the possible effects of nervousness is hyperventilation. Hyperventilation blows off carbon dioxide from the lungs and therefore decreases the acidity of the plasma: at the higher pH the ionised calcium concentration may fall below the level necessary to stabilise the cell membranes of excitable cells and these become more permeable to sodium ions. The hypopolarisation induced renders the cells more excitable and spontaneous muscle contraction can occur. This condition is termed tetany. Neuromuscular transmission is impaired but both nerve and muscle become hyperexcitable. Spasmodic flexion of the wrist or thumb is often seen and tapping the facial nerve at the angle of the jaw causes ipsilateral contraction of the facial muscles.

As only the ionised calcium is able to diffuse across the capillary walls to any significant extent, the concentrations in interstitial fluid mirror those in plasma. They may vary locally when cells are secreting or taking up calcium and there will be a local equilibrium with the calcium salts of calcified tissues.

Calcium stores in the body

Bone is the main body store of calcium

The main body store of calcium is in the skeleton. The bone of an adult male contains a total of about a kilogram of calcium, and exchange of ions can occur at hydroxyapatite surfaces bathed in interstitial fluid. In practice, this means that about 100 mmol of calcium are available for exchange (Fig. 1.1). Dentine and cementum do not take part in this exchange and enamel is separated from the circulation by the dentine. The bone crystals are in equilibrium with the tissue fluid and this in turn with the capillary blood. Simple diffusion of ions into and out of bone has little effect on the plasma calcium levels or on the overall calcium balance even though it amounts to around 500 mmol/day. It is only when the cells of bone are involved – the osteoblasts laying down bone and the osteoclasts resorbing it – that the reservoir function of bone becomes operative. However, there is a slow remodelling of bone going on all the time: some 7.5 mmol of calcium per day is mobilised and redeposited. These processes are under local control and are responses to changes in strains on the bone: larger scale responses whose object is to stabilise blood calcium concentrations are under hormonal control. Passive exchange of ions at the crystal surface is not confined to calcium: other positively and negatively charged ions may substitute at the crystal surface. Thus strontium is taken up into bone by exchange for calcium and strontium levels in bone give an indication of exposure to the ion. Radio-strontium acts as a marker for exposure to radioactivity resulting from testing of atomic bombs. Lead is also taken up and its concentrations in bone and dentine are indicative of exposure to pollution, particularly that from leaded petrol in motor vehicle exhaust fumes. Fluoride substitutes for hydroxyl ions in the hydroxyapatite crystal and so is incorporated particularly into growing bones. Fluorapatite is less readily soluble than hydroxyapatite and so resorbs less readily and accumulates in the bone as it does in forming dental tissues. In young children excretion of fluoride is a much lower proportion of the ingested dose than in adults because it is so readily taken up by the calcifying tissues.

Calcium excretion

Calcium is excreted in the faeces and in urine

Calcium is lost from the body in the desquamated cells of the gut lining and in non-reabsorbed secretions. This, together with the unabsorbed dietary calcium adds up to a daily loss in the faeces of around 0.5 g (12.5 mmol)/day. Although this figure will depend upon the dietary intake and the substances interfering with calcium absorption in the gut, it is not directly subject to control except inasmuch as there is some control over actual calcium uptake by the duodenal cells. Urinary calcium excretion, on the other hand, can be controlled by hormonal effects on the kidney. On a typical Western diet urinary calcium loss is around 100 mg (2.5 mmol)/day. Most of the filtered load is absorbed in the proximal tubule of the kidney by an active process involving calcium-ATPase on the basal membranes of the cells. In the distal tubule parathyroid hormone increases reabsorption of calcium ions from the tubular fluid.

Control of calcium balance

Plasma calcium concentrations are controlled by two hormones – parathyroid hormone from the parathyroid glands and calcitonin from the ultimobranchial tissue forming the parafollicular cells (the C cells) in the thyroid gland in the human – and by vitamin D, which effectively acts as a third hormone in this system (Fig. 1.2).

Parathyroid hormone (parathormone, PTH)

Parathyroid hormone controls calcium excretion by the kidneys and activates vitamin D to increase intestinal absorption of calcium

Parathormone is a large peptide with 84 amino acid residues (Fig. 1.3) which is synthesised in the parathyroid glands as a preprohormone of 115 amino acid residues. The gene encoding the preprohormone is situated on chromosome 11. In the endoplasmic reticulum a 25 amino acid sequence is removed from the N-terminal and a further sequence of 6 amino acids is removed from the same terminal in the Golgi apparatus to leave the peptide to be secreted. The hormone has a half-life of around 10 min. It is broken down in the liver to smaller peptides (which may retain some biological activity) and these are excreted via the kidneys.

Parathormone probably normally exerts its control over calcium metabolism by regulating absorption from the small intestine and excretion in the urine. If there is a major fall in blood calcium concentrations the hormone increases calcium mobilisation from bone by acting on osteoblasts and osteoclasts. There is a low resting concentration (10–50 pg/ml) of parathormone in blood, but when plasma ionised calcium concentrations fall below 1.2 mmol/l the parathyroid glands are stimulated to secrete parathormone at a greater rate. The cells of the parathyroid gland have surface receptors for calcium. Occupation of the receptor sites activates the G-proteins and causes inositol trisphosphate production and molibilisation of intracellular ionic calcium, inhibiting parathormone release. The secretion of parathormone is completely inhibited at a plasma total calcium concentration of 3.0 mmol/l and increases linearly with falling calcium concentrations. In the absence of parathormone the plasma total calcium concentration remains at 1.75 mmol/l and the proportion of ionised calcium is greatly reduced.

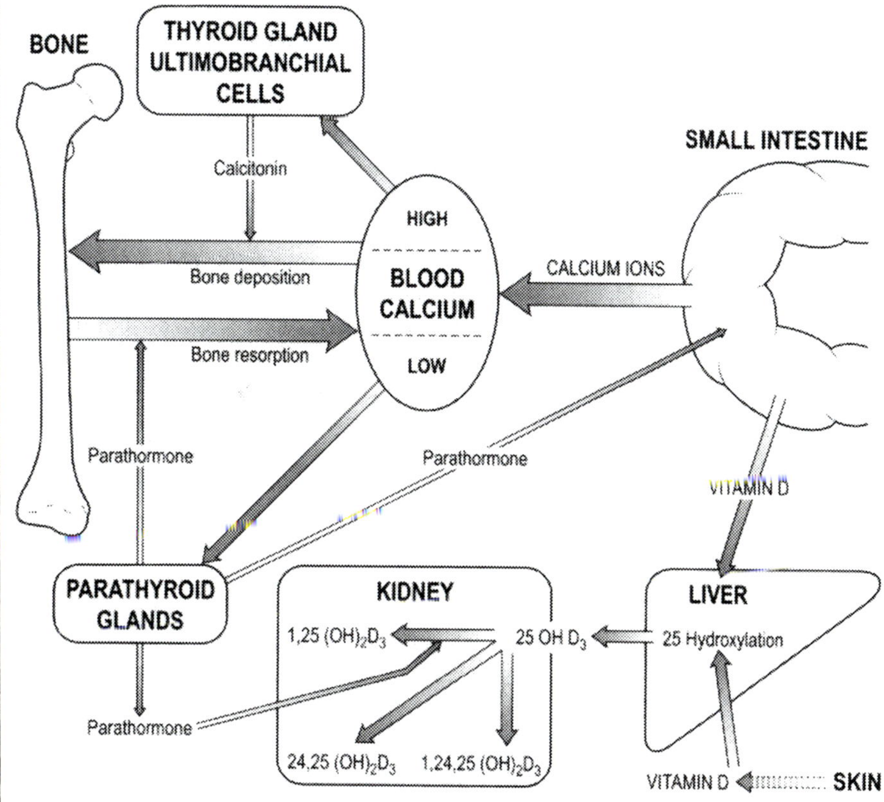

Fig. 1.2
Control of calcium balance. Heavy arrows indicate calcium transfer, medium arrows indicate calcium effects on endocrine glands and the early metabolism of vitamin D, and light arrows indicate hormonal effects on target tissues.

S-V-S-E-I-Q-L-M-H-N-L-G-K-H-L-N-S-M-E-R-V-E-W-L-R-K-K-L-Q-D-V-H-N-F-V-A-L-G-A-P-L-A-
5 10 15 20 25 30 35 40
P-R-D-A-G-S-Q-R-P-R-K-K-E-D-N-V-L-V-E-S-H-E-K-S-L-G-E-A-D-K-A-D-V-D-V-L-T-K-A-K-S-Q
45 50 55 60 65 70 75 80 84

Parathyroid hormone

S——S (disulfide bridge between residues 1 and 7)
C-G-N-L-S-T-C-M-L-G-T-Y-T-Q-D-F-N-K-F-H-T-F-P-Q-T-A-I-G-V-G-A-P-NH_2
5 10 15 20 25 30 32

Calcitonin

Fig. 1.3
Structure of the parathyroid hormone (parathormone) and calcitonin. (Amino acid residues are given in single-letter notation.)

The active form of vitamin D, 1,25-dihydroxycholecalciferol, inhibits parathormone synthesis. Increased plasma phosphate concentrations lower the concentration of ionised calcium in the blood, and hence stimulate parathormone secretion. The phosphate also inhibits the hydroxylation of vitamin D and allows hormone synthesis to occur. Changes in concentration of magnesium ions in the blood result in changes in parathormone secretion similar to those produced by changes in calcium concentration.

As a polypeptide hormone, parathormone acts on cell membrane receptors to produce its effects on target cells. Three different receptors have now been identified. The first, PTH1-R, is a member of the large family of receptor molecules which include receptors for most of the polypeptide hormones. Binding of the hormone to the receptors results in activation of adenyl cyclase and generation of cyclic adenosine monophosphate (cAMP). This causes the opening of calcium channels in the cell membranes. The receptors are found in the kidney and on bone cells. A second receptor, PTH2-R, similar in structure and mode of action, is found in a number of non-calcified tissues, and another, CPTH-R, binding the C-terminal has been reported. The significance of these latter two receptors is unclear.

When parathormone passes to the kidneys it has two effects. The first is to cause increased reabsorption of calcium in the distal tubules and inhibit renal phosphate reabsorption. The second is to stimulate the kidney cells to hydroxylate further the 25-hydroxycholecalciferol formed in the kidney from vitamin D and produce 1,25-dihydroxycholecalciferol. This second effect results in increased absorption of calcium in the small intestine (see the vitamin D group of vitamins, later).

Parathormone can also stimulate osteoclasts to mobilise bone calcium

If there is a serious and prolonged fall in calcium concentrations, or if the hormone is administered in pharmacological doses, parathormone acts on osteoblast receptors to cause them to secrete messenger molecules which stimulate the osteoclasts to resorb bone and release calcium into the extracellular fluids. The simultaneous release of phosphate has only a transitory effect on plasma phosphate concentrations because of the increased kidney excretion of phosphate ions also induced by the hormone. In addition to stimulating existing osteoclasts into resorbing bone, the osteoblast signals stimulate development of osteoclasts from their blood cell precursors.

Parathormone acts on both osteoblasts and osteoclasts via the cAMP intracellular pathway, resulting in an increased permeability of the cells to calcium ions by opening calcium channels. The indirect effect on osteoclasts appears to be similar. The calcium-ATPases of the cells do not appear to be stimulated directly by parathormone, although their activity is enhanced when 1,25-dihydroxycholecalciferol is present.

Another biologically active peptide which binds to parathormone receptors PTH1-R and PTH2-R has been described. It has 140 amino acid residues and is known as parathyroid hormone-related protein, PTHrH. It stimulates chondrocyte proliferation in cartilage and inhibits cartilage mineralisation. It appears to act as growth factor for some epithelial tissues such as skin.

Calcitonin

Calcitonin is a 32 amino acid peptide (Fig. 1.3) synthesised in the parafollicular, or C, cells of the thyroid gland as preprocalcitonin. The mRNA transcribed from the calcitonin gene is also processed in the brain and a number of neural tissues to form two peptides differing from each other in only one amino acid. These peptides are known as calcitonin gene-related peptides (CGRF). They appear to act as neurotransmitters and are involved in the transmission of impulses related to taste sensation. They are also found together with substance P in the terminals of primary afferent neurones and their release causes vasodilatation. The secretion of calcitonin occurs when plasma calcium concentrations rise above 2.38 mmol/l and increases linearly in proportion to calcium concentration. The hormone has a half-life of less than 10 min. Its mode of action is to reduce the number of active osteoclasts and to inhibit bone resorption. Unlike many factors affecting osteoclasts activity, it appears to act directly on these cells. It also increases urinary excretion of calcium, possibly by inhibiting reabsorption in the distal tubules. The role of calcitonin in the normal control of plasma calcium concentrations in the human has been questioned. It may exert a protective influence on bone formation in the foetus and in growing children; it may also protect maternal bone during pregnancy. It is secreted during food intake and calcium absorption and may therefore have a rapid and transitory stabilising effect on sudden rises in calcium concentration. Its release is triggered by a number of gastrointestinal hormones – gastrin, cholecystokinin-pancreozymin (CCK), secretin – and glucagon. The concentration of calcitonin in the blood of male subjects is higher than in female subjects and it has been suggested that this may be of significance in the greater susceptibility of women to osteoporosis. Treatment with calcitonin, however, has not produced any consistent improvement in patients with osteoporosis.

Calcitonin can reduce plasma concentrations of calcium but its physiological importance is doubtful

The vitamin D group

Vitamin D is traditionally considered as a dietary factor. However, the term is used somewhat loosely to describe a group of sterols which result from the conversion of provitamins to active agents (Fig. 1.4). The usual dietary provitamin is 7-dehydrocholesterol, which is converted into cholecalciferol, or vitamin D_3, by sunlight. This is almost the only vitamin D found in mammals although fish oils contain other substances with vitamin D activity. It is present in milk and dairy products (Table 1.2), but the amount of activated vitamin varies in summer and winter milk because of the sunlight effect. Irradiation of ergosterol and its derivatives yields calciferol and similar substances which have vitamin D activity and these are given distinguishing numerical suffixes. Steroids are lipid-soluble rather than water-soluble and hence are carried in the bloodstream bound to carrier globulins, that for vitamin D and similar compounds being termed vitamin D-binding protein or DBP. A second unrelated function of this protein is to bind excess actin in the blood.

In the liver, vitamin D_3 is converted into 25-hydroxycholecalciferol, or $25(OH)D_3$. This in turn is converted in the kidneys into 1,25-dihydroxycholecalciferol, $1,25(OH)_2D_3$, which acts as a hormone. Some other tissues can also produce small amounts of this compound. Like other steroid hormones, $1,25(OH)_2D_3$ enters the target cells and binds to an intracellular receptor, exposes a DNA-binding region and changes the types of protein synthesised by the cell. The receptors are typical of the superfamily of steroid receptors which bind other steroids and thyroid hormones.

Cholecalciferol (vitamin D_3) is activated by hydroxylation, first in the liver and then in the kidneys

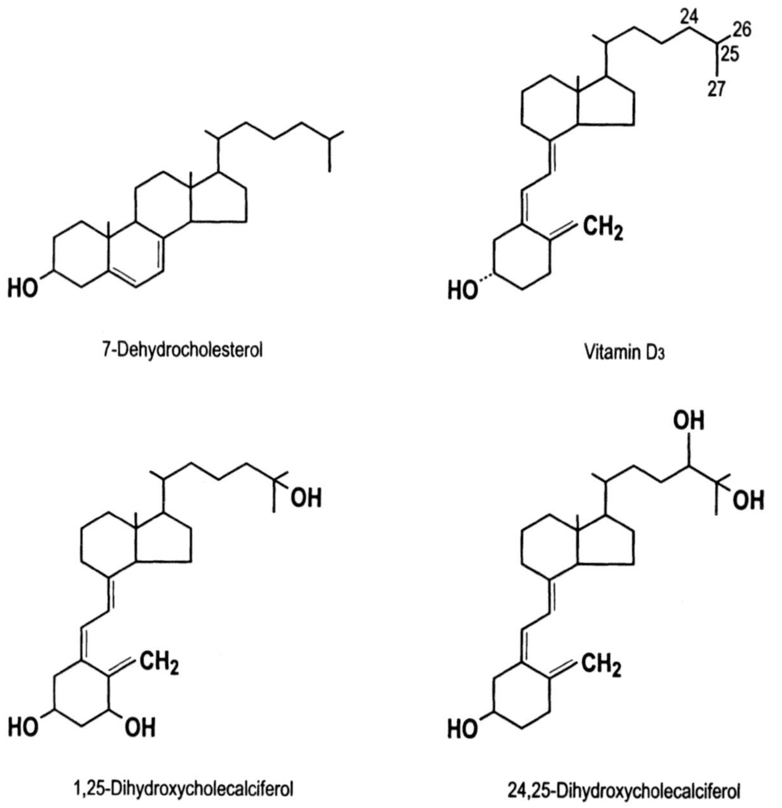

7-Dehydrocholesterol

Vitamin D3

1,25-Dihydroxycholecalciferol

24,25-Dihydroxycholecalciferol

Fig. 1.4
Structures of the vitamin D group of vitamins.

Specifically, $1,25(OH)_2D_3$ enforces the synthesis of two calcium-binding proteins, calbindin-D_{9K} and calbindin-D_{28K}. Increases in intracellular concentrations of these two calcium-binding proteins are associated with increased calcium transport across the cells. $1,25(OH)_2D_3$ also enhances the activity of calcium-ATPases in the basolateral membranes of epithelial cells and increases the turnover of some plasma membrane components (Fig. 1.5). The main target cells are those of the small intestine, but the hormone can also stimulate renal reabsorption of calcium and increases mobilisation of calcium and phosphate from bone. However, in normal circumstances it is the absorption of calcium in the duodenum that is mainly affected, and the resultant increase in plasma calcium concentration favours deposition of bone rather than the mobilisation which is seen if vitamin D acts directly on bone.

$1,25(OH)_2D_3$ increases intestinal absorption of calcium

Hydroxylation of $25(OH)_2D_3$ is controlled by plasma calcium and by parathormone

Hydroxylation of vitamin D in the liver occurs spontaneously but the second hydroxylation of cholecalciferol which occurs in the kidney is carefully controlled. Low plasma calcium concentrations stimulate 1-alpha hydroxylase activity whereas high calcium concentrations inhibit the enzyme and cause the much less active $24,25(OH)_2D_3$ to be formed instead. Parathormone secreted when blood calcium concentrations are low enhances the activity of 1-alpha

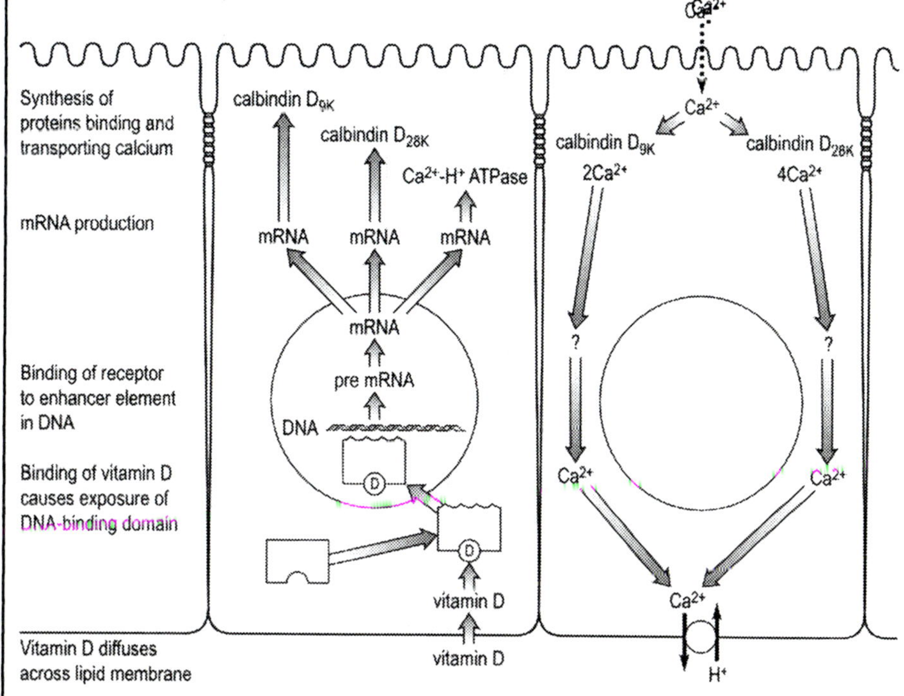

Fig. 1.5
The effects of active vitamin D on the epithelial cells of the small intestine and the resultant movement of calcium ions across the cells.

hydroxylase. There is a direct feedback control, with $1,25(OH)_2D_3$ exerting a negative feedback on its own synthesis and a positive feedback on $24,25(OH)_2D_3$ synthesis. Phosphate ions inhibit the hydroxylase and introduce a further control. Other hormones can also affect the hydroxylation: prolactin stimulates it while thyroxine decreases it. Oestrogens, growth hormone and calcitonin all increase the circulating $1,25(OH)_2D_3$ concentrations.

Although the active forms of vitamin D are usually considered as being specifically involved in calcium metabolism, there is increasing interest in their ability to stimulate differentiation of immune cells and keratinocytes in the skin.

Phosphate

Phosphate has many roles in soft tissues as well as in calcified tissues

The major store of phosphate in the body, like that of calcium, is in the skeleton. Over 85% of phosphate is in the bones (Fig. 1.6). The remainder is widely distributed in cells, usually as organic phosphates, as phosphate is present in the high energy phosphates and the creatinine phosphate of muscle, in the intracellular messengers cAMP and inositol trisphosphate, and in the phosphorylated intermediates of the metabolic pathways. Removal or

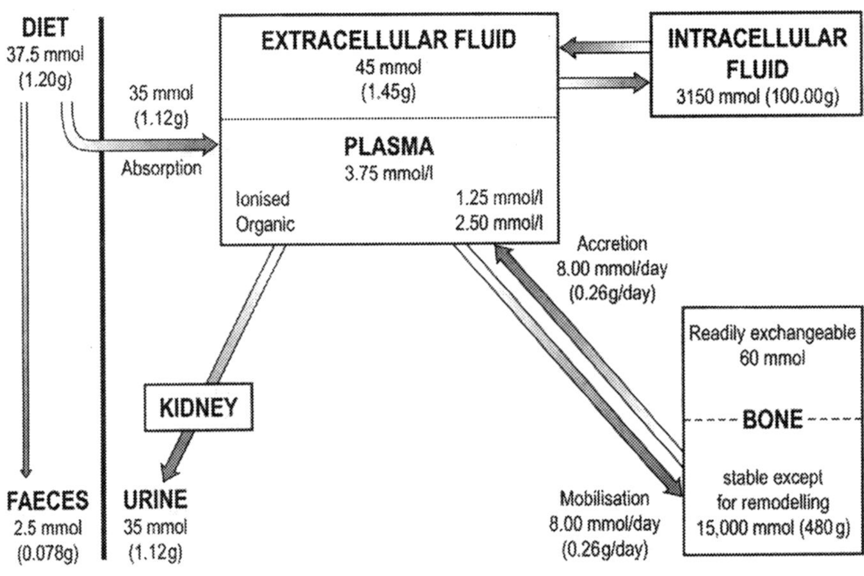

Phosphate metabolism in a young adult.

Phosphate concentrations are usually controlled in conjunction with calcium concentrations but there may be a control hormone

addition of phosphate groups to enzymes is an important means of modifying their activity. The phosphate concentration in plasma is around 4 mmol/l, with only about a third of this in an inorganic form as monohydrogen phosphate at the normal blood pH.

In general, phosphate metabolism is not under the same degree of control as that of calcium despite often being linked with it. Thus the phosphate taken in the diet from meat, vegetables and dairy products (Table 1.2) is absorbed both actively and passively in the duodenum and the jejunum as inorganic phosphate in almost direct proportion to the total intake. However, factors increasing calcium absorption, including 1,25-dihydroxycholecalciferol, usually increase phosphate absorption also. As with calcium, there is a turnover of phosphate in bone, with some 100 μmol/kg/day being removed and redeposited. The main excretory route is via the kidneys. Inorganic phosphate ions pass through in the glomerular filtrate, but around 90% of the filtered load is actively reabsorbed in the proximal convoluted tubules. The phosphate ion acts as one of the buffers in the tubular fluid and may be excreted as either dihydrogen monophosphate or monohydrogen phosphate. It is one of the characteristic ions of urine: the early chemists used urine as a source of phosphorus.

There is some control of phosphate excretion since its reabsorption in the kidney is inhibited by parathormone although this is actually incidental to the control of calcium excretion and it is plasma calcium concentrations, not phosphate, which stimulate parathormone secretion.

It has also been postulated that there may be a specific hormone controlling phosphate metabolism and that the site of action of this hormone would again be the kidneys.

Other hormones affecting calcium metabolism and bone turnover

Several hormones other than parathormone, calcitonin and 1,25-dihydroxycholecalciferol have already been mentioned because of their interactions with these three major influences on calcium metabolism. A summary of the actions of hormones not primarily involved in calcium metabolism is an appropriate ending to this section (Table 2.1 identifies some of these effects at the cellular level).

Growth hormone

Hormones involved in regulation of growth and sexual development and in stress can affect calcium balance

Growth hormone increases absorption of calcium in the small intestine and also its excretion in the urine. The net effect of these processes is an increase in total body calcium – a positive calcium balance. In bone, the hormone stimulates production of an insulin-like growth factor (IGF1) and this in turn stimulates protein synthesis in bone.

During growth, growth hormone stimulates increase in the length of the long bones by its action on cartilage via somatomedin C, but overproduction of the hormone in the adult characteristically causes selective growth of those bones in which remodelling is most active – the mandible being one of these. One of the most noticeable effects of a pathological increase in growth hormone in the adult (acromegaly) is the thickening and lengthening of the body of the mandible with consequent changes in facial appearance, and spacing of the teeth or alteration in the fit of a lower denture.

Insulin

Insulin is an anabolic hormone: it favours bone formation and may be an important factor in bone growth during foetal and childhood development.

Testosterone and other androgenic hormones

Although the effects of androgenic hormones on growth of bone are rarely referred to, they may be important during foetal and childhood development. Certainly testosterone produces differential effects on cartilage and it is these effects which result in the increased growth of the shoulders in the male. Presumably other secondary sexual characteristics apparent in the skeleton, such as the more developed supraorbital ridges and the tendency to greater mandibular growth and prognathism, are also due to localised effects on bone growth.

Oestrogens

Oestrogens affect bone growth in two ways. During pubertal development they have very selective actions on cartilage, usually inhibiting its growth and accelerating its conversion to bone; they also promote local growth to increase the relative size of the pelvis and the pelvic opening. Thus the ratio of shoulder width to hip width is high in the male and low in the female.

When oestrogen secretion ceases at the menopause, the balance of calcium deposition and mobilisation in bone shifts to the side of mobilisation and loss of calcium from the bone may result in osteoporosis. This is seen in the mandible as well as in the long bones. Oestrogen administration can halt development of osteoporosis. The hormones act on the osteoblasts to stimulate their activity.

Human placental lactogen and prolactin

During pregnancy there is maternal requirement for calcium to support the calcification of the bones of the foetus. This is met by increasing the absorption of calcium from the diet by stimulating hydroxylation of 25-hydroxycholecalciferol in the kidneys and by mobilising calcium from bone. Human placental lactogen is probably the hormone stimulating vitamin D hydroxylation, although oestrogens may contribute to the effect on intestinal absorption. During the period of lactation there is a need for calcium to be secreted in the milk. Prolactin acts by stimulating both intestinal absorption and calcium mobilisation from bone, again by favouring the hydroxylation of vitamin D. Whether there is a more specific effect of these hormones on osteoclasts is unclear.

Thyroid hormones: thyroxine and tri-iodothyronine

The effects of thyroid hormones on growth presumably include stimulation of bone growth (the hypothyroid infant is typically dwarfed), but in the adult increased thyroid gland activity leads to increased bone metabolism which favours calcium mobilisation. There is, therefore, hypercalcaemia and hypercalciuria. This may lead to osteoporosis.

Glucocorticoids

The glucocorticoid hormones exert a number of effects on bone metabolism. They have an anti-vitamin D action, decreasing absorption of calcium and phosphate in the small intestine, and increasing renal excretion of calcium. The resultant decrease in plasma calcium concentrations stimulates parathormone secretion and causes bone resorption. In addition to this, the glucocorticoids actually inhibit osteoclast formation as well as reducing the activity of osteoclasts already present – again lowering plasma calcium concentrations. The catabolic actions of the hormones have a direct effect on bone: they inhibit DNA replication and protein synthesis and so decrease bone formation. The combination of these effects when corticosteroid drugs are administered over long periods of time results in osteoporosis. The manifestations of this in the bones of the jaws can add a further hazard to the problems of oral surgery in these patients.

2 Calcified tissues

Introduction

Calcified tissues are specialised connective tissues made up of a matrix with embedded fibres, cells and apatite crystals

Most of the calcified tissue in the body can be classed as a connective tissue – that is to say, a tissue with relatively few cells dispersed in an extracellular matrix which fills the spaces between protein fibres. In the soft connective tissues the matrix holds the extracellular fluid, but in the hard connective tissues insoluble calcium salts are laid down in the matrix and only small amounts of extracellular fluid remain. Connective tissues in general originate in the mesoderm and so three of the hard tissues of the body – bone, cementum and dentine – are of mesodermal origin. The fourth, dental enamel, is an exception: it is of ectodermal origin.

Each of the tissues derived from mesoderm has all the components of calcified connective tissue: cells which synthesise matrix and protein fibres and also transport calcium and phosphate to the forming tissue, crystals of a slightly calcium-deficient hydroxyapatite, fibres principally of the protein collagen, and between them the components of the matrix. However, the ectoderm-derived dental enamel is very highly calcified: no obvious fibrous network exists in it; its unique matrix, which occupies only 2% of its volume, appears rather as a fine reticulum when the tissue is decalcified.

The cells which form enamel stay on its surface during its formation and are lost from the mature tissue, in contrast to those of bone and cellular cementum which remain in the mature tissue, and those of dentine which remain in contact with, and have processes extending into, the calcified dentine.

Matrix is first laid down and then calcified

In the process of formation of the calcified tissues, fibres and matrix must first be laid down and calcium salts then deposited into the matrix. In bone and cementum the specialised matrix is termed osteoid and cementoid and is evident as a layer over bone and cementum surfaces where new deposits of calcified material may be laid down. In dentine the equivalent layer is known as predentine. There is no direct equivalent in enamel because of the rapid calcification of the matrix. It must be added, however, that enamel has at first only some 37% inorganic salts but progressively accumulates calcium salts to reach some 95% inorganic matter as it matures.

The cells associated with calcified tissues

There are three possible types of cell associated with a hard tissue: a cell which lays down matrix, transports calcium and phosphate into the matrix, and may be directly involved in the process of mineralisation; a cell present in, or in contact with, the calcified tissue, maintaining metabolic activity in it; and a cell which is able to remove calcified tissue. The formative cells are termed blast cells with the appropriate prefix: osteoblast, ameloblast, odontoblast, cementoblast. The cells embedded in bone or cementum are termed osteocytes or cementocytes (no cells remain in contact with mature enamel and the cells whose processes remain within the dentinal tubules are the odontoblasts themselves). The cells which resorb bone, dentine and cementum, although similar multinucleate cells probably all derived from a leucocyte line, are termed osteoclasts, odontoclasts and cementoclasts. No resorbing cells have been described for dental enamel.

Physical characteristics of the hard tissues

Bone

As bone is a tissue forming the rigid support of the whole body, it cannot be considered as a specifically oral tissue and is perhaps not an appropriate topic in this volume. However, some aspects of bone physiology are dealt with, and in the context of this chapter some comparison with the dental hard tissues is useful.

The bone of the jaws is similar to that elsewhere

The bone of the jaws is similar to the compact bone found elsewhere in the body. It can be regarded as having two zones: the mandible or maxilla proper and the superimposed alveolar processes which carry the teeth. The alveoli are the tooth sockets (Fig. 2.1). They are lined by a thin layer of compact bone, the lamina dura, perforated by minute foramina for the access of blood vessels and nerves to the periodontal ligament, and at the tooth apex to the dental pulp. The tooth is attached to the alveolar bone by collagenous fibres of the periodontal ligament which are inserted either into the bone or into the cementum of the tooth; some fibres extend across the ligament to be inserted into both. Bone is usually subject to remodelling as the stresses on it change according to the action of the muscles which are attached to it; alveolar bone has no muscles attached and its function is solely to support the teeth. The development of alveolar bone, therefore, is governed by the development and growth of the teeth: movement of the teeth will demand resorption when the tooth moves toward the wall of the socket and deposition on the opposite side; and when the teeth are lost by extraction or periodontal disease the alveolar bone will begin to remodel and resorb. In older edentulous patients the alveolar bone may be lost completely, leaving only the ridge of basal bone of the jaw on which it was situated. The provision of dentures may be difficult, not only because of the sensitivity of the thin layer of mucosa covering the ridge, but also because the denture will be limited in size and retention by the proximity of the mandibular and maxillary muscle insertions.

Alveolar bone is part of the tooth support apparatus

Bone responds to stress by remodelling

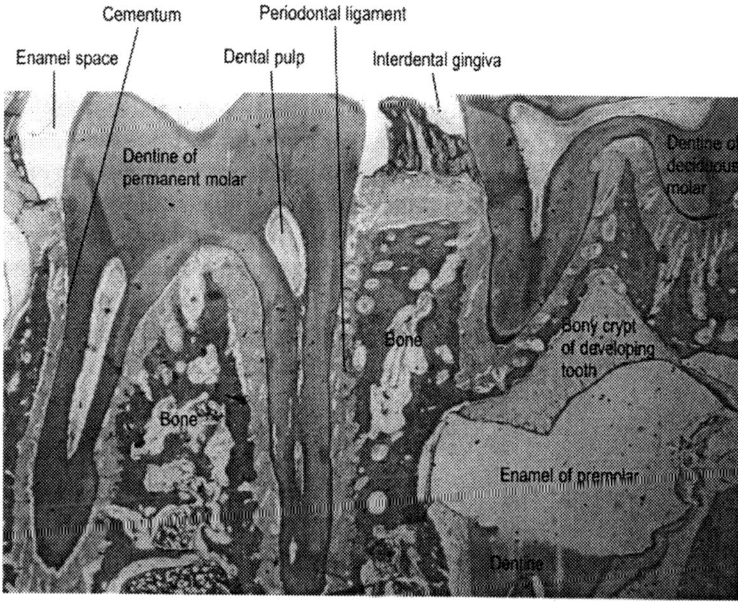

Fig. 2.1
The hard tissues of the oral cavity as seen in a section through a permanent molar, a resorbing deciduous molar and the erupting premolar. The teeth are held in their bony sockets, or alveoli, by the periodontal ligaments.

Bone is approximately one-third organic and two-thirds inorganic

Bone contains some 25% organic material by weight (35% by volume) and some 15% of water by weight (28% by volume); its mineral content is less than that of dentine and cementum at around 65% (36% by volume). The apatite crystals are small (25 × 3 nm) and contain much more carbonate and sodium than either dentine or enamel; the magnesium content is midway between that in enamel and dentine. Bone has a calcium:phosphate ratio of 1.7:1; this is higher than that for enamel or dentine or pure hydroxyapatite and suggests that other calcium salts are present in bone.

As a tissue which is not situated on the body surface and therefore not subject to wear, bone is one of the less hard of the hard tissues. It can be cut relatively easily with steel saws and steel burs. Its strength is critically dependent upon its structure: the hard cortical layer resists both compressive and tensile forces – particularly the former – but trabecular bone can resist such forces only in a direction along the lines of the trabeculae.

The bone of the jaws has a good blood supply and is readily permeable to dyes

Bone is an active tissue, constantly changing in response to the stresses and strains upon it. Even when apparently completely formed and at its adult size, bone can thicken by apposition. The bony walls of the alveolus in which a tooth sits adapt to the movement of the tooth. Deformation occurs even under the stresses of mastication. This becomes important when considering the stresses involved when an implant is inserted and becomes functional.

As an active tissue, bone has a good blood supply, with small blood vessels passing into the canaliculi and providing nutriment for the bone cells. The marrow spaces of bone in younger subjects are occupied by blood sinuses which form the bone marrow. In older subjects the marrow will no longer be the red, erythrocyte-forming marrow, but even in the adult the small marrow spaces of the mandible and even maxilla may continue to form white blood cells. Bone is a highly permeable tissue which allows ready penetration of small molecules and dyes unless these are bound either by the calcium salts or the matrix molecules, although the denser cortical bone presents more of a barrier to diffusion. Dyes which bind to calcium salts can be injected into the bloodstream and these will then 'label' newly forming bone. Several fluorescent dyes and the tetracyclines can be used in this way as bone markers.

Nerve fibres in bone are usually limited to the periodontium but may also be found in the larger canals of the mature tissue.

The bone cells

The cells associated with bone are the preosteoblast–osteoblast–osteocyte cell line which is responsible for bone formation and maintenance, and the osteoclasts, which are responsible for the removal of one crystals and matrix in bone resorption.

Preosteoblasts

The cells which differentiate into bone-forming cells are fibroblast-like in appearance. They develop membrane-associated alkaline phosphatase activity and synthesise osteonectin and proteoglycans. These properties are retained as they develop into osteoblasts. Although most preosteoblasts proceed along this developmental pathway, those forming the endosteum within the bone marrow eventually become adipocyte-like and fill with fat globules.

Osteoblasts

Osteoblasts are the bone-forming cells: they are influenced by both systemic and local factors

The osteoblasts (Fig. 2.2) are the cells which lay down bone matrix as osteoid and calcify it to form bone. They are usually described as plump cells. They have an extensive rough endoplasmic reticulum and Golgi apparatus. The cell membranes show alkaline phosphatase activity. In addition to the synthesis of osteonectin and small proteoglycans they begin to synthesise bone sialoprotein, osteopontin and osteocalcin. The osteoblasts have other functions in relation to bone metabolism. They form a layer of cells on the thin osteoid layer at the bone surface which protects the osteoid and bone from resorption. When the cells move away from an area of the osteoid surface osteoclastic cells can gain access and begin the resorptive process. Further, the osteoblasts have surface receptors for most of the chemical substances which stimulate bone deposition and resorption, and they are necessary for the transmission of signals to the osteoclasts to cause resorption (Table 2.1). Thus parathormone and prostaglandin E_2 bind to receptors not on the osteoclasts but on the osteoblasts, and the osteoblasts secrete messenger molecules which diffuse to the osteoclasts to activate them. Another property of the osteoblasts is their ability to produce tissue inhibitors of metalloproteases (TIMPs) which will prevent collagenases from attacking the bone matrix.

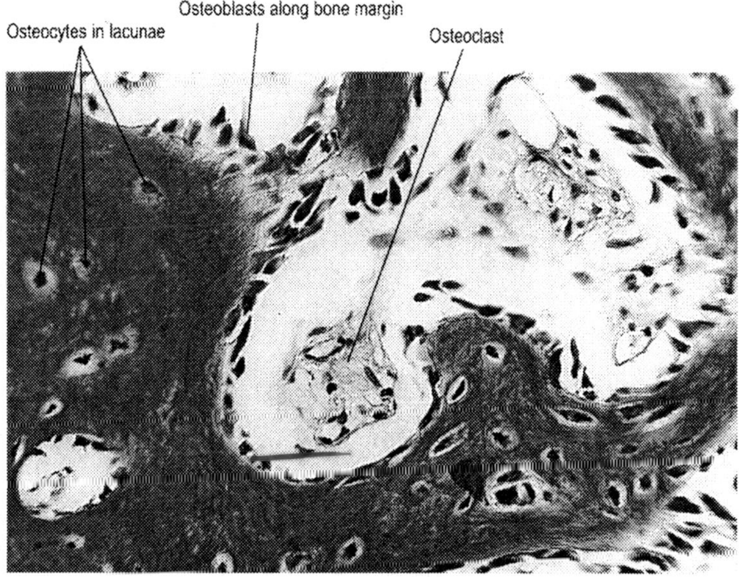

Fig. 2.2
A section through bone to show the osteocytes embedded in the bone, the osteoblasts on the bone margin and the multinucleate osteoclasts.

Table 2.1
Factors affecting osteoblast and osteoclast activity

	Osteoblasts	Osteoclasts
Stimulatory	Parathyroid hormone	Parathyroid hormone
	1,25 DHC	1,25 DHC
	Interleukin 1 (IL-1)	Interleukin 6 (IL-6)
	Thyroxine	Interleukin 11 (IL-11)
	Tri-iodothyronine	
	Growth hormone	
	Insulin-like growth factor-1	
	Prostaglandin-E_2	
	Tissue necrosis factor	
	Oestrogens?	
Inhibitory	Corticosteroids	Calcitonin
		Oestrogens (inhibit IL-6)
		Transforming Growth Factor beta(TGFb)
		Interferon alpha (IFN alpha)
		Prostaglandin E_2

Osteocytes

Formation of bone around the osteoblasts results in their becoming surrounded by calcified tissue. They remain within lacunae in the bone, connected to each other by narrow processes which pass along canaliculi through the bone (Fig. 2.2). They lose their alkaline phosphatase activity. They are thought to be responsible for the maintenance of the bone around them.

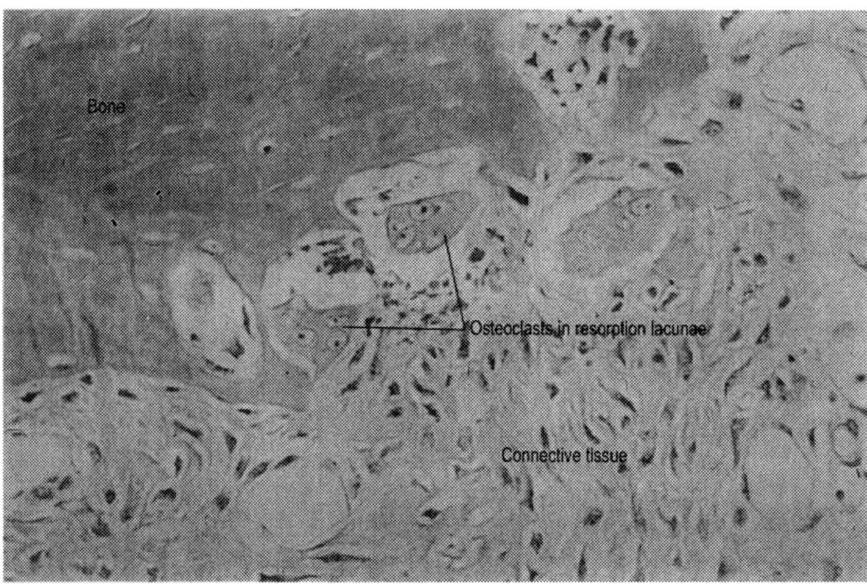

Fig. 2.2
A section through bone to show osteoclasts in the lacunae they have produced by resorbing bone.

The tendency for the outer layers of bone to dissolve in tissue fluids is countered by the maintenance of high levels of calcium by the osteocytes. These cells may be able to respond to stresses in the surrounding bone crystals – possibly by a piezo-electric effect – and are able to transmit stimuli to the osteoblasts on the bone surface. Remodelling of bone in response to stress occurs in this manner.

Osteoclasts

Osteoclasts are monocyte-derived multinucleate cells which resorb bone

The osteoclasts are large cells with many nuclei (Figs 2.2, 2.3). Their origin is completely different from that of the osteoblasts: they are thought to arise from monocytes. They attach to the bone surface around their periphery so that a minute microenvironment is created between the cell and the bone. The cell membrane adjacent to the bone becomes 'rough' by developing many short blunt processes. The cells contain lysosomes and they produce organic acids which can dissolve the apatite crystals, and metalloproteinases which can digest the collagen fibres of the bone. Collagenases are inactivated at low pH and hence some temporal specialisation of activity must occur. Matrix proteins can also be phagocytosed by the osteoclast and exposed to the action of lysosomal enzymes.

Cementum

Cementum is a tissue found only in the teeth. In the human it covers the root dentine, rarely extending over the cervical edge of the dental enamel. It is the

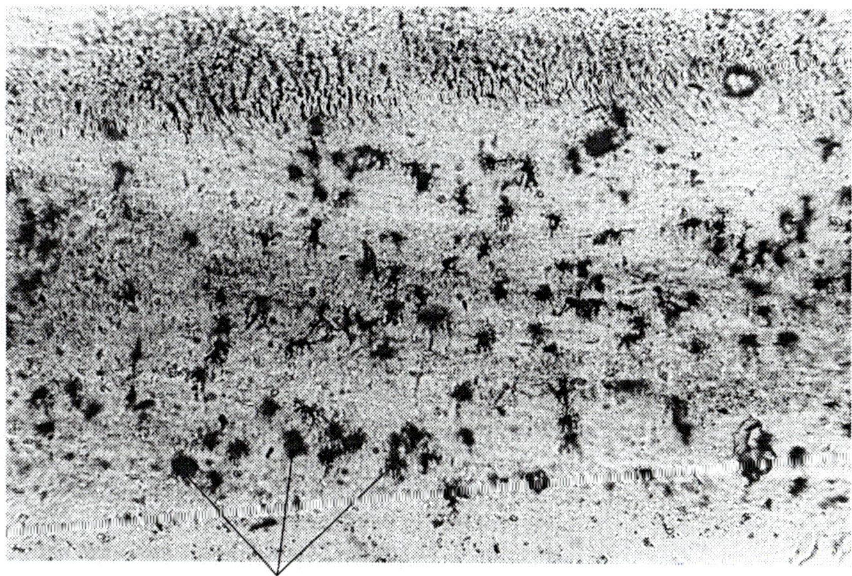

Fig. 2.4
A section of cellular cementum showing the cementocytes.

Cementum is a thin layer of bone-like material covering the root dentine

softest of the dental hard tissues, readily worn away by the abrasive action of foodstuffs and toothbrushing. Its role is to provide anchorage for the fibres of the periodontal ligament and thus through them to attach the tooth to its bony socket. Of all the dental tissues it is most like bone, although it has no blood supply of its own and depends on the periodontal ligament for its nutrition, and it has no nerve supply.

Histologically, cementum has been described as being of two types: cellular and acellular. The acellular cementum is formed around the dentine: it is covered in the apical third of the root by the cellular cementum which has incorporated cementocytes lying in lacunae connected by canaliculi in a similar fashion to osteocytes in bone (Fig. 2.4). More recently cementum has been reclassified according to the origin of the collagen fibres making up its matrix into intrinsic fibre cementum with collagen fibres laid down by the cementoblasts and extrinsic fibre cementum whose fibres are derived from the periodontal ligament. Acellular cementum is first formed as extrinsic fibre cementum and later layers may have either intrinsic or extrinsic fibres, whilst the earliest cellular cementum has only intrinsic fibres and the later layers have both extrinsic and intrinsic fibres.

There is little information on the composition of cementum, probably because it forms a layer on the root surface only 20–50 μm thick at the neck of the tooth and at most about 200 μm thick at the apex, and because its density is so similar to that of dentine that it is difficult to separate.

Around 70% of the weight of cementum is inorganic material and this occupies just under half (47%) of its volume. The organic content of cementum is a little over 20% by weight, or 30% by volume, with the acellular cementum being closer in composition to dentine and the cellular cementum to bone. It is made up principally of type I collagen.

The apatite of cementum has a crystal size similar to that in dentine and, as in dentine, there is a relatively high proportion of carbonate and magnesium substitution. The fluoride content of cementum is similar to that of dentine, ranging from as low as 50 ppm to as high as 800 ppm. Accumulation of the trace elements strontium, lead, zinc, copper and iron is essentially similar to their accumulation in dentine.

The tissue resembles bone in its resistance to compressive and tensile forces. The permeability of cementum to dyes differs according to the type and age of the cementum. Acellular cementum is almost impermeable to dye molecules, whilst cellular cementum is readily permeable along the channels linking the embedded cementocytes from both the dentine and the periodontal ligament aspects in young teeth. As the tooth ages the cementum becomes progressively less permeable from the dentinal side although it remains permeable from the periodontal ligament side. The amount of cementum towards the apex of a tooth root increases throughout life. Normally cementum does not undergo resorption in response to pressure in the same way as bone, but application of excessive forces during orthodontic movement can cause it to do so. During resorption of the deciduous teeth cementum and dentine are resorbed by osteoclast-like cells (cementoclasts or odontoclasts).

Dentine

Dentine forms the bulk of a tooth. It is formed by cells from the future pulp

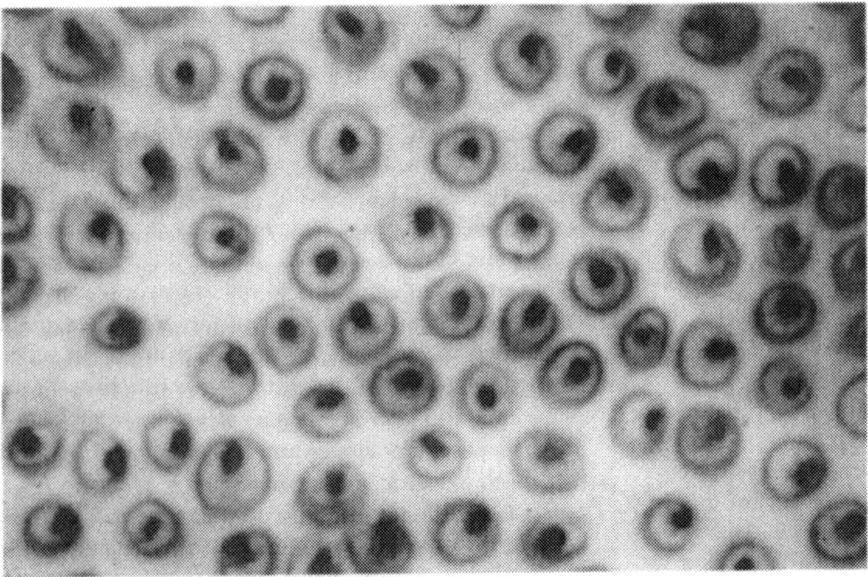

Fig. 2.1
Cross-section of dentine showing dentinal tubules and the odontoblast processes inside them.

Dentine consists of calcified tubules which originally contained odontoblast processes. It makes up the bulk of the tooth

In adults the odontoblast process extends less than one-quarter of the tubule length

and hence surrounds the pulp; in the crown of the tooth it is covered by the hard protective layer of dental enamel and in the root it is surrounded by cementum with its fibres attaching the tooth to the bone of the socket.

Once enamel is formed and the tooth has erupted there is no further addition to it. The tissue may, however, be lost by wear (attrition) or acid dissolution (either in erosion or in dental caries). Dentine, on the other hand, can form throughout life. Different terms are used to describe dentine formed at different times and in different circumstances. The dentine formed before the tooth erupts consists of a calcified collagenous matrix penetrated by the processes of the odontoblasts to give a tubular structure (Fig. 2.5). The tubules are around 2.5 μm in diameter near the pulp and taper down to just under 1 μm as they approach the amelodentinal junction. The number of tubules in a given volume of dentine increases towards the pulp as the odontoblasts become crowded together and the thickness of calcified material between them decreases. Each tubule has short lateral branches which are presumably formed from lateral extensions of the odontoblast process, but there is no evidence of connection between these branches. In the first formed layer of dentine, the mantle dentine, there is more extensive branching. At eruption, therefore, two types of dentine can be distinguished: the first formed mantle dentine; about 150 μm wide, and then the primary dentine, a few millimetres wide. When the root of the tooth is complete the rate of dentine apposition slows and the dentine formed is less regular, although the tubules are continuous with those of the primary dentine: this more slowly formed dentine continues to be laid down throughout life and progressively narrows the pulp chamber. It is known as secondary dentine. In areas where there is noxious stimulation of dentine – by caries, by damage, or by the presence of foreign substances in the dentinal tubules – a protective layer of dentine is formed relatively rapidly in the localised area. The more rapidly it is formed the less regular it appears: the tubular pattern may be irregular and there may be cellular inclusions. This type of dentine is termed tertiary dentine or reparative dentine. Within dentine the calcified part of the tissue between the tubules is sometimes termed intertubular dentine. In the dentine of the root small areas of hypocalcified dentine may be seen immediately below the mantle dentine. These occur when the globules of calcified material expanding from nuclei of calcification fail to fuse and are therefore referred to as interglobular dentine.

As dentine forms the odontoblast process retreats from the amelodentinal junction and in mature dentine extends only some 0.7 mm along the tubule. In cat dentine there is a variation at different sites in the tooth, with the odontoblast process reaching two-thirds of the way to the outer surface of dentine in the cervical region but only about a quarter of the way in the crown and at mid-root level. There is still some doubt about the length of the tubule filled by the odontoblast process because small amounts of cell-associated proteins such as tubulin have been detected near the amelodentinal junction. The remainder of the tubule is filled with the dentinal tissue fluid. Electron microscopy has demonstrated a thin layer of organic material lining the tubules but it is not known what this is composed of, nor how it is laid down. Collagen has also been demonstrated in the dentinal tubules as well as in the odontoblast processes. The dentinal fluid has a high calcium concentration: calcification can therefore continue along the inner wall of the tubule throughout life. The resultant homogeneous layer of calcified material lining the tubule is confusingly referred to peritubular dentine although modern histologists prefer to call it intratubular dentine. Eventually this continuing process leads to obliteration of the tubules and the dentine in that area becomes translucent. This is most often seen in the apical third of the root, but also in the crown where it appears midway through the thickness of the dentine. Such dentine is termed sclerosed.

Some nerve fibres enter a short way into dentinal tubules

It is now agreed that some nerve fibres pass from the subodontoblastic plexus (the plexus of Raschkow) between the odontoblasts to enter the predentine in close association with the odontoblast processes. Most of the nerve fibres terminate in the predentine, but about 10% continue on to extend some 0.2 mm into the dentinal tubules. This occurs mainly towards the tip of the cusps. In the cervical area there are very few nerve fibres in the dentinal tubules.

Dentine is approximately 70% inorganic material by weight (47% by volume)

Dentine is much less highly calcified than enamel with only some 70% of inorganic material by weight (Table 2.2). The remaining fraction comprises approximately 20% organic and 10% water. As in enamel the different densities of these fractions mean that the proportions by volume are different: 47% inorganic, 33% organic and 20% water. Type I collagen is the most abundant organic molecule but the remaining 10% of the organic material, termed the non-collagenous proteins, has been extensively studied to try and evaluate its role in the mineralisation of dentine.

Table 2.2
Chemical composition of hard tissues

	Bone	Cementum	Dentine	Enamel
% tissue weight				
Total inorganic	65	61	70	97.0
Total organic	25	27	20	0.6
Water	10	12	10	3.4
% ash weight				
Calcium	34.8	35.2	35.1	36.5
Phosphorus	15.2	16.1	16.9	17.7
Ca:P molar ratio	1:1.71	1.71	1.61	1.63
Crystal size	25 x 0.3	No data	20 x 4	130 x 30
Index of crystal regularity	33-37	33-37	33-37	70-75
% of ash weight				
Sodium	0.9	No data	0.6	0.5
Magnesium	0.72	0.73	1.23	0.44
Potassium	0.03	No data	0.05	0.08
Fluoride	0.03	No data	0.06	0.01
Chloride	0.13	No data	0.01	0.30
% dry weight carbonate	7.4	5.5	5.6	3.5

The apatite crystals of dentine are smaller than those in enamel (approximately 20 × 4 μm) and the crystallinity index (a measure of the regularity of crystal structure) is about half that in enamel. This difference in size may arise from the ease of growth of crystals during the maturation of enamel compared with the constrained growth in collagen fibre rich tissues, but it also relates to the higher carbonate and magnesium content of dentine and bone apatites.

There are few data on the distribution of inorganic ions in dentine except for fluoride. Fluoride concentrations in bulk dentine are similar to those in bulk enamel (about 300 ppm), but they rise towards the pulpal side. This is probably due to the slower deposition of dentine after tooth eruption and hence the longer period available for incorporation of fluoride from the diet and water into the forming crystals. In an area with over 1 ppm fluoride in its water supply the concentration of fluoride in dentine may be around 300 ppm.

Dentine is highly permeable to small molecules but becomes less so as it ages and undergoes further calcification

With its tubular structure dentine is highly permeable to water, small ions and dyes: application of dyes to the cut surface results in rapid permeation. Dyes placed in the pulp are less likely to penetrate because they have difficulty in passing the tight junctions between cells in the odontoblast layer. As dentine ages and intratubular dentine is laid down the permeability decreases. There is no evidence of any circulation of dentinal fluid in and between the tubules, but if dentine is exposed, as for example after gingival recession when the cementum covering the neck of the tooth has been worn away, the dentinal tubules may be open to the oral fluids. Under these circumstances an outward flow of dentinal fluid has been demonstrated. Pulpal blood flow is relatively high at some 0.4 ml/min/g, and the tissue fluid pressure amounts to some 1.5 kPa in the pulp. Calculations of the flow of dentinal fluid through open dentinal tubules and its loss by evaporation give figures of around 18 μl/cm^2/min. This figure is increased if the open tubules are exposed to toothpastes or to osmotically active solutions. Noxious stimulation of the pulp through the dentine causes an inflammatory reaction which increases the blood flow, the tissue pressure and the driving force for outward flow of dentinal fluid. It is suggested that this is a protective mechanism to remove harmful substances from the dentine surface.

Odontoblasts

Odontoblasts arise from undifferentiated pulp cells; they lay down dentine matrix, assist in its calcification and maintain the vitality of the tissue

Although located around the periphery of the dental pulp (see Fig. 4.1), the odontoblasts are intimately associated with dentine. They are the cells which form dentine: they define the dentinal tubules and their processes remain at least partially within them (Fig. 2.6). They arise from undifferentiated mesenchymal cells of the pulp, large polyhedral cells with centrally placed nuclei. During tooth development the differentiation of odontoblasts is triggered by the epithelial cells of the internal enamel epithelium or the root sheath of Hertwig, but the mechanism by which new odontoblasts are recruited in response to irritation or exposure of the pulp does not involve epithelial cells and is still unexplained.

The mature odontoblast varies somewhat in shape in different parts of the tooth, ranging from columnar in the crown, to cuboidal at mid-root level, and flattened at the root apex. The nucleus is situated basally and the cell contains a well-developed Golgi complex and rough endoplasmic reticulum when actively engaged in laying down dentine. The active cells have many secretory

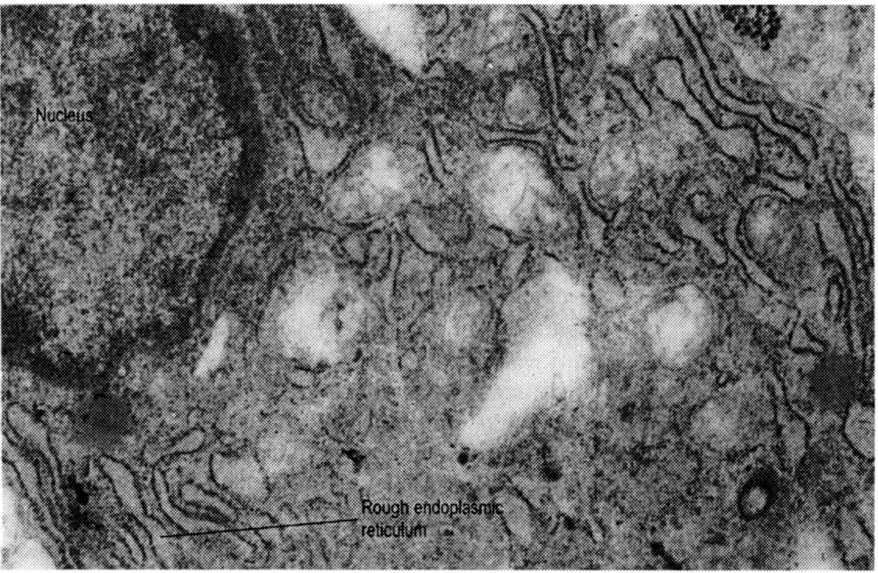

Fig. 2.6a
Electron micrograph of an odontoblast cell body.

vesicles and membrane-bound organelles, filaments and microtubules. The odontoblast process extends from a narrowing of the cell body as it enters the predentine and passes through this tissue to reach the dentine itself. The process contains few organelles: there are microtubules and filaments and some coated vesicles. There is evidence of both exocytosis and endocytosis at the junction of the cell body and the process. As the odontoblast ages and becomes less functional it loses its rough endoplasmic reticulum and the Golgi apparatus becomes reduced in size; the nucleus then adopts a more central position. The odontoblasts form a regular continuous layer of cells on the pulpal face of the predentine. In the crown of the tooth there are estimated to be some 45 000 cells/mm^2, and the crowding of these cells gives an impression of several layers; in the root the numbers are less and they can be clearly seen to form a single layer. The cells are attached to each other by tight junctions, gap junctions and desmosomes.

Enamel

Dental enamel forms the hard outer surface of the tooth crown: it is made up of highly calcified prisms of apatite crystals

Dental enamel forms the covering of the crowns of the teeth (Fig. 2.7), varying in thickness from around 2.5 mm at the tip of the unworn cusps to a feather edge where it ends at the neck of the tooth. Dental enamel is the hardest of human tissues, being made up of large crystals of apatite arranged in columns which extend from the amelodentinal junction in a predominantly perpendicular manner almost to the surface of the tooth. These columns were named prisms but their cross-sectional shape has been variously described as keyhole or fishtail; they are also termed rods (Fig. 2.8).

The organic content of enamel in the erupted tooth is around 1% by weight and 2% by volume. This contrasts with the enamel formed in the earliest

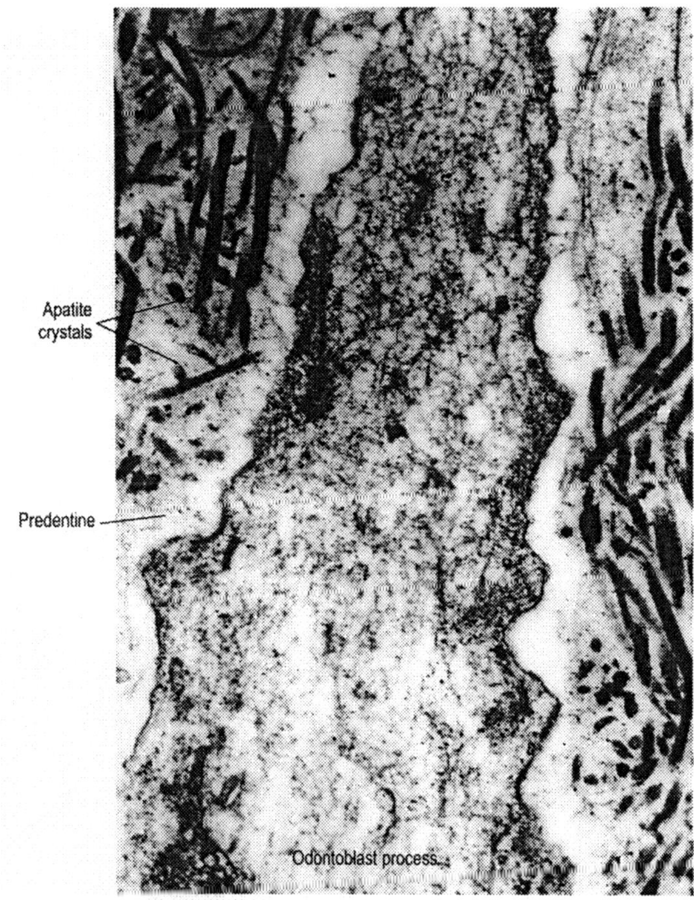

Fig. 2.6b
Electron micrograph of an odontoblast process in calcifying predentine.

stages of amelogenesis which has some 20% of organic material and 15–30% inorganic.

Enamel is only 1% organic material by weight (2% by volume)

Although originally formed in an organic matrix, fully formed enamel contains only some 1% by weight (2% by volume) of organic material, arranged as a fine reticulum around the enamel crystals and as lamellae – thin sheets of material where enamel has failed to calcify between the prisms. The organic material consists mainly of enamelins, some of the original matrix proteins which are closely associated with the crystals. The water content of the tissue is around 11% by volume although this represents only 3% by weight. Each prism or rod is made up of enamel crystals with their long axes lying longitudinally. To the cervical side of the rod the direction of crystal orientation becomes progressively more oblique until they are almost at right-angles to the rod when they meet the next more cervically placed rod. This forms the tail of the rod shape. The abrupt changes of crystal direction at the rod boundaries result in larger intercrystal spaces, giving the appearance of a prism sheath. Acid etching removes the centre of the rods first because there is less protective protein in these sites: this results in a regular series of pits on

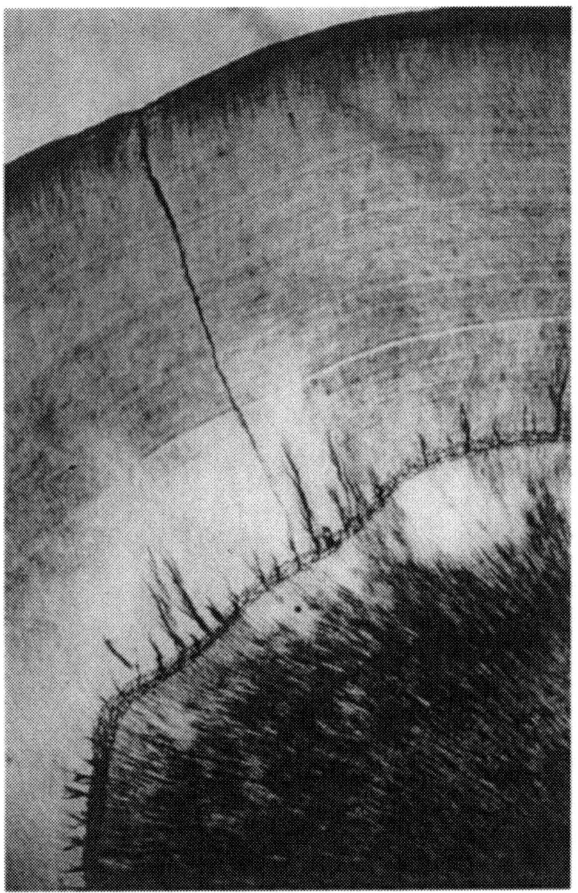

Fig. 2.7
Ground section of a tooth to show the enamel covering the dentine.

the etched surface. The adhesion of resin composite filling materials depends upon the mechanical interlocking of the resin with the uneven surface of enamel produced by etching. Despite, or because of, its hardness, enamel is extremely brittle and splits readily along the prism or rod edges if unsupported by dentine – hence the recommendation to remove unsupported prisms at the edge of cavity preparations.

The physical properties of enamel therefore are its hardness, its compressive strength, its translucency and its thermal conductivity (Table 2.3). An ideal restorative material would be capable of mimicking all these. The hardness of enamel is only slightly less than that of steel so that steel burs rapidly blunt when cutting enamel. Measurement of hardness by the Vickers or Knoop method involves the use of measured heavy forces to force a diamond-shaped diamond tip into the test substance. Standard Knoop hardness values for intact enamel are between 300 and 350 kg/mm^2. The method is used experimentally to determine the degree of decalcification and

Enamel is hard and of high compressive strength

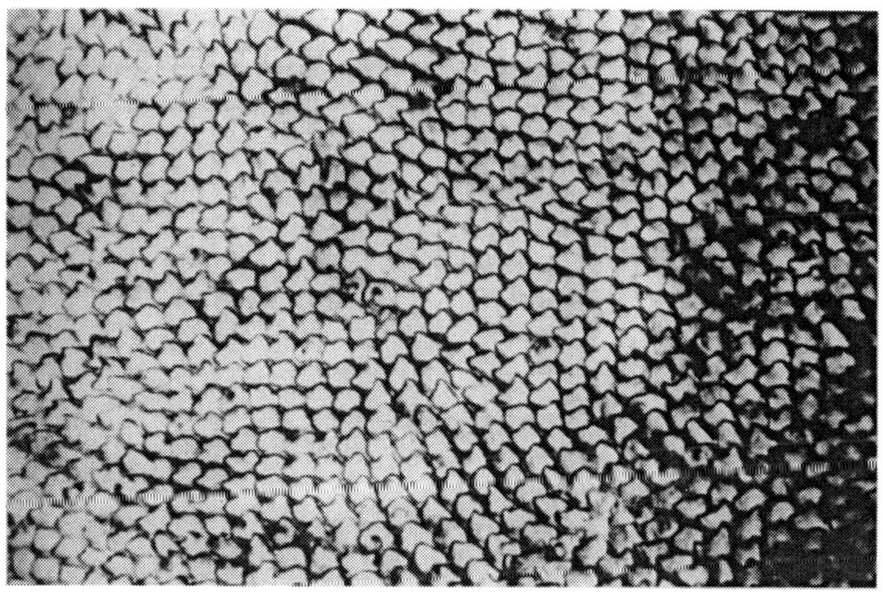

Fig. 2.8a
Transverse ground section of enamel etched to show the prism cross-sections.

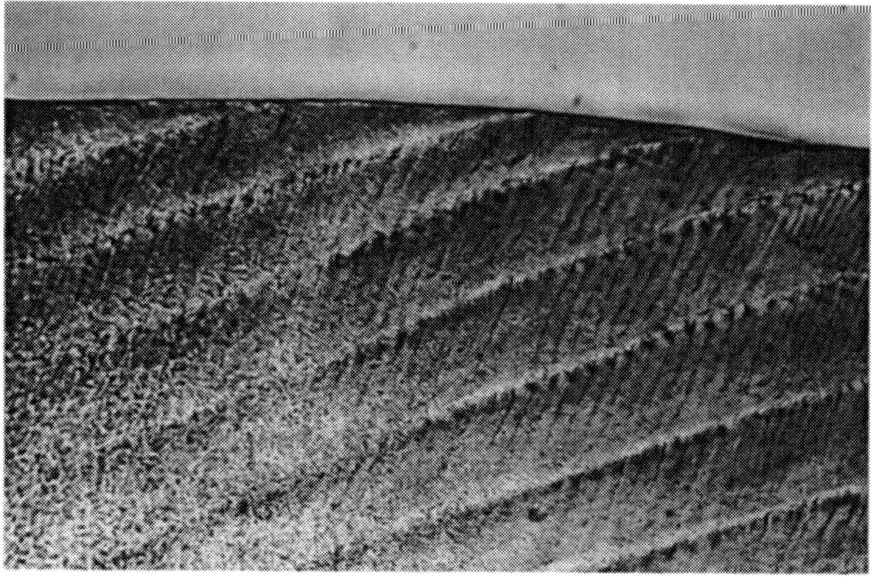

Fig. 2.8b
Longitudinal section of enamel etched to show prisms running at right-angles to the enamel surface.

Table 2.3
Properties of dental tissues and replacement materials

Thermal properties	
Thermal conductivity	(W/mK)
Enamel	0.90
Dentine	0.60
Amalgam	23.00
Composite resin	1.0
Acrylic	0.21
Porcelain	1.65
Gold	291.0
Thermal expansion ($\times 10^{-6}$/°C)	
Enamel	11.4
Amalgam	25
Composite resin	28
Acrylic	81
Porcelain	4–14
Gold	12–15

Physical properties	Knoop hardness (kg/m²)	Compressive strength (MN/m²)	Tensile strength (MN/m²)	Elastic modulus (MPa)
Enamel	300	400	35	4.8×10^4
Dentine	70	300	50	1.4×10^4
Cementum	43			
Bone (cortical)		150	90	1.38×10^4
Amalgam	110	400	55	1.4
Composite resin		250	55	1.4×10^4
Acrylic	20	97	28	
Porcelain	460	280	70	
Gold	85		600	7.7
Ca-P ceramic		300–900	70–110	$3.5–10.3 \times 10^4$

remineralisation of enamel specimens under different conditions as the hardness is a good measure of the apatite content. The compressive strength of enamel is around 300 MN/m^2. It is salutary to compare the values for hardness and compressive strength with those of restorative dental materials. Hardness, in particular, gives some idea of the resistance of a tissue to wear or abrasion. The translucency of enamel is due to its high crystal content. Enamel is slightly bluish in colour but when over its natural dentine base the yellow of the dentine shows through. Restorations can mimic only the total appearance of graded shades of yellowish white. The thermal conductivity of enamel is important because it protects the dental pulp from undue stimulation by hot foods in the mouth – and even some of the heat generated during cavity preparation. Restorative dental materials which have some of the other properties of enamel usually have greater thermal conductivity, and cavity linings have to be used to protect the pulp from thermal insult.

The high inorganic content (around 96%), the low organic and water content (about 1% and 3–4%, respectively), the lack of cells and the separation from blood vessels or tissue fluid by the intervening dentine layer give a tissue which appears to be physiologically dead. The only contrary evidence to this conclusion is the observation that, when teeth were covered in oil in an anaesthetised cat, small droplets of fluid were seen to form on the tooth surface beneath the oil layer. This enamel fluid has never been satisfactorily explained, although it was suggested that this might represent a movement of fluid down a pressure gradient from the dental pulp to the oral cavity. This would presuppose a continuous pathway through dentine. There is no histological evidence for this. However, calculation of the composition of enamel on a basis of volume rather than weight suggests that some 11% of the volume of enamel might be water. Enamel has been shown to be porous to small molecules such as urea but less so to organic dyes, which penetrate largely through defects in the enamel (the enamel lamellae with their greater protein content). Polarised light microscopy after exposure of enamel to fluids of different molecular weight gives an estimate that pores make up some 0.1% of intact enamel and this rises to around 4% in an early carious lesion. Enamel is therefore able to act as a semipermeable membrane – which permits water to cross – and even as a selectively permeable membrane – which permits some ions and small molecules to cross.

Enamel is porous to small molecules

Even if enamel is not a vital tissue it does undergo change. Its composition is not even throughout its thickness. As a result of the manner of its formation (see later) with a maturation stage in which proteins and water are removed and replaced with calcium salts, the layer nearest the amelodentinal junction has the highest protein content and therefore the lowest density. It is probable that the water content is also high in this region. The cells which form enamel, the ameloblasts, are at their most active in the early stages of enamel formation and so the carbonate content of enamel is highest at the amelodentinal junction, as is that of sodium which is usually incorporated into apatite at the same time as carbonate to balance the ionic charge. Magnesium ions are also incorporated into the apatite at an early stage of formation. There is therefore a downward gradient of concentration of these components from the amelodentinal junction to the enamel surface. Before eruption, the outer surface of enamel is exposed to tissue fluids, and, when the tooth has erupted, enamel comes into contact with the oral fluids. The apatite crystals on the enamel surface can pick up ions from the saliva, and possibly food and drink; these are taken into the outer hydration layer of the crystals and then incorporated into the crystal structure. Once within the crystal structure they can be passed on between crystals by ionic exchange. The composition of enamel does change throughout life, however, because of metabolic events in the dental plaque on its surface and because of the normal process of wear or attrition. Acid production in dental plaque selectively dissolves apatite crystals high in carbonate and, to a lesser extent, magnesium, and the

The composition of enamel varies because of the ease with which ions in the apatite structure can be substituted

remineralisation process tends to replace these with fluorapatite, thus altering the composition of the enamel surface. Attrition removes the outer layers of enamel and distorts the previously established concentration gradients: the surface fluoride concentration may be quite low when the outer layers have been worn away. Abrasion – the wear resulting from forces other than those of occlusion – and erosion – the dissolution of the tooth surface by food, drink, or even atmospheric acids – will produce more dramatic results.

The fibres of calcified tissues

The fibres of bone, dentine and cementum are collagen; enamel has no obvious fibres

Bone, dentine and cementum contain collagen as their major protein component – some 90% of the organic matrix is collagen. It is mainly type I (with two alpha-1(I) chains and one alpha-2(I) chain making up the triple helix). In predentine there are some trimeric type I helices (with three alpha-1(I) chains).

Although the term collagen is loosely used as if it referred to a single protein, it actually describes a family of some 20 proteins encoded by at least 30 genes. All collagens contain at least one region with a triple helix conformation. In the triple helix, three alpha chains, each with a left-handed helix, are wound around each other and linked by hydrogen bonds into a right-handed helix. The polypeptide chains have a repeating structure with glycine as every third residue and one in five of the remaining residues is either proline or hydroxyproline. After secretion from the fibroblast the collagens form a variety of supramolecular structures. In the case of the so-called fibrillar collagens – types I, II, III and V – the fibrils consist of tropocollagen molecules aligned with each other, the heads and tails of successive molecules in a line being separated by a 40-nm gap, and the molecules in adjacent lines being displaced by 64 nm relative to each other; this arrangement is described as a quarter stagger because it corresponds with a quarter of the 285 nm length of the tropocollagen complex (Fig. 2.9). Other collagen types do not form fibrils but are arranged in a meshwork (type IV, found in basement membranes), or may link collagen fibrils to other molecules in the matrix (the fibril-associated collagens with interrupted helices such as IX, XII and XIV). Cross-linking occurs between collagen molecules in type I fibres at lysine and hydroxylysine residues and increases slowly throughout life. The cross-linking confers strength on the molecule, but as the number of cross-links increases with age the collagen-containing soft tissues become stiffer and lose their elasticity.

Enamel proteins are small in quantity and do not provide an obvious fibrous framework.

The extracellular matrix in calcified tissues

The extracellular matrix of mesodermally derived tissues consists of glycoproteins and proteoglycans

In connective tissues generally the extracellular matrix forms a gel holding the extracellular fluid. In specific situations the components of the gel hold greater volumes of fluid and may exert pressure on neighbouring structures. The matrix contains proteins and proteoglycans which mediate attachment between different cells and between extracellular fibres and cells.

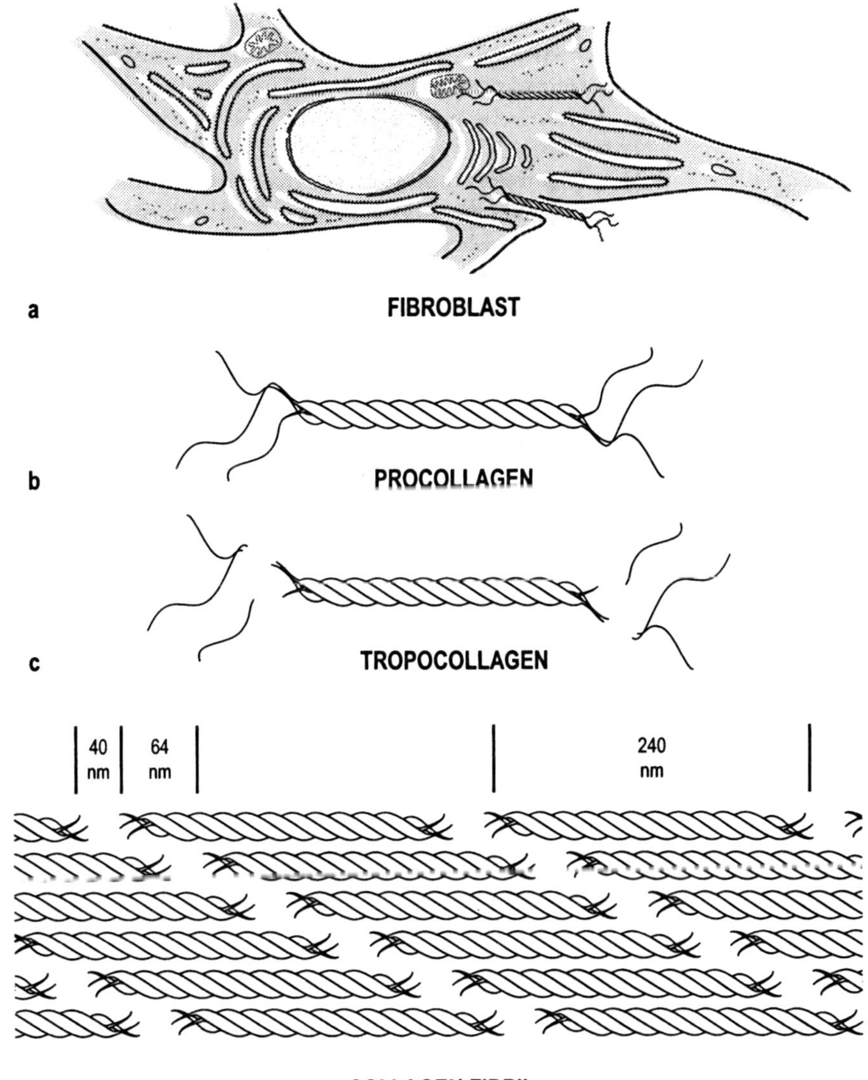

Fig. 2.9
Sequence of formation of collagen fibres. Hydroxylation of precursor peptide chains by 3-proline hydroxylase, 4-proline hydroxylase and lysine hydroxylase results in the helical procollagen peptides within the fibroblast. These are then wound in threes to form the triple helix of procollagen. At this stage terminal peptides prevent further aggregation. After secretion from the fibroblast the terminal peptides are split off by exopeptidases to form tropocollagen molecules which can then aggregate to form collagen fibrils. The tropocollagen molecules link along their long axes so that each molecule is displaced by one-quarter its length (64 nm) in relation to its neighbour, and separated from the next molecule in line by 40 nm. The resulting periodicity is observable in electron micrographs as a 64-nm cross-banding on the collagen fibres. The separation between one molecule and the next in line gives the so-called 'hole' regions in the fibre. The earliest crystals of hydroxapatite are often seen in the hole regions of collagen fibres in calcifying collagenous tissues.

The molecules of the matrix also have signalling functions and can influence cell shape, movement and multiplication by binding to cell-surface proteins known as integrins. The extracellular matrix of the calcified tissues performs the special function of allowing crystallisation of calcium salts to occur.

The main components of the matrix of tissues derived from mesoderm are glycoproteins and proteoglycans. The glycoproteins are described as adhesive molecules as they often function to bind together other matrix components with each other or with the tissue cells. The gene products are diverse because of alternative splicing. Thus fibronectin, the most studied of the glycoproteins, appears in a number of isomeric forms. Parts of its molecule are specialised, with sequences of amino acids that allow it to bind to cell membrane integrins, and other sequences which can bind to bacterial cell walls or to other proteins in the matrix. Other glycoproteins in the matrix share common amino acid sequences found in fibronectin: laminin, thrombospondin and tenascin are examples. Another amino acid sequence in these glycoproteins can bind to receptors for epithethial growth factor, suggesting some kind of signalling role for these components. The proteoglycans are a family of molecules consisting of a protein core with one or more glycosaminoglycan chains attached. The glycosaminoglycan chains consist of alternating amino sugars (*N*-acetylglucosamine or *N*-acetylgalactosamine) and uronic acids (glucuronic or iduronic acid, or galactose). Many of these are sulphated. The glycosaminoglycans include hyaluronic acid, chondroitin sulphate, dermatan sulphate, keratan sulphate and heparan sulphate, as well as the very large hyaluronan. Many matrix proteoglycans are small molecules (decorin, biglycan and fibromodulin), but others form very large aggregates – such as aggrecan present in cartilage.

Cartilage

The extracellular matrix of cartilage contains the proteoglycans aggrecan, decorin, biglycan and fibromodulin

The major proteoglycan of cartilage (5–10% wet weight) is aggrecan. This is a large proteoglycan with keratan sulphate and chondroitin sulphate side-chains. It binds to hyaluronate to form a meshwork which takes up and swells with water. The pressure of this against the collagen fibre framework gives the tissue great resistance to compression. The small proteoglycans, decorin, biglycan and fibromodulin, are present in similar molar quantities but their much smaller molecular size means that they represent only 1–2% of the proteoglycan by weight. The other proteins described in cartilage are anchorin CII, cartilage matrix protein, cartilage oligomeric high molecular mass matrix protein (COMP), chondrocalcin, Ch21, fibronectin, and a 48-kDa protein. Although some of these proteins have interesting binding properties, little is known of their function in cartilage matrix. However, mutations in COMP are associated with some forms of chondrodysplasia.

When bone mineralisation takes place in cartilage, there is a clear association of proteoglycans with the formed crystals and calcium and proteoglycans are co-located at the first sites of crystallisation.

Bone

The extracellular matrix of bone contains acidic glycoproteins and small proteoglycans. Gamma-carboxyglutamate-containing proteins are also found in the matrix

The organic component of bone is largely collagen, but other components are present in small amounts – acidic glycoproteins, serum proteins and small proteoglycans.

In the matrix of forming bone the attachment glycoproteins thrombospondin and fibronectin are present, together with the acidic glycoprotein osteonectin. One group of acidic glycoproteins is the phosphoproteins, which exhibit strong calcium-binding properties and can also bind to collagen. Such proteins might themselves act as seeds or may be able to do so when linked to collagen. In supersaturated solutions of calcium and phosphate many of these proteins inhibit crystal formation, but when they attach to an immobilised layer of collagen they promote crystal formation.

Gamma-carboxyglutamate-containing (GLA) proteins in bone

Proteins containing the unusual amino acid gamma-carboxyglutamate, formed from glutamate by a vitamin K-dependent posttranslational modification, are found in bone. Two types are described: osteocalcins and matrix GLA proteins. Osteocalcins are very small proteins which make up most of the GLA protein in bone. Although osteocalcins bind calcium relatively poorly, they can induce some mineral formation in calcium phosphate solutions and they can bind to hydroxyapatite. However, they inhibit growth of seeded apatite crystals. Interestingly, serum levels of these proteins increase during bone formation and in patients with metabolic bone disease. Another of these proteins demonstrated in bone is simply known as matrix GLA protein. When the genes coding for osteocalcins or GLA proteins are removed from, or are unable to function in, experimental animals, there is excessive deposition of bone or widespread ectopic calcification, suggesting that their normal function is to regulate bone growth and calcification.

Other acidic non-collagenous proteins of bone

Osteonectin and osteopontin (bone acidic sialoprotein) are two of the acidic proteins of bone

Many other proteins of bone contain aspartic, glutamic and sialic acids so that they are acidic in nature. Osteonectin is the major non-collagenous protein of bone. It binds strongly to hydroxyapatite and has a non-specific binding to collagen. After its demonstration in extracellular matrix in other tissues it was found to be identical with SPARC, a glycoprotein in basement membrane. It seems unlikely that osteonectin plays any role in calcification although it is known to inhibit growth of apatite seeds in vitro. Other major members of this group are termed bone acidic sialoprotein I or osteopontin and bone sialoprotein II (BSPII). Several other acidic glycoproteins and some serum proteins such as albumin have been also identified.

Bone contains a number of growth-related proteins and peptides, such as bone morphogenetic protein, transforming growth factor beta and insulin-like growth factors IGF1 and IGF2.

Proteoglycans of bone

Adult bone contains the proteoglycans biglycan and decorin. The main glycosaminoglycan is chondroitin 4-sulphate

The proteoglycans form the second major group of non-collagenous macromolecules in bone. The proteoglycan versican is observed at an early stage in bone formation but is subsequently replaced by biglycan and decorin. Mineralised bone contains the small proteoglycans biglycan with two side-chains, and decorin with one. The side-chains are galactosaminoglycans, the principal one being chondroitin 4-sulphate. There are also reports of chondroitin 6-sulphate and small amounts of dermatan sulphate. The protein core is small – around 36 kDa. The role of the proteoglycans is unclear. It has been suggested that they can initiate collagen fibre formation by providing a nucleus for the molecule. Later, however, they retard fibre formation and they can stabilise a collagen fibre network. These properties suggest that they may be controlling factors in the organisation of the collagen network. Their properties in relation to apatite crystallisation are apparently contradictory: in solution they inhibit crystallisation but when immobilised on a solid support they promote crystallisation. It is possible that the meshwork of proteoglycan molecules may inhibit diffusion of ions and this would account for the inhibitory effect on crystal formation. These diverse properties may, however, be useful in the control of mineralisation.

Cementum

Cementum contains osteopontin and other proteins found in bone matrix. The matrix close to dentine also contains amelogenin-like proteins

Cytochemical studies with antibodies against osteopontin, osteocalcin, osteonectin (SPARC), bone sialoprotein, bone acidic glycoprotein-75, serum albumin and alpha-2 HS-glycoprotein have given detailed information as to the occurrence of these proteins in cementum. In the layer next to mantle dentine there is a higher concentration of non-collagenous proteins, particularly osteopontin. Osteopontin is thought to bind to mineral, and to type I collagen and osteocalcin; it can also cross-link to fibronectin. This suggests that it has an important function in the binding of cementum to dentine and in tissue cohesion. It is found at the cementum lines and bone cement lines where a new layer of hard tissue has been laid down on an existing hard tissue surface, and in the first layer of bone formed against prosthetic implants of titanium and hydroxyapatite. Other organic molecules in cementum include fibronectin, tenascin, cementum-derived attachment protein and a number of growth factors.

The cementum matrix laid down next to dentine contains collagen fibres, amelogenin-like proteins, osteopontin, bone sialoprotein, osteocalcin and alpha-2 HS-glycoprotein. Bone acidic glycoprotein is not found in cementum matrix.

Dentine

The distribution of proteoglycans in dentine differs from that in bone, and dentine matrix contains the unique highly

Analysis of dentine matrices, like those of bone, reveals many non-collagenous proteins: the acidic highly phosphorylated phosphoproteins, GLA proteins such as osteocalcins, acidic glycoproteins like osteonectin, serum proteins and proteoglycans. The highly phosphorylated phosphoproteins are thought to be unique to dentine, and the distribution of the proteoglycans is not the same as that in bone. Many of these non-collagenous proteins have been shown to

phosphorylated phosphoproteins such as phosphophoryn

promote apatite crystallisation, whilst some proteoglycans inhibit it. It is likely that they are important in controlling the growth and orientation of the apatite crystals.

Other organic materials in dentine include lipid (about 0.1%) and citrate (about 0.9%).

Phosphoproteins in dentine

The largest group of non-collagenous proteins in dentine are phosphoproteins. More than half the total amount of phosphoprotein in dentine is termed highly phosphorylated phosphoprotein or phosphophoryn. This is not found in bone. It contains more than 20% phosphate, probably as phosphoserine since serine makes up 50% of the amino acid residues. Another acidic amino acid, aspartic acid, accounts for a further 40% of residues; it is not surprising, therefore, that phosphophoryn is one of the most acidic phosphoproteins known, with an isoelectric point of 1.1. Because of the unusual composition, the molecular weight has been difficult to measure and varying figures have been put forward. There is evidence that some of the highly phosphorylated phosphoprotein is linked to collagen and this may have some significance in the mineralisation process. The distribution of this protein in dentine is not uniform – in bovine dentine there is more in dentine taken from the crown than that in the root – and it is not present in predentine. The properties of the highly phosphorylated phosphoprotein suggest that it may be significant in the mineralisation process since it binds calcium ions strongly, it is able to bind phosphate in a ratio of 8:3 with calcium (a ratio observed in amorphous calcium phosphate) and it can induce hydroxyapatite formation when present in low concentrations and stabilised on some solid support.

The other phosphoproteins of dentine are much less highly phosphorylated. They are found in predentine as well as dentine and they resemble those found in bone.

Proteoglycans of dentine

The proteoglycans of dentine are similar to those of bone

The proteoglycans form the second major group of non-collagenous macromolecules in dentine. Mineralised dentine contains the small glycoproteins biglycan with two side-chains, and decorin with one. As in bone the side-chains are galactosaminoglycans. The main glycosaminoglycan is chondroitin 4-sulphate with some chondroitin 6-sulphate, hyaluronic acid, dermatan sulphate and keratin sulphate. The protein core is small – around 36 kDa. Dentine and predentine have differing glycosaminoglycan compositions. In predentine the free glycosaminoglycan hyaluronate is present and the proteoglycans themselves seem to be larger.

Gamma-carboxyglutamate-containing (GLA) proteins in dentine

Osteocalcin is absent from dentine

Osteocalcins, which make up most of the GLA protein in bone, appear to be virtually absent from human dentine forming in tooth germs. In rat incisors, osteocalcins are synthesised by the odontoblasts before calcification begins.

They are present in vesicles in the odontoblast process, but not in predentine itself. Matrix GLA protein has been demonstrated in dentine.

Other acidic non-collagenous proteins of dentine

Many other proteins of dentine contain aspartic, glutamic and sialic acids, so they are acidic in nature. Osteonectin, the major non-collagenous protein of bone, represents about 5% of the protein in bovine dentine and is present in predentine and in the odontoblasts to a greater degree than in the intertubular dentine. It is not present in rat incisor dentine. The bone acidic sialoprotein osteopontin has been found in predentine but may be absent from dentine.

As in bone, several other acidic glycoproteins and serum proteins have been identified in rat incisor dentine. Dentine, like bone, contains bone morphogenetic protein, transforming growth factor beta and IGF1 and IGF2. The bone and dentine morphogenetic factors have been studied with a view to using them as stimulants of dentine formation across small traumatic exposures of the pulp and some success has been claimed for this treatment.

Enamel

The proteins of enamel are known as amelogenins and enamelins. The former are largely lost during the maturation stage of enamel formation but the latter persist in the adult enamel

The protein content of enamel in its first formed state is approximately 90% amelogenin and 10% enamelin. The amelogenins are lost preferentially during the process of maturation when the matrix is removed and replaced by the growth of the apatite crystals. The amelogenins are high in proline, leucine, histidine and glutamine, but unlike collagen or keratin they contain no hydroxyproline or cystine. One of the smaller amelogenins with a molecular mass of around 5 kDa is rich in tyrosine and is therefore known as TRAP (tyrosine-rich enamel peptide). The enamelin, however, has a molecular mass between 50 and 70 kDa. It contains less proline, glutamine and histidine but more aspartate, serine, glycine, alanine and arginine. It is glycosylated with some 4% hexosamine and 4% sialic acid. Recent work suggests that one enamelin protein is identical with, or at least very similar to, serum albumin. It remains after maturation and appears to be bound to the enamel crystals where it is located with its long axis perpendicular to the length or c-axis. It is possible that the enamelins play some part in determining the shape and size of enamel crystals. Mature enamel contains acidic proteins, low molecular weight lipids, and some carbohydrate and organic acids such as citrate and lactate.

The mineral component of calcified tissues – apatite

With the exception of the calcite otoliths of the middle ear, all mammalian calcified tissues are made up of calcium phosphate salts. The process of calcification in the mineralised tissues is therefore a transition from soluble calcium and phosphate ions to crystalline calcium phosphates and must be governed by the solubility products of those crystals. Similar considerations apply both to bone and to the dental tissues.

Three simple combinations of cations and phosphate can exist in solution according to pH, and phosphates are able to provide buffering power for this reason. They are orthophosphate, monohydrogen phosphate and dihydrogen phosphate. In plasma at pH 7.4 the monohydrogen phosphate is the more likely to exist. However, there are at least eight crystalline calcium phosphates reported in calcified tissues (Table 2.4). The simplest of these is monetite – a monohydrogen salt often referred to as dicalcium phosphate. It is, however uncommon in calcified tissues: the hydrated form, brushite ($CaHPO_4 \cdot 2H_2O$), is more likely to crystallise from biological solutions. Between pH 4 and pH 7 brushite will crystallise from supersaturated solutions such as plasma. As the pH approaches 7, a new crystal form, octacalcium phosphate, appears. This has a unit cell of $Ca_8(PO_4)_4(HPO_4)_2 \cdot 5H_2O$. At pH values above 7 the crystal product depends upon the degree of supersaturation. In the presence of some other ions, particularly magnesium, whitlockite $Ca_9(PO_4)_6$ may be formed. Supersaturated solutions yield apatite $Ca_{10}(PO_4)_6(OH)_2$, whilst less supersaturated yield imperfect apatites – typically $Ca_9(PO_4)_5(HPO_4)(OH)$. An amorphous calcium phosphate with no clear X-ray diffraction pattern is thought to precede and transform into apatite during calcification in many tissues, and a crystal form intermediate between apatite and octacalcium phosphate – tricalcium phosphate – may exist but transforms spontaneously into apatite. Apatite itself shows many minor variations, of which the substitution of carbonate ions for hydroxyl is one.

Human bone is made up of 20% magnesium whitlockite, 15% non-carbonate-containing apatite and 65% carbonated apatite. Dental enamel is a

Table 2.4
Crystal forms of calcium phosphate found in hard tissues

Calcium phosphate	Structure	Occurrence
Apatite	$(Ca,w)_{10}\,(PO_4,x)_6(OH,y)_2$	Bone, dental enamel, dentine, dental calculus
Carbonate apatite	$(Ca_{10-x}Na_x)(PO_4)_{6-x}(CO_3)_x(OH)_2$	As above
Fluorhydroxyapatite	$Ca_{10}(PO_4)_6(F,OH)_2$	As above
Fluorapatite	$Ca_{10}(PO_4)_6F_2$	Fluorosed bone
Brushite, dicalcium phosphate dihydrate	$CaHPO_4 \cdot 2H_2O$	Dental calculus
Octacalcium phosphate	$Ca_8H_2(PO_4)_6 \cdot 5H_2O$	Dental calculus
Whitlockite, tricalcium phosphate	$(Ca,x)_9(PO_{4,x})_6$	Dental calculus, dental caries
Amorphous calcium phosphate	$(Ca,Mg)_?(PO_4,z)_?$	Calcification sites

w may be Na, Mg, K, Sr, etc.
x may be CO_3, HPO_4, etc.
y may be Cl, F.
z may be P_2O_7, CO_3.

mixture of carbonated and non-carbonated apatite with a small proportion of magnesium whitlockite, whilst dentine contains some 20% non-carbonated apatite and about 30% magnesium whitlockite.

The key crystal in all these is apatite. The unit cell of apatite has a hexagonal arrangement of phosphate ions with the hydroxyl ions forming a core within this (Fig. 2.10). Calcium ions are arranged on a screw axis forms around the phosphates.

The most usual form of crystalline calcium phosphate in human tissues is hydroxyapatite, although other forms may also occur

Ion substitutions can occur within the unit cell if the substituent ion is of similar size (ionic radius) to the normal ion. Thus carbonate substitutes for hydroxyl but more rarely for phosphate. Fluoride can substitute for hydroxyl. Since fluoride is smaller than hydroxyl the column of hydroxyl ions is dislocated and the *a*-axis of the crystal is decreased in size from 0.947 nm to 0.938 nm if both hydroxyls are substituted. This shorter *a*-axis is associated with a decrease in solubility of the crystal: such substitution will affect the properties of structures built up from the crystal; thus dental enamel with a high proportion of hydroxyapatite will dissolve more slowly in acid than will enamel with a low fluorapatite content. Properties such as hardness depend upon the proportion of the tissue made up by the hard crystals; hydroxyapatite and fluorapatite crystal structures are too similar to affect the hardness of the tissue.

The phosphate ions are the largest ions in the crystal. They can be regarded as spheres packed tightly together. Each ion is therefore in contact with six others in each plane. The next plane of phosphate ions fit into the hollows between spheres and so on. This results in a structure in which each phosphate ion is immediately above or below a phosphate ion in the next but one plane. The spaces between the spheres are filled by the smaller ions. Of the spaces in a hexagon of phosphate ions two are filled by a column of calcium ions and one by a column of hydroxyl ions. The columns of calcium ions contain 40% of the calcium: the remainder line the channel containing the hydroxyl ions.

Substituents

Hydroxyapatite often contains ions which have substituted into the crystal lattice (e.g. carbonate and fluoride)

Biological apatites differ from pure synthetic crystals in several ways. Firstly, they are microcrystalline and may be mixed with other crystal forms; secondly, the proportions of ions present depart from the 1.67 calcium:phosphate molar ratio of pure apatite (with enamel and dentine having slightly lower proportions and bone slightly higher); and thirdly, there are many elements other than calcium and phosphorus present in trace amounts. These impurities may be present in the apatite lattice, on the crystal surfaces or in other non-apatite crystals.

The main substituents in human apatite are: HPO_4 and CO_3 for PO_4; Sr, Ba, Pb, Na, K and Mg for Ca; and F, Cl, Br and I for OH. Crystallographers describe two types of carbonate apatite: one with the carbonate substituting for hydroxyl ions and the other with carbonate substituting for phosphate ions. The former is rare in biological apatites whilst the latter occurs frequently, usually in association with a sodium for calcium substitution. As the substituent ion is not exactly the same size as the one substituted for, the dimensions of the crystal axes will be modified and the properties of the crystal will be altered. This may

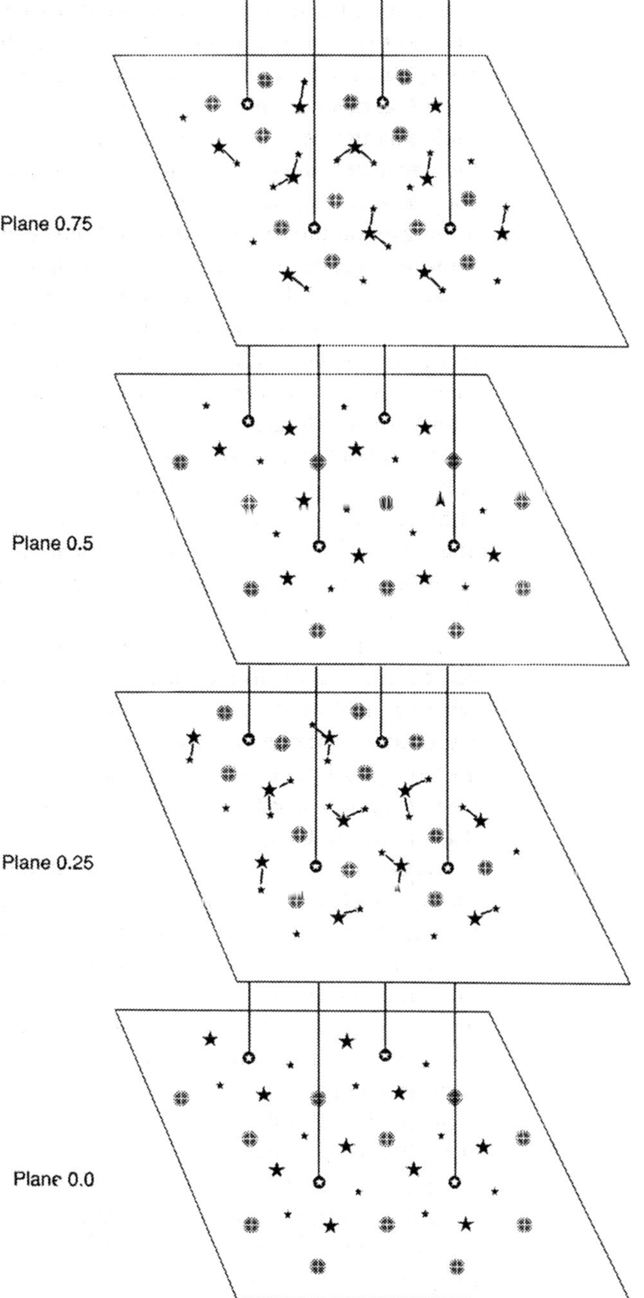

Fig. 2.10
The ionic arrangement in hydroxyapatite. The diagram shows the 0.0, 0.25, 0.50 and 0.75 planes in the unit structure. The column of hydroxyl ions ✪ extends up through these planes. A triangle of calcium ions ⊕ surrounds the hydroxyls at the 0.25 and 0.75 planes and more widely spaced calcium ions ⊕ form a hexagon around each hydroxyl column on the 0.0 and 0.50 planes. The oxygen atoms are those of the phosphate ions: on the 0.25 and 0.75 planes these lie on the plane ★, but they are slightly above ⋆ or slightly below the 0.0 and 0.5 planes.

be important in diseases which affect the calcified tissues. The ions present in dental enamel may influence dental caries both by affecting the dissolution of the apatite crystals and by affecting the remineralisation process which repairs the initial defect. Thus boron, copper, fluoride, lithium, magnesium, molybdenum, strontium and vanadium have all been identified as inhibiting the development of carious lesions, whilst carbonate, cadmium, chloride, copper, lead, magnesium, potassium, selenium and silicon have been identified as promoting the carious attack. Of these, fluoride and carbonate seem to be the most important. The appearance of magnesium in both lists reflects the fact that magnesium may be incorporated together with either fluoride or carbonate, as well as the different measures which have been used to assess cariogenicity. The processes of calcification and remineralisation can also be affected by ions present in the calcifying solution: pyrophosphate, magnesium, fluoride and strontium are all known to influence mineralisation.

Fluoride in appropriate concentrations promotes bone formation and enhances calcification and remineralisation by increasing the rate of hydrolysis of amorphous calcium phosphate, brushite and octacalcium phosphate to apatite, and by promoting apatite formation even in acid or high magnesium solutions. At the crystal level, fluoride fits neatly between calcium ions so that the crystal is smaller in the *a*-axis and more stable; this permits the growth of larger crystals with less intracrystal strain and results in a more stoichometric composition closer to the ideal 1.67 calcium:phosphate molar ratio. All these effects contribute to a decreased solubility in acid. However, the application of high concentrations of fluoride to the surface of a calcified tissue will result in the precipitation of calcium fluoride rather than the incorporation of fluoride into the apatite crystals and this will therefore have little effect on acid dissolution of the apatite.

Carbonate causes a decrease in the *a*-axis and a lengthening of the *c*-axis; the crystals become more like hexagonal plates than needles, they are smaller, have greater intracrystal strain, and are more soluble. Sodium ions increase carbonate substitution whilst strontium ions decrease it. After exposure to acid the carbonate content of apatite decreases, either because the carbonate apatite dissolves more readily or because any remineralisation results in an apatite with a lower carbonate content.

Magnesium decreases the *a*-axis and the crystallinity of apatite and increases its solubility. Most other cations with the exception of sodium are larger than calcium and cause expansion of the *a*- and *c*-axes. Strontium increases solubility.

Where fluoride and other substitutions occur together, the protective effect of fluoride dominates: thus fluoride reduces or eliminates the effects of carbonate, magnesium and strontium on crystal size, crystal stress and solubility.

Minor variations in the composition of the hard tissues

Characteristic variations in apatite substitution occur in different hard tissues

Although the composition of each of the hard tissues of the body shows little variation in its major components from site to site, or even between individuals, there may be considerable variation in the minor components depending upon the age of the tissue and its local environment, which in turn may be influenced by the environment and nutrition of the body as a whole. Thus bone will accumulate fluoride throughout life but the actual amount will depend upon the fluoride content of the water supply. In a low fluoride area the bone of a 5-year-old has some 250 ppm of fluoride whereas that from an 80-year-old will have increased to 2000 ppm. In an area where the water supply contains around 1 ppm (0.05 mM) the corresponding figures will be 500 ppm and 4000 ppm.

The distribution depends upon the plasma and extracellular fluid concentrations of ions and on the ability of these to exchange with the apatite of the bone. In dentine and, more particularly, enamel, the possibility of ion exchange is more limited. The first formed dentine and enamel are similar in fluoride content to each other and to young bone; up to the time of eruption there is slow accumulation of fluoride in both tissues. After tooth eruption dentine continues to accumulate fluoride from the interstitial fluid of the pulp and the limited exchange with already formed dentine gives an increase from 100 ppm at 5 years to 700 ppm at 80 years. Enamel of the erupted teeth, however, is exposed to the fluoride ions in saliva (similar to interstitial fluid) and in the water and food and drink – usually in excess of extracellular fluid concentrations. As a result, the fluoride content of the surface enamel increases markedly and there is a steep downward gradient of concentration in the outer few micrometres of the enamel. The concentration in the outer layers may be several thousand parts per million compared with a few hundred at the amelodentinal junction. This is evident in Table 10.2.

As well as fluoride, zinc, lead, tin and iron are all found in higher concentrations in surface enamel than in the deeper layers, and there is again a gradient of concentration downwards into the deeper enamel, although the effects are less marked. Ions which are incorporated into the forming crystal structure throughout amelogenesis and which are low in concentration in saliva will remain evenly distributed through enamel: strontium and copper are examples.

Other elements may be present in enamel or dentine as a result of systemic uptake from the environment. Lead is a good example: its steady incorporation into dentine as it forms throughout life makes this tissue a good marker of exposure to lead. Until the introduction of lead-free fuels, teeth from urban and rural areas could be distinguished by this characteristic.

Brief exposure to some substances during the formative period of calcified tissues may result in clearly defined lines in those tissues. The earliest report of this was that of Brash, who fed the dye madder to pigs and then was able to identify stained lines within bone. From this he was able to quantitate accurately the amount of bone formed between two periods of madder feeding and so study bone growth. The tetracyclines are incorporated into hard tissues and produce discoloration. This can be more readily seen in ultraviolet light which causes the tetracycline to fluoresce. Treatment with these antibiotics will have no visible effect in adults but if they are administered to young children they may be taken up into forming enamel and produce an unsightly grey line or patch on the teeth. Apart from the dental interest in demonstrating which parts of the tooth enamel in different teeth were formed at the same time, the consequent markings, particularly on incisors and canine teeth, may cause the patient to seek cosmetic treatment such as veneers over the anterior surfaces.

Significance of apatite substituents in relation to dental caries

Dental enamel is less susceptible to dental caries if fluoride is substituted into the apatite crystals, but more susceptible if the carbonate content is increased

The effects of ions substituted into the apatite crystal on its solubility in acid already described might explain some of the variation in the susceptibility of enamel to dental caries. There has been extensive analysis of enamel to see whether the presence of any particular elements or radicals in the apatite is associated with greater or lesser susceptibility to dental caries. The only clear-cut correlations are with fluoride, which reduces susceptibility, and carbonate, which increases it. Currently there are investigations into the treatment of enamel with low power lasers which can heat the surface of the enamel to temperatures of around 600°C and break down carbonate apatites so that hydroxy- or fluorapatite remains. In the laboratory such treated enamel is resistant to acid dissolution and yet, by treating small areas at a time, the temperature of the dental pulp remains within safe limits. Analysis of carious lesions in enamel usually shows high levels of fluoride together with appreciable levels of magnesium. This is thought to be due to the rapid uptake of these ions by the newly exposed layers of apatite. Magnesium seems to have an anti-caries effect, reducing the spread of the lesion. Other elements which are associated with reduced susceptibility to caries are molybdenum and vanadium, but there is no evidence of their localisation in enamel. Similarly, selenium, associated with increased caries susceptibility, has not been demonstrated to show significant variation in dental enamel.

Further reading

Standard texts in dental anatomy and histology

Mineral Aspects of Dentistry. Driessens, F.C.M. Monographs in Oral Science, Vol. 10. Karger, Basel, 1982

Calcium Phosphates in Biology and Medicine. LeGeros, R.Z. Monographs in Oral Science, Vol. 15. Karger, Basel, 1991

3 Calcification

Problems of calcification: how, why and where

It is not difficult to explain why calcium phosphate crystals appear in a test-tube when sufficiently concentrated solutions containing calcium and phosphate ions are mixed together: in biological situations it is difficult to explain why a complex crystal form such as apatite should appear, why, if calcium and phosphate ion concentrations in body fluids appear to be sufficient, calcification does not occur throughout the body, and why, if calcium and phosphate concentrations in body fluids are not sufficient, calcification should occur at all or, even more surprisingly, in very specific locations. The problem can be approached by considering the physicochemical constraints on crystallisation of apatite, or its possible precursor crystals, by looking at the specificity of biological calcification, and finally by considering the calcification of the individual hard tissues.

Physicochemical considerations

Crystallisation from a solution is seen as occurring in two steps: nucleation and crystal growth. In any solution there is constant movement of solute and solvent particles. For any ion or molecule in solution the energy involved in this movement will be proportional to the concentration of that ion or molecule, so that, at low concentrations, ionic activity can be expressed as concentration. In more concentrated solutions the random collision of particles results in energy loss and so the ionic activity is less than might be expected from the number of ions at that concentration. The possibility of collision between ions to form the first arrangement of ions as in a crystal depends upon the product of the component ionic activities. Two consequences follow from that: precipitation of a crystal depends upon concentrations in solution; and the more ions involved in the unit cell of the crystal, the more energy will be required. The situation is even more complex because the collision of the ions results in formation of an ion aggregate which is itself unstable – unless the forces holding the aggregation together exceed those involved in the normal movement of the ions crystal formation will not occur. The formation of an aggregation of ions as the first step in crystallisation is termed nucleation. The energy requirement for nucleation is termed the activation energy barrier and it depends upon the number of ions in the crystal, upon the ratio of the ion activity product to the solubility product (i.e. the ion

Precipitation occurs when the ionic activity product exceeds the solubility product of the crystal

Nucleation is the first aggregation of ions to form a crystal

activity product of a solution in equilibrium with formed crystals) and also upon the diameter of the ion cluster (because this is related to the energy requirement to maintain the cluster surface).

A solution is termed supersaturated when the ion activity product exceeds the solubility product: in these circumstances nucleation will take place if a sufficiently large ion cluster can form – in the case of apatite this is probably around 1 nm. Thus, as the concentrations in solution are increased, there are three stages: a stage of undersaturation, a stage of supersaturation where the formation of ion clusters is balanced by the breakdown of ion clusters, and a stage of nucleation where the formation of ion clusters exceeds their dissolution. Because nucleation can be achieved in another way if the activation energy barrier can be overcome by the introduction of other components into the solution, this simpler form of nucleation is termed homogeneous nucleation.

Calcium phosphate can crystallise in a number of forms

There are a variety of crystal forms of calcium phosphate as described in Table 2.3. These differ in the types of phosphate ion, depending upon the pH of the solution and in their content of other ions such as hydroxyl. Phase diagrams can be constructed to show how crystal forms will vary with ion activity products and pH (Fig. 3.1). In body tissues the pH would be expected

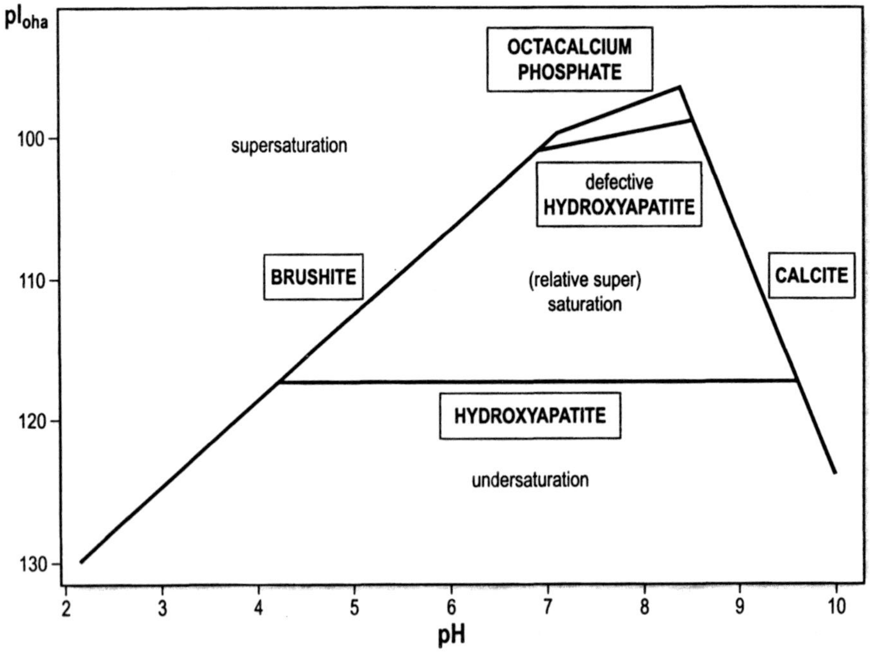

Phase diagram for calcium phosphate precipitation in the presence of carbon dioxide. pI_{oha} is here used as an index of the solubility product of the different calcium phosphate forms. Each line refers to the solubility product (or precipitation product) of the crystal form indicated on the label nearest to it. Under each line the solution is undersaturated, above each line the solution is supersaturated, with respect to that crystal form.

to be around 7.2 (nearer that of venous than arterial blood), although it might be altered by local tissue products. At such a pH the first material precipitated from a supersaturated solution of calcium and phosphate appears to be amorphous – i.e. of no defined crystal structure. Chemical analysis of amorphous calcium phosphate reveals a composition virtually identical to that of whitlockite. Amorphous calcium phosphate is more soluble than apatite but at physiological pH it tranforms into octacalcium phosphate $Ca_8H_2(PO_4)_6 \bullet 5H_2O$. These two crystals form more readily than apatite because they have lower surface energies – i.e. the ion clusters are less likely to break up. However, both these crystal forms can tranform into apatite at a later stage (Fig. 3.2).

Local increases in calcium and phosphate concentrations may cause crystallisation

In human serum, and probably in most extracellular fluids, the activity product for calcium and phosphate ions is around 1.3 mM^2, whilst the activity product required for nucleation is above 2.0 mM^2. It is possible that in localised extracellular fluid sites the ionic concentrations could be higher – as, for example, in the vicinity of cells actively pumping out calcium – but the first mineralised material in calcifying tissues is always some distance away from the cells. In tissues which calcify relatively quickly the cells bud off small membraneous sacs into the matrix. These membrane vesicles are described more fully later, but crystals are formed inside them and it seems likely that they are microenvironments in which higher levels of supersaturation may be produced and homogeneous nucleation takes place.

Seeding (epitaxy) may be necessary to initiate crystallisation

If the energy activation barrier could be partially overcome, nucleation could occur at much lower levels of supersaturation. Binding of ions to solid molecule surfaces could reduce the surface energy of an ion cluster. When this occurs, the nucleation is described as heterogeneous as a particle other than

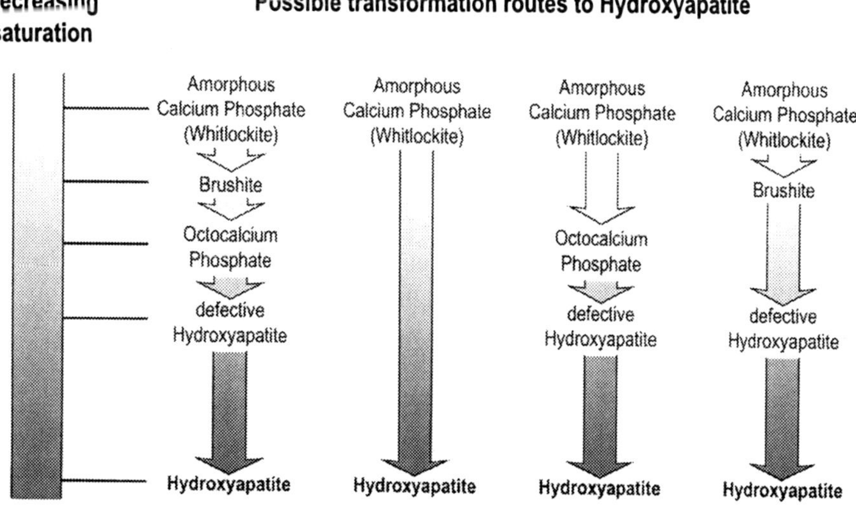

Fig. 3.2
Sequences of transformation between different crystal forms of calcium phosphate showing the tendency for them to convert into hydroxyapatite in physiological solutions.

the ions contributing to the crystal is involved. A nucleator of this kind is termed a seed, and the process of heterogeneous nucleation is often referred to as seeding or epitaxy. It must be able to bind the ions which form the initial cluster and the binding must be spatially suitable and the charge relationships correct for the formation of a stable crystal nucleus. Even if its affinity for the ions is high, nucleation cannot occur in the absence of the correct spatial arrangement. However, it is likely that, in the biological situation, more than one molecular type may be found in juxtaposition so that together they fulfil the requirements for nucleation.

Collagen may be a possible seeding substance but non-collagenous proteins may be needed by themselves or with collagen

A number of different molecules have been proposed as heterogeneous nucleators in calcifying tissues. The presence of collagen in all calcifying tissues except enamel and the apparent close proximity of early small crystals specifically to the 'hole' regions of the molecules (Fig. 2.9) led to the hypothesis that collagen must be the seeding molecule in these tissues. Although it binds phosphate ions well, collagen is a poor calcium-binding agent, and the conformation of the ions bound differs from that in apatite crystals. When other bone-derived proteins are present on a collagen surface in the test-tube, nucleation can occur. This could mean that the non-collagenous bone proteins are the nucleators (although they are ineffective in free solution) or that they and collagen together provide the right combination of properties to permit nucleation. In the biological situation there is also the possibility of other molecules acting as inhibitors of nucleation; selective breakdown of such molecules by enzymes might be necessary to allow nucleation to take place.

Crystal growth

Once the ion cluster has reached an adequate size it can itself act as a seed: ions can attach to its surface in an appropriate conformation. This usually constitutes growth by accretion and may occur uniformly round the crystal or, as on enamel crystals, may be limited to particular crystal faces. A second type of growth is by screw dislocation but this is probably not seen in bone crystal growth.

Nucleation by an already formed crystal may result in the initiation of new crystals rather than enlargement of the existing one. This seems to occur by localised growth producing a projection which then separates off. Another way in which multiple crystal formation can occur is thought to be during the conversion of octacalcium phosphate to apatite. This process is not always uniformly progressive, and so layering of apatite and octacalcium phosphate may occur and the strains between the two crystal lattices may result in fracture of the crystal into smaller fragments.

Once the crystals begin to grow, their shape, size and final orientation must be closely controlled to give the final remarkable consistency seen in each of the calcified tissues. This control must be exerted by the matrix components: collagen fibres may be an influence in bone, dentine and cementum and the enamelins (including serum albumin) in dental enamel. Bone with crystals of 10–50 nm oriented along the collagen fibres is completely different from enamel with its 56-nm wide crystals and a highly defined pattern of crystal orientation resulting in the rod structure of mature enamel.

Molecules associated with calcifying tissues

Collagen

Collagen is one of the most abundant body proteins. Although a characteristic component of three of the four calcifying tissues, it is also present in almost all other tissues in the body. Even if the different collagen types are considered as conferring different properties on tissues, this does not distinguish the calcifying tissues because collagen type I, the major type in bone dentine and cementum, is also the major type in other tissues. It is now thought that there are no differences in the properties of collagen in calcifying and non-calcifying tissues. Nonetheless, electron microscopic observations of calcifying bone consistently show the earliest crystals in the portions of the collagen fibrils where four rather than five molecules overlap – the so-called hole regions, which are recognisable in the cross-banding pattern characteristic of collagen fibrils (Fig. 2.9). This suggests that the hole regions may act as seeding sites. Collagen binds phosphate well but calcium poorly and so, of itself, would not fulfil the requirements of a seeding substance for apatite crystals. In fully formed bone, apatite is said to be present in two forms: an amorphous or finely crystalline form in the hole regions of collagen fibres, and thin elongated extrafibrillar crystals which are associated with other matrix proteins.

Non-collagenous proteins

Non-collagenous proteins are found in the matrices of bone, dentine and cementum

Analysis of bone and dentine matrices has revealed a number of proteins, mainly acidic phosphoproteins, which exhibit strong calcium-binding properties and can also bind to collagen. Such proteins might themselves act as seeds or may be able to do so when linked to collagen. In supersaturated solutions of calcium and phosphate many of these proteins inhibit crystal formation, but when they attach to an immobilised layer of collagen they promote crystal formation. The gama-carboxyglutamate-containing proteins (GLA proteins) osteonectin, osteopontin and bone sialoprotein II have also been considered as candidates for seeding molecules (but see the comment on animals with gene knockouts in Ch. 2).

Proteoglycans

When bone mineralisation takes place in cartilage, there is a clear association of proteoglycans with the formed crystals, and calcium and proteoglycans are co-located at the first sites of crystallisation. However, it should also be realised that at the stage of bone formation there is a major reduction in the amount of proteoglycan in the cartilage.

Lipids

The role of lipids in calcification is still unclear

Since the observation in 1959 of lipids at the developing front of mineralisation in bone, evidence for their role has been sought. As phospholipids are normal cell membrane components and are also now known to be important in intracellular signalling, their presence in calcifying tissues may not be directly relevant to the process. The membrane-bound vesicles found in early calcification in bone, however, could be the source of lipids at the developing front. The vesicles appear to arise from specialised areas of the cell membrane which contain phosphatidylserine and other acidic calcium-binding lipids, phospholipid–calcium-phosphate complexes and specific proteolipids. Alkaline phosphatase is bound to cell membranes by lipid bonding. Phosphatidylserine can act as a calcium ionophore – i.e. it can mediate calcium transport. It is possible that these membrane components are either seeding substances or can assist in raising local calcium and phosphate concentrations to allow crystallisation to take place; the first crystals in the membrane-bound vesicles are observed to lie immediately next to the membrane.

Lipids are certainly associated with signalling mechanisms within and between the cells of forming bone. Thus parathyroid hormone and prostaglandin E_2 cause release of inositol trisphosphate and diacylglycerol in osteoblasts. Prostaglandins and leucotrienes have variously been shown to stimulate or inhibit osteoblast proliferation.

Matrix vesicles

Matrix vesicles are formed as intracellular vesicles which are then extruded from the cell. They contain high concentrations or actual crystals of calcium phosphate

Membrane-bounded vesicles were first described in calcifying cartilage in 1967. They were seen as buds on the chondrocyte cell membranes which broke off to form closed vesicles of about 100 nm in diameter. They are seen in cartilage and in bone, including maxilla and mandible, in cementum and in reparative dentine as well as in healing bone. In primary dentine itself they are seen only during the formation of mantle dentine. The membrane of the matrix vesicles differs from the cell membrane chemically, in having high concentrations of alkaline phosphatase and phosphatidylserine. There are differences between individual matrix vesicles, possibly between those produced at different stages of tissue activity, and their composition changes as they mature. Immediately after release the vesicles contain relatively little calcium and phosphate but they rapidly accumulate these ions. Calcium enters the vesicle down concentration gradients, the proteolipids acting as ionophores. A phospholipid–calcium-phosphate complex can be identified. Calcification begins at a point on the internal surface of the membrane and is followed by the growth of, usually, a single crystal inside the vesicle. As this increases in size, the vesicle ruptures and releases it. Crystals from several vesicles stick to each other and form centres for further calcification. The cluster of initial crystals and those that form round them constitute the globular structures termed calcospherites.

Matrix vesicles contain enzymes capable of breaking down or modifying matrix proteoglycans and inhibitors of calcification. Changes in matrix vesicle activity have been observed when isolated vesicles have been treated with vitamin D metabolites and growth factors such as transforming growth factor beta.

Bone formation

Bone formation begins in two different ways: in membrane (intramembraneous) or in a cartilage template (endochondral). The maxilla and most of the mandible are formed intramembraneously, but part of the ascending ramus of the mandible is formed by endochondral ossification of the condylar and coronoid cartilages.

Intramembraneous calcification

Bone formation in the mandible begins in a fibrous template in which some cells differentiate into osteoblasts

In bones such as the mandible a template of fibrous tissue is laid down. Fibroblast-like cells begin to proliferate in one or more specific zones. Despite many studies on cells in tissue culture it is not clear what growth factors are involved in this process in the body. Once a group of cells have sufficiently differentiated into pre-osteoblasts or early osteoblasts they begin to lay down a matrix of collagen types I and III, together with the attachment glycoproteins thrombospondin and fibronectin, and osteonectin. The proteoglycan versican is observed at an early stage but is subsequently replaced by biglycan and decorin. The glycosaminoglycan portion of these proteoglycans is chondroitin sulphate. Cell proliferation slows down and the more mature osteoblasts begin to express alkaline phosphatase rather than collagen. Finally the cells begin to secrete other bone matrix proteins including osteopontin, bone sialoprotein and osteocalcin. The vitamin D metabolite 1,25-dihydroxycholecalciferol stimulates production of all these proteins, including alkaline phosphatase. Budding of matrix vesicles from the osteoblasts initiates calcification, although there is also the appearance of crystal formation within the collagen fibrils. Even fully formed bone is not uniform in its crystallinity: there are areas of fine, almost amorphous crystals within collagen fibrils and larger coarser crystals between the fibrils. Of the bone matrix proteins some may participate in seeding but osteocalcin is thought to appear after calcification has begun. Once calcification has begun it spreads rapidly throughout the volume defined by the fibrous template (Fig. 3.3). Crystal size and orientation are presumably governed by the matrix proteins.

Endochondral ossification

In most bones and in parts of the mandible, bone formation is preceded by formation of a cartilaginous template and this is replaced by bone

In most of the bones of the body a template of cartilage is first produced. In the mandible only the part of the ramus above the mandibular notch is produced in this way although the later growth of the mandible is concentrated in this part. Cartilage consists of large cells (chondrocytes) separated by a hydrated matrix of collagen, proteoglycans (largely aggrecan as previously described) and some non-collagenous proteins.

The development of cartilage can be most easily described from the series of events occurring in the epiphyseal plates at the end of developing and growing long bones (Fig. 3.4). The condylar cartilage of the mandible has a

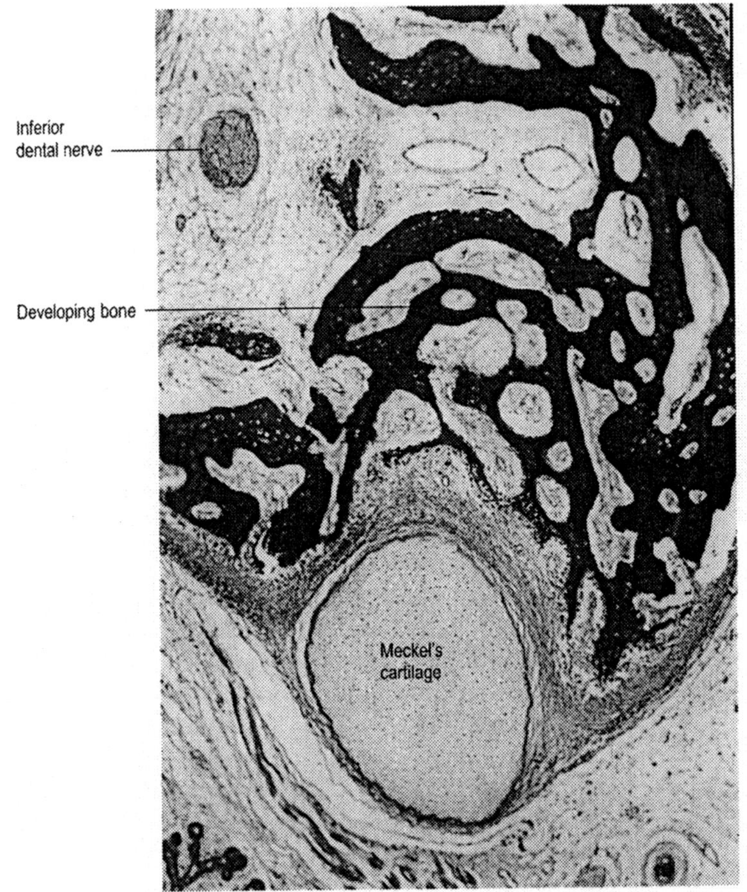

Fig. 3.3
Intramembraneous calcification in the mandible. Note that calcification occurs in a site clearly separate from Meckel's cartilage.

similar pattern of development but differs in the degree of organisation of the changes. A resting zone or reserve zone is described in the epiphyseal plate of long bones but is either very narrow or forms part of the inner layer of the fibrous articular layer of the condylar cartilage. In this zone, extracellular matrix is the main component (about 85% of the volume) in the epiphyseal plate, with scattered rounded cells of about 700 μm^3. These cells are mesenchymal cells which have begun to differentiate and move into the zone during development. They are directly affected by growth hormone and somatomedin C (IGF1). 1,25-Dihydroxycholecalciferol also modulates chondrocyte differentiation. The chondrocytes are responsible for the secretion of the matrix which consists of collagen type II and cartilage proteoglycans. It is not surprising that ascorbic acid (vitamin C) should be a necessary factor to promote growth and activity of these cells. In the proliferative zone, cell division results in an increased number of cells, now wedge-shaped, which

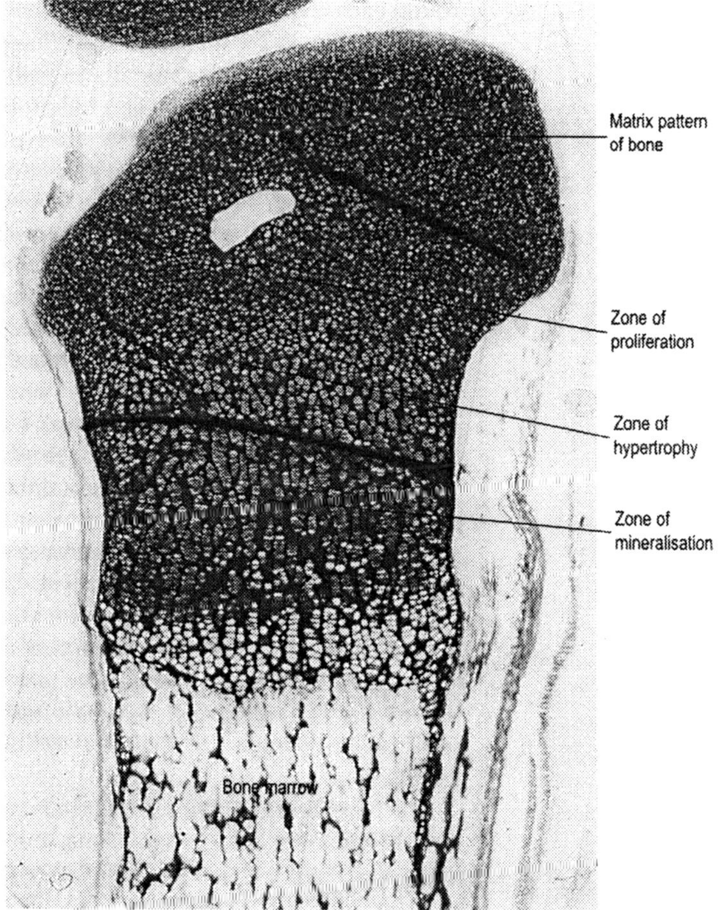

Fig. 3.4
Endochondral ossification: the epiphysis of a long bone. The structure is first laid down in cartilage and this is then replaced by bone.

become arranged in columns in the long axis of the long bones. In the mandibular cartilage this columnar arrangement is absent; instead, there is a more general proliferation of cells. The cells are metabolically active and secrete more matrix so that some two-thirds of the volume of the zone is matrix. The number of cells in unit volume is some 20% greater than in the resting zone. The cells have an extensive endoplasmic reticulum and Golgi apparatus, demonstrating that they are highly metabolically active in protein synthesis. Proliferation of these cells is increased by basic fibroblast growth factor (bFGF) and by transforming growth factor beta. The matrix forms columns between the cell columns and thin layers separating cells within them. The proliferative zone gives way to the hypertrophic zone, in which the columnar arrangement is maintained but the cells become taller and more rounded, their size increasing by a factor of ten, and the amount of matrix round each cell triples. This is the zone which contributes most to growth in length. Again, in the mandibular cartilage the cells remain randomly oriented and so growth can occur laterally as well as in the long axis of the ramus. The cells contain many vacuoles and the proportion of rough endoplasmic reticulum is less than in the cells of the proliferating zone. The chondrocytes in both the proliferative and the hyperplastic zones are stimulated by growth hormone to produce somatomedin C and this acts in paracrine fashion to stimulate clonal expansion. The zone furthest away from the articulation is the calcifying zone, clearly identifiable by the presence of calcified material. Calcification occurs between the cell columns and not between the cells within them. When the hypertrophied chondrocytes reach the layer of tissue rich in capillaries and osteoblasts on the surface of already calcified bone – the periosteal layer – they disintegrate. Their death may be due to the increased availability of oxygen from the greater blood circulation in this area. The hypertrophic and calcifying zones are relatively anaerobic since they derive their nutriments from blood vessels at the periphery of the cartilage. The onset of calcification involves loss of aggrecan and breakdown of the matrix vesicles – processes which require precise changes in the activity of enzymes and their inhibitors. In the calcifying zone of cartilage, apatite is laid down only in the columns of matrix; the matrix between the cells in the chondrocyte columns is not calcified. The initial nucleation probably takes place in the matrix vesicles, although this does not eliminate the possibility of seeding by molecules present in the matrix itself. A mineralisation front is seen in the condylar cartilage but there is no pattern of calcification similar to that in the epiphyseal cartilage.

The extracellular matrix of cartilage consists of collagens, some non-collagenous proteins, proteoglycans and water – the last amounting to between two-thirds and three-quarters of the volume. In all zones the principal collagen type is type II. Its fibres are laid down parallel to the cell columns and form a soft tissue framework for the tissue. In the proliferative zone collagen types IX and XI as well as type II predominate, together with a small amount of type VI. In the hypertrophic zone there is a progressive switchover to producing collagen type X, which may be important in matrix turnover, or even in the process of calcification. The major proteoglycan of cartilage (5–10% wet weight) is aggrecan. This is a large proteoglycan with keratan sulphate and chondroitin sulphate side-chains. It binds to hyaluronate to form a meshwork which takes up and swells with water. The pressure of this against the collagen fibre framework gives the tissue great resistance to compression. The small proteoglycans – decorin, biglycan and fibromodulin – are present in cartilage (see comment in Ch. 2). The other proteins described in cartilage are anchorin CII, cartilage matrix protein, cartilage oligomeric matrix protein (COMP), chondrocalcin, Ch21, fibronectin and a 48-kDa protein; although some of these have interesting binding properties, little is known of their function in cartilage matrix, although mutations in the cartilage oligomeric matrix protein are associated with some forms of chondrodysplasias.

Matrix vesicles are seen in cartilage matrix in all zones, with the highest concentration in the resting zone, least in the proliferative zone, and increasing concentration in the hyperplastic zone and a rapid decline in concentration in the mineralising zone. In the proliferative, hyperplastic and mineralising zones of epiphyseal cartilage they are found in the matrix columns, but appear more randomly distributed in the mandibular cartilages. They are typically around 70 nm in diameter. Although they are thought to arise by active budding off from the chondrocytes it is also possible that they are fragments of dead cells and result from apoptosis.

Conversion of cartilage to bone

Osteoclasts break down mineralised cartilage and then osteoblasts replace it with bone

In the long bones there is a periosteal layer around the shaft. Soon after the calcification of the cartilage has begun the cells of the periosteum differentiate into osteoblasts and begin to lay down bone. Matrix vesicles appear in the first formed matrix and calcification occurs. As this bone is laid down, osteoclasts develop by fusion of blood cell precursors and begin to break down the mineralised cartilage which is then replaced by bone. In the mandibular ramus a similar process occurs at the interface of the intramembraneous bone and the calcified cartilage (Fig. 3.5). In comparison with cartilage this bone is well vascularised and generates a sufficiently well-oxygenated area to cause the chondrocytes to degenerate.

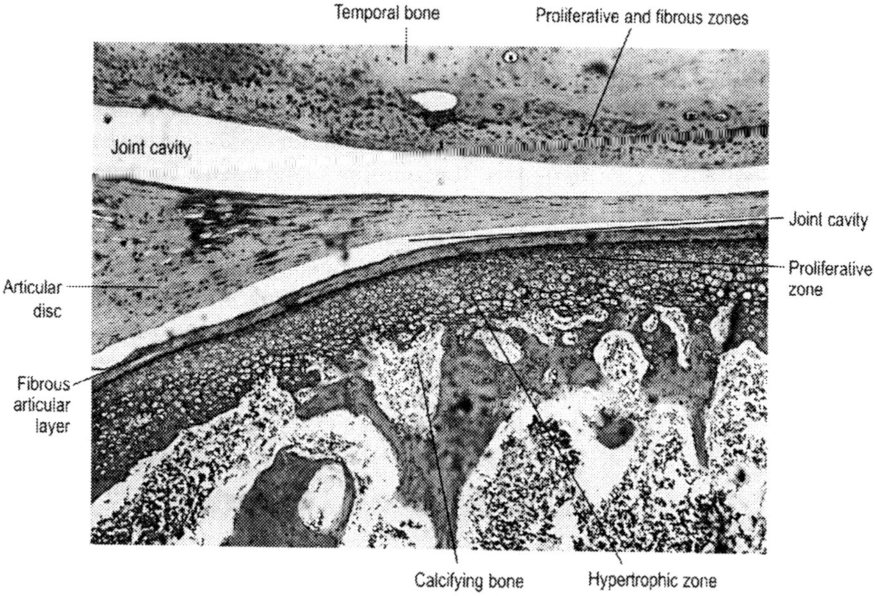

Fig. 3.5
Endochondral ossification: the mandibular condyle. The head of the condyle articulates with the temporal bone in a synovial joint. The two surfaces are separated by a synovial cavity, itself separated into two compartments by the articulating disc. The head of the condyle consists of fibrocartilage covered by a dense fibrous articular layer. The condyle does not complete its ossification until the late teens.

Maturation of bone

The initially formed bone is fibrillar but is replaced gradually to give compact and trabecular bone

The initially formed bone is coarse and fibrillar in structure and is usually described as foetal or woven bone. It is replaced gradually by osteoclastic action and then remodelling to form either compact or trabecular bone. Most of the osteoblasts become incorporated into the bone structure and remain as osteocytes, although they remain as osteoblasts on the bone surface. There they may form new bone. This appears at first as osteoid – a defined layer of uncalcified bone matrix – and calcification takes place by seeding from the existing bone as the osteoblasts maintain a supply of calcium and phosphate to the matrix.

Maxilla and mandible consist of a core of trabecular bone surrounded by compact bone. The teeth are supported and their roots surrounded by an alveolar process

The bone of the jaws consists of compact bone in the body and processes of the mandible and the body of the maxilla around the maxillary sinuses. On the tooth-bearing surface of these bones is the alveolar process, bone supporting the teeth which is resorbed after loss of the teeth. Although the alveolar process is often considered to be a separate entity from the rest of the bone, it is identical in structure and differs only in that it is the part of the jaw which responds most obviously to the functional demands of mastication. The bone of the mandible and maxilla, therefore, consists of a core of trabecular bone enclosing spaces filled with marrow in the child, but replaced with fatty tissue in the adult, and an outer layer of compact bone organised into subunits – the osteons – with concentric layers of bone surrounding a canaliculus lined with embedded osteocytes. The outer surface of the bone and the marrow surfaces are lined by a periosteum. This consists of two layers: an inner layer of bone cells and precursor cells with a rich vascular supply, and an outer fibrous layer. The fibrous layer is predominately circumferential but also contains bundles of fibres which pass through the inner layer to penetrate the surface bone lamellae. In the tooth sockets the periosteum is more developed to become the periodontal ligament. The marrow spaces are lined by the endosteum, a single layer of bone cells. The Haversian systems each have a central canal containing a blood vessel, and these are linked together by vessels in connecting canals (canals of Volkmann). Again there is a single layer of bone cells lining these canals. The collagen fibres of the bone lie in preferred orientations. The bone lamellae are arranged so as to counteract the stresses on the bone – osteons generally lying at right-angles to compressive or torsional stresses.

The periosteum is specialised around the teeth to form the periodontal ligaments

Calcification of dentine

Dentine resembles bone in being of mesodermal origin

Dentine, like bone and cementum, is a tissue of mesodermal origin and, like them, consists of an extracellular matrix of which the main component is collagen but which is given rigidity and hardness by embedded crystals of calcium phosphate. Since it is formed, like the dental pulp, from the dental papilla of the tooth germ, and derives its nutrition and nerve supply from that tissue, the two are sometimes considered together as the dentinopulpal complex. However, dentine is formed by a specific type of cell, the odontoblast, and its matrix differs from that of the pulp. The chemistry of this matrix, similar in many ways to that of bone, gives important clues as to the process of its mineralisation.

The matrix of dentine

The matrix of dentine is mainly type I collagen

The hydroxyapatite of dentine is closely associated with the main organic component of the matrix, the collagen fibres, and the crystals are arranged with their *c*-axes parallel to them.

The organic components of the matrix (about 90% collagen together with other proteins, proteoglycans and some lipids) are secreted by the odontoblasts as a network of fibres and the calcium phosphate crystals form in this network. Mineralisation occurs some distance away from the odontoblasts; the layer of unmineralised matrix between the odontoblasts and the calcified dentine is known as predentine.

Collagen in dentine

The main collagen present in dentine matrix is collagen type I. This has two alpha-1(I) chains and one alpha-2 chain in its triple helix. The long chains are in a staggered arrangement so that there are alternate zones of overlapping and non-overlapping molecules, giving the typical collagen cross-striation in electron micrographs. The non-overlap zones are referred to as hole zones, and it is in these zones that apatite crystals are usually seen. There is some debate over the other types of collagen to be found in human dentine. In the continuously growing incisor of the rat, collagen type V which contains three unique alpha chains is present and this same collagen is a minor constituent of bone matrix. It is reported that it is not present in human dentine. However, type III collagen – a major constituent of soft tissues, including dental pulp – has been reported to be present as procollagen in human predentine. Small amounts of type III collagen have been found in bone. Yet another type of collagen, type VI, has been reported in human predentine.

The cross-links between collagen chains which stabilise the collagen network are of two types: those that are reducible and those that are not reducible by borohydride. The former are hydroxylysinonorleucine-based and the latter are pyridinoline-based. In young dentine the reducible forms predominate but they slowly transform into the more rigid reducible types with ageing and so the proportions of the two types of cross-link change.

Lipids

Lipids constitute about 2% of dentine matrix

Although the lipid content of dentine is about 2% of the organic material, it is likely that much of it is from the cell membranes of the odontoblast processes. The lipids are phospholipids, cholestrerol and cholesterol esters and triacyglycerols. Acidic phospholipids such as phosphatidylserine, phosphatidylinositol and phosphatidic acid are tightly bound to the mineral. Interest in the lipid content of dentine was stimulated by the observation of acidic phospholipids at the mineralisation front in predentine and the effect of a deficiency of essential fatty acids in the diet on dentine formation. More recent work suggests that the phospholipids may be associated with the matrix in both dentine and predentine. There is evidence that one of the differences between calcifying and non-calcifying tissues is the presence of acidic phospholipid complexes with calcium and phosphate, and it is possible that these may play a role in the mineralisation of dentine.

Tooth development – the tooth germ

The process of tooth development begins with invagination of epithelium from the future oral cavity as the dental lamina. From this arise the tooth buds which develop into enamel organs with associated dental papillae

The dividing cells of the oral epithelial lining produce an ingrowth of epithelium into the ectomesenchyme in both the developing maxilla and mandible: the ingrowth splits to give the vestibular lamina, some of whose cells will degenerate to form the cleft between the tissues covering the jaws and those of the lips and cheeks – the vestibule – whilst the remainder form its epithelial covering, and the dental lamina which will give rise to the dental arch in each jaw (Figs 3.6 and 3.7). At ten defined areas in each jaw equivalent in position to the ten eventual deciduous teeth, the epithelium proliferates away from the oral cavity to give a mass of cells termed the tooth bud. At a later stage of development the dental lamina extends lingually to generate tooth buds for the anterior five permanent teeth in each quadrant of the mouth, and distally to generate the tooth buds of the permanent molar teeth.

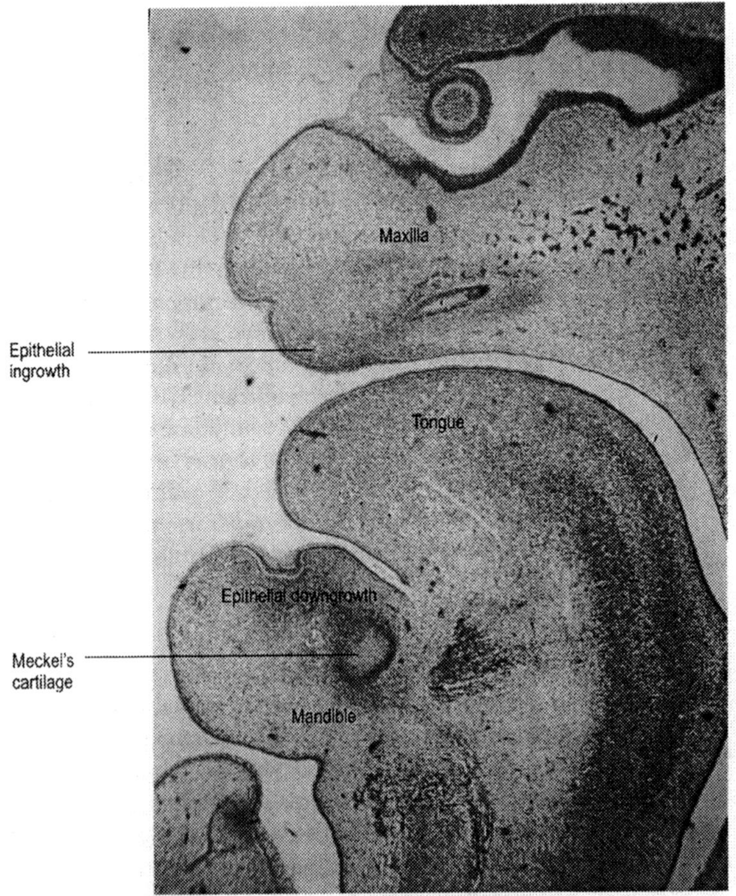

Fig. 3.6
Development of the jaws and tongue. The first invagination of the epithelium marks the future vestibule and alveolus.

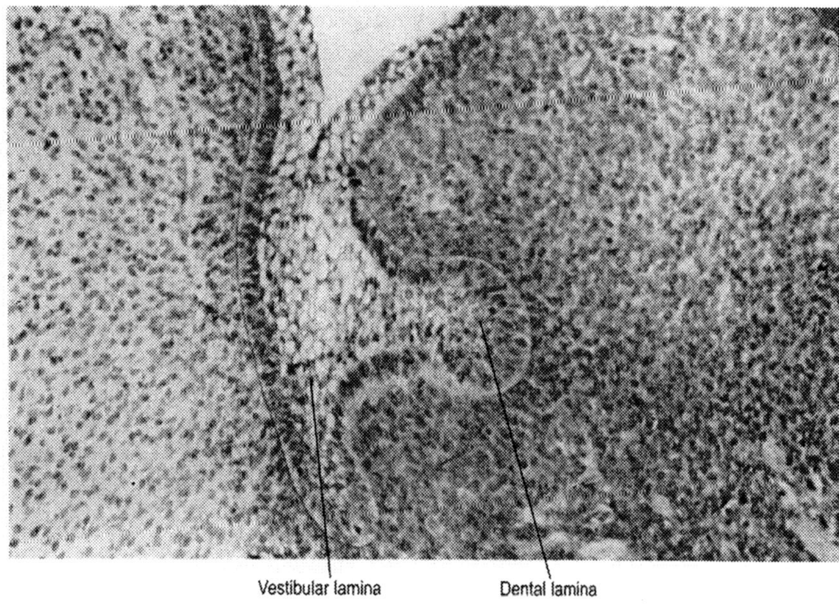

Fig. 3.7
The invagination of the oral epithelium differentiating into a vestibular lamina and the dental lamina.

Each tooth bud is surrounded by closely packed ectomesenchymal cells; indeed, it may be the division of these cells which pushes away the dental lamina rather than growth of the epithelial cells which invades the ectomesenchyme. Further division of the ectomesenchyme deep to the tooth bud and reduced production of intercellular material between the cells result in a close packing of ectomesenchyme (cellular condensation, as it is termed) which pushes the epithelium into a cap shape over the roughly spherical mass of ectomesenchymal cells. The epithelial ingrowth is now termed the enamel organ, although as it is involved not only in enamel formation but also in determining the shape of the tooth crown and initiating dentine formation (and ultimately in contributing to the junction between tooth and gingiva) some writers prefer to call it the dental organ. The condensed ectomesenchyme beneath the 'cap' will give rise to dentine and the dental pulp and hence is termed the dental papilla, whilst the condensed ectomesenchyme at its periphery which extends round the enamel organ also is the dental follicle which will form the periodontal ligament and the cementum. Whilst the dental papilla and the dental follicle are highly vascularised, the enamel organ is avascular. At this stage only the dental follicle contains nerve fibres. The three structures – enamel organ, dental papilla and dental follicle – together constitute the tooth germ (Fig. 3.8).

The cells of the enamel organ now divide and begin to differentiate. Those on the periphery on the convex surface assume a cuboidal shape, whilst those in the concavity become short columnar cells with centrally placed nuclei.

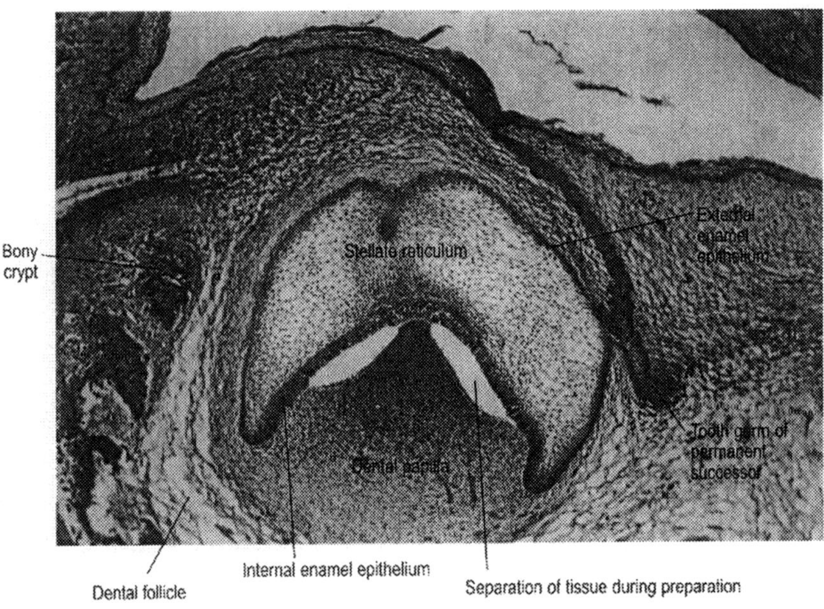

The tooth germ has now differentiated into the late-cap or early-bell stage with the inner and outer enamel epithelium surrounding the stellate reticulum. The dental papilla is still a condensation of mesenchyme below the enamel organ.

These two cell layers are termed the outer and inner enamel epithelium, respectively.

The process of dentinogenesis

The odontoblasts differentiate from cells of the dental papilla. The first layer of calcified material laid down in dentine is the mantle dentine. Matrix vesicles are seen at this stage

The differentiation of the inner enamel epithelium triggers the differentiation of the odontoblasts by a series of still poorly understood matrix signals. The odontoblasts differentiate from precursor cells in the dental papilla (Fig. 3.9). Before the odontoblasts reach their full differentiated form and before they make up a continuous layer on the pulp surface, they begin to lay down the first layer of dentine – the mantle dentine. The collagen fibres of the dental papilla are arranged circumferentially and the odontoblasts have not yet begun to synthesise a distinctive matrix. Thus mantle dentine contains type I collagen. In the rat incisor mantle dentine contains collagen type V and fibronectin; GLA proteins appear only in the odontoblasts themselves and as isolated patches in the mantle dentine whilst phosphoproteins have not been detected. The initial crystals are seen either on the surface of, or actually within, membrane-bound vesicles which have been secreted by the odontoblasts. Mantle dentine differs from circumpulpal or intertubular dentine in that the initial crystals are not closely related to particular sections of the collagen fibres and the membrane-bound vesicles are associated only with this initial stage of dentine formation. The implication is that the

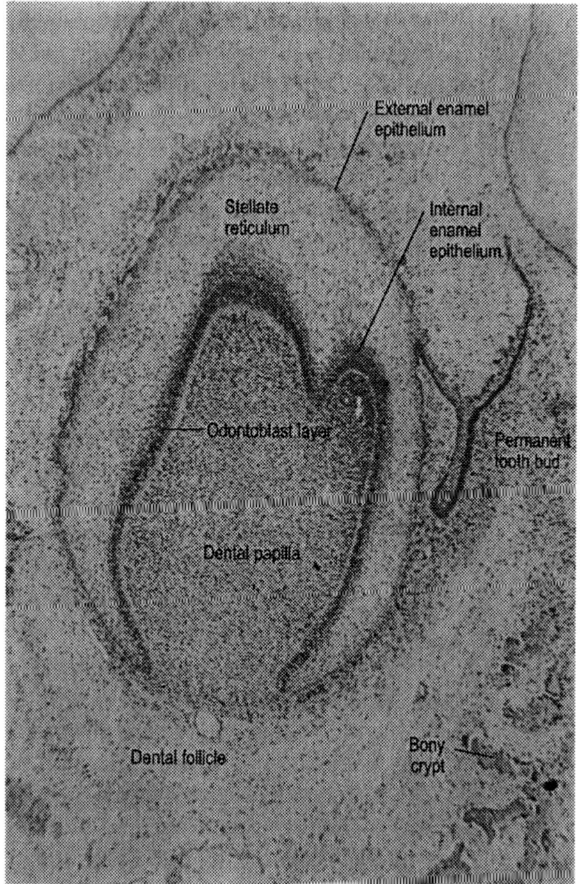

Fig. 3.9
The bell stage of tooth development with the odontoblast layer formed inside the internal enamel epithelium. Calcification of dentine has not yet commenced.

calcification of mantle dentine occurs as a result of matrix vesicles crystals seeding the formation of apatite in the matrix.

Later the odontoblasts secrete matrix components as predentine and calcification takes place in predentine

Once the initial layer of calcified material has been laid down the odontoblasts begin to secrete organic matrix in the form of predentine. This consists of collagen fibres which are arranged in a network with stabilising crosslinks. The final arrangement and linking together of this network occurs in the predentine and not until it is complete can calcification begin. A layer of predentine, therefore, always separates the odontoblasts from the calcification front.

The odontoblasts have an extensive rough endoplasmic reticulum and a well-developed Golgi system. Collagen is synthesised by the ribosomes of the endoplasmic reticulum as procollagen chains: the procollagen chains undergo posttranslational modification by prolyl hydroxylase which converts proline and lysine to hydroxyproline and hydroxylysine. Some carbohydrate is also attached at this stage. The procollagen chains are assembled in threes to form procollagen itself with its triple helix. Procollagen is then packaged into saccules in the Golgi apparatus and exocytosed into the predentine. Procollagen peptidases then remove the terminal peptides to leave the inner two-thirds of the procollagen – the actual collagen molecules. The collagen molecules aggregate into collagen fibres with their typical staggered arrangement of the molecules. Lysyl oxidase initiates the formation of covalent crosslinks. In some species a proportion of the type I collagen is present as a trimer with three alpha-1(I) units instead of the more usual two alpha-1(I) and a single alpha-2 unit.

Phosphophoryns are also synthesised by the odontoblasts and appear in the newly calcifying dentine but are not otherwise distributed in the predentine.

Predentine matrix is not identical with that of dentine

The predentine contains collagen type I with a relatively high proportion of reducible cross-links; in dentine there are a significant number of pyridinoline type cross-links and it is possible that the change occurs during the mineralisation stage. The highly phosphorylated protein, phosphophorin, is not found in predentine, but appears to be transported along the odontoblast process to be secreted next to the mineralisation front. Similarly, the gamma-carboxyglutamate containing osteocalcins are absent in predentine but have been detected in the vesicles of the odontoblast processes and in the mineralised tissue. The proteoglycan composition of predentine and the mineralised dentine appears to be different, some of the sulphated fractions apparently being lost during mineralisation. The parts of the odonblast processes close to the mineralisation front contain enzymes such as cathepsin D which break down proteoglycans, and there is evidence of removal of glycosaminoglycans from, and breakdown of the protein core of, proteoglycans during mineralisation. A possible explanation of these observations is that the proteoglycans are mainly concerned with collagen fibrillogenesis and the organisation of the collagen network, whilst their role in apatite crystallisation is actually inhibitory. Another protein which may be involved in the organisation of the collagen reticulum is osteonectin (SPARC). This protein is present in bovine and porcine dentine and odontoblasts.

When the dentine matrix has been laid down and modified at the mineralisation front, calcium must also be accumulated there to begin and continue mineralisation. It is clear that calcium passes from the rich vascular network which lies on the pulpal side of the odontoblasts – a few capillaries may sometimes be seen extending even between odontoblasts – across the odontoblast layer into the area where crystallisation will take place. The mature odontoblasts form a continuous cell layer with tight junctions between the cells; transport of calcium could occur either through the cells or between them if calcium can pass the tight junctions. It is not clear how the odontoblasts could produce a unidirectional flux of calcium ions from the interstitial fluid at the base of the cells to the fluid in the calcifying region.

The odontoblasts control the movement of calcium ions into the calcifying area

Odontoblasts involved in active mineralisation have high concentrations of calcium-ATPase localised in vesicles derived from the Golgi apparatus and in their cell membranes. Vesicles in the odontoblasts have been shown to demonstrate an ATP-dependent accumulation of calcium. Sodium–calcium exchanger proteins have been detected in odontoblast cell membranes and mitochondria. Measurements of ionic calcium in predentine show higher concentrations than in the dental pulp, and phosphate concentrations are much higher in predentine than in extracellular fluid.

The actual process of mineralisation of dentine depends upon the arrangement and immobilisation of calcium and phosphate ions by specific seeding molecules and the removal of molecules which inhibit seeding or crystal growth. In this latter group, pyrophosphate, nucleotides and some of the proteoglycans are included. Removal of proteoglycans may also create space for crystal deposition and growth. The characteristic relationship of the new hydroxyapatite crystals with the hole zones of the collagen fibres strongly suggests that collagen may fulfil a seeding role. The fact that the bulk of collagen in the body does not calcify weakens this hypothesis, although some researchers think that the answer may lie in the different arrangement of crosslinks. It now seems much more likely that the collagen matrix governs the position of the non-collagenous proteins and that these are more likely candidates as seeding substances. In dentine the transport of phosphophoryns and some proteoglycans to the mineralising front in the odontoblast processes suggests that these may have a key role, and the observation that phosphophoryn can act as a seed when immobilised on a solid or gel support makes it likely that this is so. The ability of higher concentrations of these proteins to inhibit crystal growth may be important in regulating crystal growth. The high binding capacity for calcium of the very acidic phosphophoryn may also help to maintain the gradient for calcium ions into the mineralising front and help in calcium accumulation, rendering crystallisation more likely.

Although the relationship of new crystals to collagen suggests a seeding role for collagen, other organic molecules are also necessary

The calcification of enamel – amelogenesis

Enamel differs from the other calcified tissues in being a product of epithelial cells rather than of mesenchymal cells.

The enamel organ

The early development along the dental lamina of the tooth germs with enamel organs and dental papillae and the subsequent differentiation of the enamel organ into a convex outer enamel epithelium with cuboidal cells and a concave inner enamel epithelium with short columnar cells has been described above.

Both the inner and outer enamel epithelium synthesise small amounts of type IV collagen and the glycosaminoglycan necessary to form a surrounding basal lamina for the enamel organ. The inner enamel epithelium begins to store glycogen. The main bulk of the cells within the enamel organ secrete proteoglycans into the extracellular matrix, and this, together with the large amounts of tissue fluid usually associated with matrices rich in glycosaminoglycans, pushes the cells apart between the points where they are linked by desmosomal attachments. They therefore appear in the two-dimensional view of a histological section as star-shaped, and the tissue is termed the stellate reticulum. The layer of cells between the stellate reticulum

The enamel organ consists of an inner and an outer enamel epithelium, meeting at

the cervical loop and enclosing the stellate reticulum

and the inner enamel epithelium adopt a flattened appearance, and is termed the stratum intermedium. The cells characteristically contain alkaline phosphatase. The growth and differentiation of the enamel organ changes its overall appearance from that of a flat cap to a bell shape. The edge of the bell, where the inner and outer enamel epithelia meet, is the cervical loop.

The evidence suggests that the eventual tooth shape is determined by the cells of the dental papilla, but the actual mechanism by which this is achieved is by the maturation of inner enamel epithelial cells. In the specific areas where the tooth cusps or tips will develop, the inner enamel epithelium cells mature – i.e. they cease to be able to divide further. Continuing division of the remainder of the cell layer between the high pressure of the closely packed cells of the dental papilla and the low pressure of the fluid-filled stellate reticulum causes the inner enamel epithelium to fold into the future tooth form.

As the enamel organ differentiates, the epithelial link to the oral cavity, the dental lamina, undergoes apoptosis and breaks up, although it still continues on the lingual side of the deciduous tooth germs, where it forms the tooth buds of their permanent successors, and it extends further round the horseshoe shape of the jaws to form tooth buds for the permanent molars which have no deciduous predecessors.

Maturation of the cells of inner enamel epithelium causes them to pass through a pre-ameloblast stage to become secretory ameloblasts

At the stage of determination of the crown shape, the cells of the inner enamel epithelium are still cuboidal with centrally placed nuclei and the Golgi apparatus is at the end of the cell proximal to the stratum intermedium. Other organelles are apparently randomly distributed. As the cells mature and lose the capability of further cell division they become pre-ameloblasts and begin a life cycle which will take them through the stages of presecretory ameloblast, secretory ameloblast, maturation-stage ameloblast and finnaly protective-stage ameloblast immediately before cell death. In the pre-ameloblast stage the cells become elongated to adopt a tall columnar shape, the nucleus moves towards the side closest to the stratum intermedium, mitochondria localise to this part of the cell, the Golgi apparatus moves to a central position, and the rough endoplasmic reticulum increases in amount and occupies a considerable portion of the remainder of the cell. All this is characteristic of a cell that is to become secretory in function. As these changes are occurring the outer enamel epithelium becomes more flattened and the capillary network around it increases in density. The pre-ameloblasts are responsible for the transformation of the pre-odontoblasts of the dental papilla into odontoblasts. As these lay down the first layer of calcified dentine – the mantle dentine – the basal lamina disintegrates and disappears.

Enamel matrix formation

After formation of the initial layer of enamel, the ameloblasts develop Tomes' processes and begin to secrete amelogenins and enamelins

The pre-ameloblasts have been shown to synthesise and secrete protein material which is seen both on the future enamel side of the basal lamina and within the outer layers of mantle dentine matrix between the collagen fibres. It appears granular in nature; chemically it appears to be high molecular weight amelogenin-like protein. The early appearance of this protein in the lamina fibroreticularis of the basal lamina has suggested that it may be involved in the redistribution of the fibronectin in this layer, and the fibronectin may be one of the signal molecules which cause the final stages of odontoblast differentiation. The presence of the protein in the outer layers of mantle dentine may contribute to the strength of the bond between enamel and dentine. When the basal lamina disappears the high molecular weight enamel proteins on either side become continuous and calcify as an initial structureless layer of enamel. The hydroxyapatite crystals formed are randomly orientated. There is no evidence that the enamel protein present at this time has any seeding property, and it seems most likely that the initial calcification results from seeding of hydroxyapatite by the already formed crystals of the mantle dentine. The ameloblasts move outwards from this first formed enamel and develop a short conical process containing secretory granules and vesicles; this process was first described by Tomes and is still known as the Tomes' process (Figs 3.10 and 3.11).

The enamel organ in the secretory stage consists of the inner enamel epithelium, now made up of secretory ameloblasts, the outer enamel epithelium, the stellate reticulum and, between the stellate reticulum, the stratum intermedium, made up of two to three layers of cuboidal cells with many microvilli. These cells contain many mitochondria, coated pits and vesicles, polyribosomes, some rough endoplasmic reticulum, lysosomes and Golgi complexes. They are linked to the ameloblasts by macular tight junctions, gap junctions and desmosomes. Their membranes contain non-specific alkaline phosphatase, calcium-ATPase, sodium–potassium-ATPase and hydrogen–potassium-ATPase. These enzymes are also present in the ameloblast layer but not in the stellate reticulum or the outer enamel epithelium. The cell characteristics are therefore those of a transport

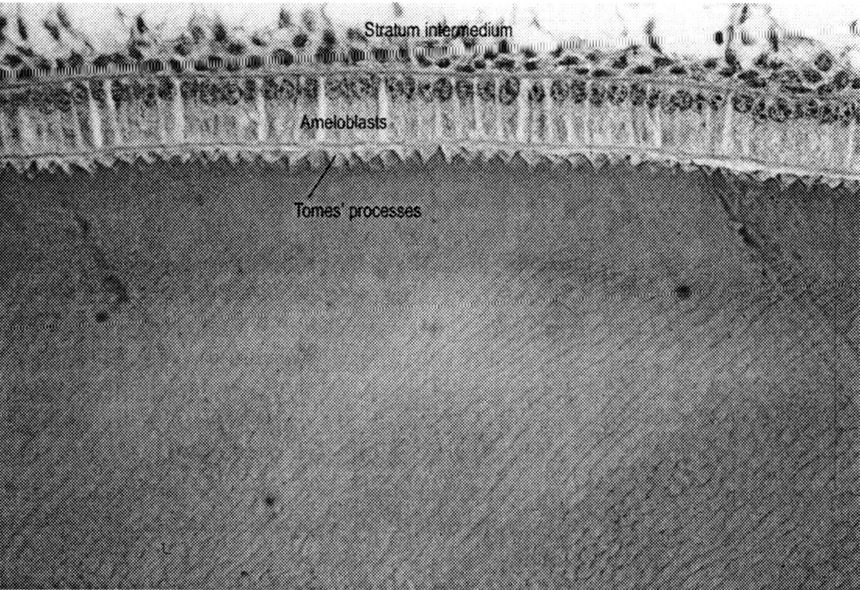

Fig. 3.10
Ameloblast layer with the Tomes' processes forming the enamel rods. The distal terminal web gives the 'picket fence' appearance.

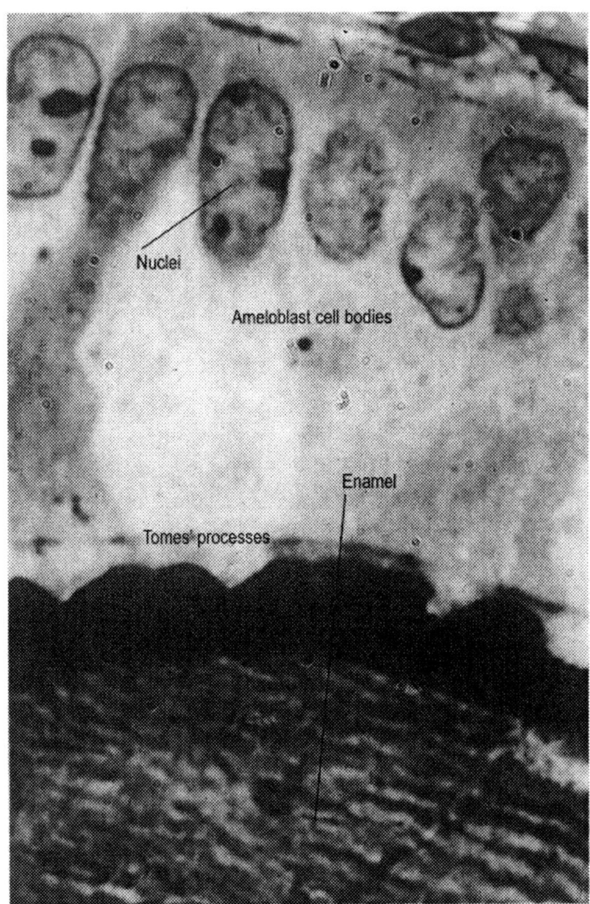

Fig. 3.11a
High power micrograph of ameloblasts.

epithelium. The calcium-binding protein calmodulin is present throughout the enamel organ prior to secretion but the 28-kDa calcium-binding protein appears only when secretion beings and is found only in the ameloblasts and stratum intermedium. Parvalbumin has a similar distribution to that of the 28-kDa calcium-binding protein. Calmodulin causes activation of protein kinase C, which is involved in the opening of calcium channels in mitochondria and the endoplasmic reticulum; it is likely that protein kinase C plays an important role in the transfer of calcium between intracellular compartments. Calcium itself is present in mitochondria, particularly at the basal end of the ameloblasts, in the endoplasmic reticulum, in the Golgi saccules and in the cytoplasm immediately below the distal cell membrane. It is possible that the Golgi apparatus may package calcium together with the enamel proteins: this would explain the rapid calcification of enamel matrix immediately after its secretion. However, calcium can also be detected between the ameloblasts and in the matrix and this may be a result of transfer across the cell membranes by calcium-ATPase.

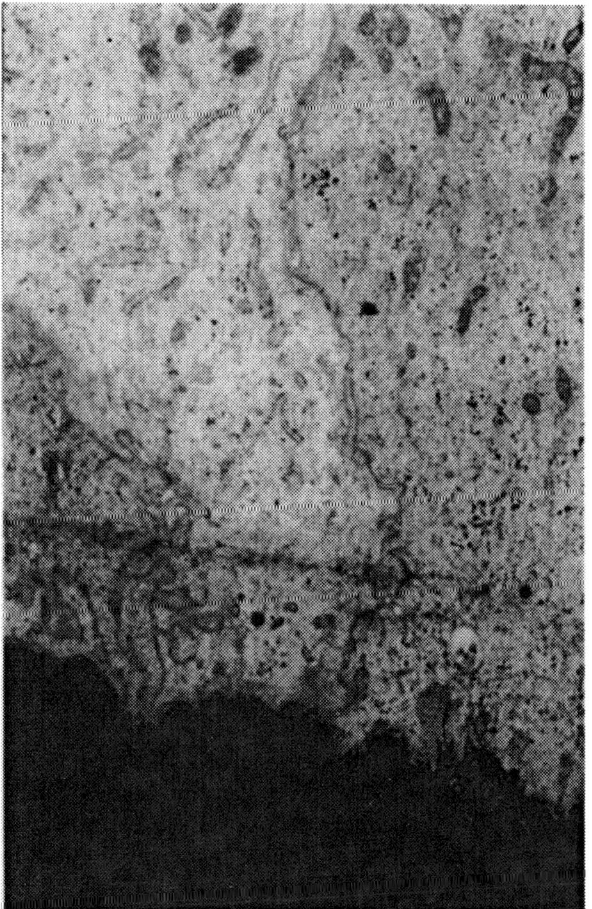

Fig. 3.11b
Electron micrograph of ameloblasts. Note the wide intercellular space and the distal terminal web.

During the secretory stage, the outer surface of the enamel organ is surrounded by a meshwork of blood capillaries. The cells of the outer enamel epithelium are cuboidal with large nuclei and many mitochondria. They have a well-developed Golgi apparatus but little endoplasmic reticulum, and they contain vesicles of different kinds, together with ribosomes and glycogen granules. The cells are narrower distally where they are linked to the basement membrane by hemidesmosomes. Proximally they have gap junctions and desmosomes linking them together and extend processes through a wide extracellular space filled with a complex carbohydrate and lipid gel to link with the cells of the stellate reticulum via desmosomes and gap junctions. The cells of the stellate reticulum resemble the outer enamel epithelium in having a high nucleus:cytoplasm ratio and many mitochondria and ribosomes, but they have no Golgi apparatus or rough endoplasmic reticulum. The long thin processes between cells are linked together via desmosomes and gap junctions. The gap junctions between the cells of the enamel organ permit transfer of ions across the structure. In addition, amino acids have been seen to pass across and from one cell to another. The wide intercellular spaces filled with proteoglycans allow larger molecules to pass through.

The secretory ameloblasts are long narrow cells (35–50 × 5 μm in the human) arranged perpendicular to the forming dentine surface. The nucleus and mitochondria lie distally and the cytoplasm in the proximal two-thirds of each cell is filled with rough endoplasmic reticulum above and around a well-developed Golgi system. Glycogen granules tend to lie in the proximal part of the cell. At each end of the cells is a terminal bar apparatus; this is a web of cytoplasmic filaments approximately 6–7 nm in diameter, oriented perpendicular to the long axis of the cell and in contact with a narrow specialised area of cell membrane which forms part of a tight junction with the neighbouring cells. The tight junctions are leaky at the proximal ends but much less so at the distal ends – an arrangement which prevents leakage of the secreted enamel proteins away from the forming enamel surface. The cells are separated by some 20–30 nm and are linked between the terminal bars by desmosomes and gap junctions. The proximal surfaces of the cells have many projections which interdigitate with similar projections from the cells of the stratum intermedium, to which they joined by desmosomes and gap junctions. This arrangement permits movement of small molecules and ions between the cell layers.

The outer enamel epithelium and the pre-ameloblasts have a uniform distribution of prokeratins from which 50- and 63-kDa keratins are formed. In the secretory ameloblasts these proteins are located distally. Vimentin is present in the outer enamel epithelium but not in the ameloblasts. Actin, which is important in cell adhesion, exocytosis and endocytosis and in maintaining cell shape (as in the microvilli and in the Tomes' process), is localised in the terminal webs and in the Tomes' process. Microtubules in the ameloblasts map out pathways for granule transport and maintain the polarisation of the cell.

Secretion of matrix begins immediately after commencement of dentine mineralisation and at first occurs from the flattened proximal end of the ameloblast: the lack of the orientation which will later result in the production of enamel prisms from the Tomes' processes results in an aprismatic layer of enamel next to the mantle dentine. When the Tomes' process forms, it secretes matrix from its distal and proximal portions and calcification of the matrix results in differences in crystal orientation, the proximal portion of each process giving rise to interrod enamel and the distal portion forming the prism or rod. The interrod enamel arises from many adjacent ameloblasts whilst the rod arises from only one. The smooth non-secretory zone between the two secreting zones of the ameloblast is represented in the finally formed enamel by the so-called enamel sheath.

Protein synthesis occurs in the rough endoplasmic reticulum. The new proteins are transported to the Golgi apparatus where glycosylation and phophorylation can occur; the packaged proteins are then transported to the cell surface and exocytosed. Energy for these processes is derived from the glycogen stored in the stratum intermedium. The proteins are of two types: the more rapidly formed amelogenins, which are of lower molecular weight and

In addition to the amelogenins the

ameloblasts secrete enamelins. These remain in the mature enamel but most of the amelogenin is lost

rich in proline and are largely removed during the next stage of maturation, and the enamelins which largely remain in the final enamel. The newly formed protein is subject to turnover; the ameloblast secretes not only the protein but also a protease which breaks it down. This process seems to be necessary for the simultaneous calcification of the matrix. Small amelogenin fragments are endocytosed by the ameloblasts.

The Tomes' process is demarcated from the ameloblast cell body by the terminal web: in addition to the secretory granules it contains only those organelles necessary for exocytosis and for endocytosis.

Calmodulin is widely distributed in ameloblasts although there is more in the cell body than in the Tomes' process. Together with protein kinase C it seems to be involved in balancing calcium distribution in the cell and possibly in modulating the activity of the membrane calcium-ATPase. It may also have some function in enamel protein synthesis. Other calcium-binding proteins in the cell are endonexin, chromobindin, calpactin and phospholipids and actin-binding proteins.

The sodium–potassium-ATPase and the hydrogen–potassium-ATPase in both ameloblasts and the stratum intermedium cell membranes probably demonstrate the high metabolic activity of the cells.

Maturation of enamel

During maturation, enamel loses proteins and water as the crystals grow in size

As the enamel reaches full thickness the morphology of the enamel organ changes and the functions of its cells alter. Enamel at this stage has a mineral content roughly the same as dentine; in order to reach the final 98% mineral of mature enamel it has to undergo a maturation stage in which protein and water are removed from the matrix and more calcium and phosphate are incorporated by crystal growth. The differentiation between the cells of the outer enamel layer, the stellate reticulum and the stratum intermedium disappears and these layers are replaced by a several layers of cells of similar morphology making up what is termed the papillary layer (Fig. 3.12). The papillary layer is extensively infolded on the surface distal to the formed enamel, and the ameloblasts and the invaginations contain an extensive network of anastomosing blood capillaries. The capillaries do not reach the ameloblasts but are separated from them by at least one papillary cell thickness. They arise from a network of small arterioles around the cervical region which sends out branches parallel to the long axis of the future crown, giving off capillaries as they go and ending in capillaries at the tips of the cusps. The capillaries have a fenestrated endothelium and molecules up to the size of small proteins can pass through the fenestrations. Additionally, there is evidence of pinocytotic transport across the cells although intercellular passage is blocked by tight junctions. The cells of the papillary layer are typical of cells engaged in the transport of water and ions: they have outer membranes with infoldings and microvilli, resulting in a large surface area, the membranes are rich in enzymes associated with transport – both acid and alkaline phosphatase, calcium-ATPase, sodium–potassium-ATPase and hydrogen–potassium-ATPase – they have many mitochondria and intense cytoplasmic cytochrome *c* activity signifying a high energy usage, and they have extensive links with each other and with the ameloblasts via gap

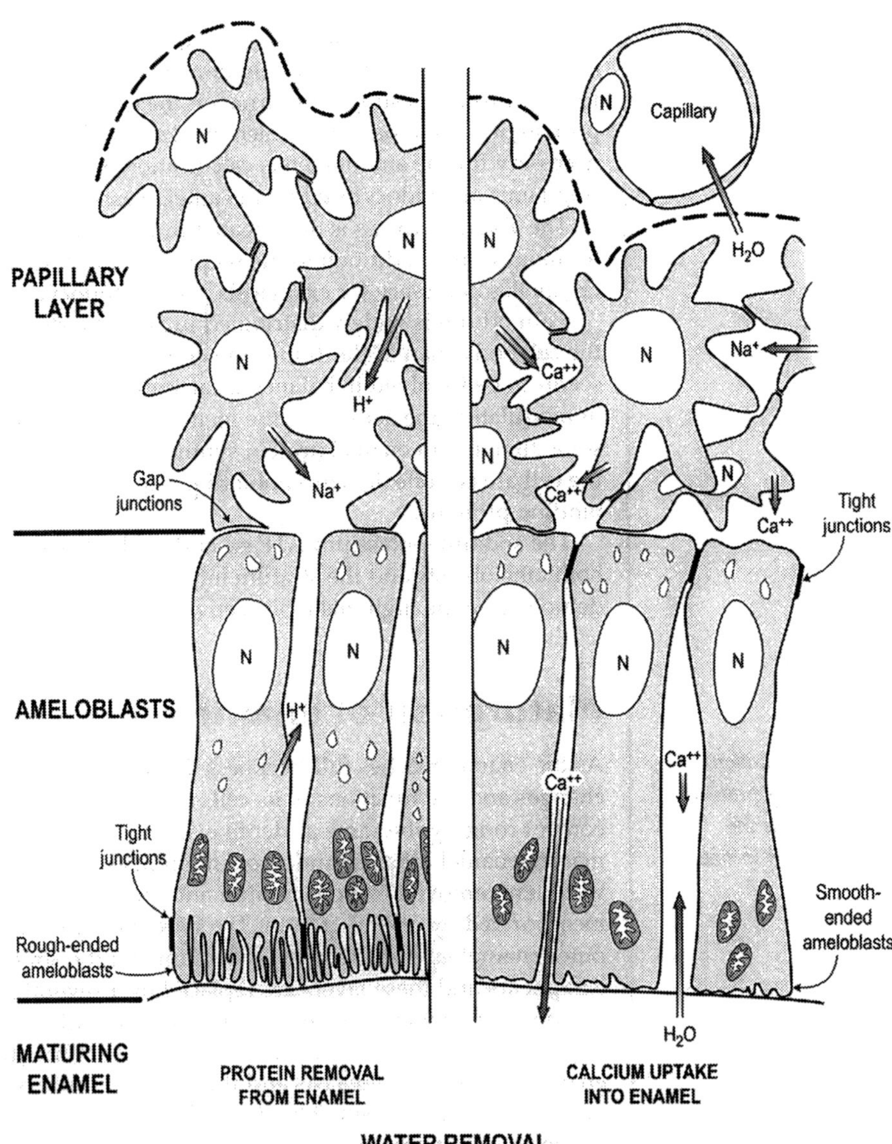

Fig. 3.12
Diagram of the maturation-stage ameloblasts showing the movements of ions and water.

junctions. The Golgi apparatus and the rough endoplasmic reticulum are minor cell components, but the cells do contain lysosomes and vesicles and can digest small proteins.

Maturation ameloblasts remove protein and water from enamel

The maturation ameloblasts lose their Tomes' processes but their final secretory products are exocytosed from their flat surfaces to form a final layer of rodless enamel some 10–15 μm thick on the surface of the tooth. A

matrix and transport calcium into it

basement membrane is then laid down on the enamel surface. The cells shorten to become cuboidal in shape and separate from each other – possibly due to death of some cells – to give wide intercellular spaces. The morphology of the cell membrane next to the enamel surface now undergoes a rhythmic change between two forms – the so-called ruffled end and the smooth end (Fig. 3.12). The ruffled border is made up of numerous deep invaginations which are wider towards the cell than at the surface. Beneath the ruffled border are many endocytotic vacuoles and the cells stain readily with anti-amelogenin reagents. The cells are very active, as shown by the many mitochondria and the large amounts of cytochrome *c* and hydrogen–potassium-ATPase. The nucleus is still proximally situated but is only about two-thirds of the way down the cell instead of being at the proximal end as in the cell's secretory ameloblast precursor. Laterally there are still proximal and distal tight junctional complexes, the proximal ones being macular rather than zonular and therefore allowing molecules to pass into the intercellular spaces, but the distal ones are tight zonulae occludens which restrict the passage of molecules even as small as EDTA (ethylenediamine tetra-acetic acid). There are a few desmosomes and gap junctions between the cells. The base or distal end of the cells is undulating and interdigitates with the cells of the papillary layer with which they have many gap junctions and desmosomes. At any one time approximately one-fifth of the maturation ameloblasts are ruffle-ended: the remainder are smooth-ended or in transition between the two forms. In the smooth-ended ameloblasts the nuclei vary in position, the Golgi apparatus is situated either above or below the nucleus and the infranuclear mitochondria and rough endoplasmic reticulum are aligned parallel to the long axis of the cells. The metabolic markers indicate a continuing high level of activity and there remain many lysosomes. There is, however, a major change in the lateral cell junctions; whilst the proximal tight junctions are still macular, the distal junctions cease to encircle the cells and also become macular so that movement of molecules between the cells is much less restricted.

Although classically the secretion phase of enamel formation was regarded as the time at which matrix was laid down and the maturation stage the time at which the bulk of the matrix was removed, it is now clear that enamel protein secretion begins even in the pre-ameloblasts and continues into early maturation. Similarly, secretion of proteolytic enzymes by the ameloblasts occurs during the secretion phase and there is breakdown of enamel proteins in the forming matrix. The breakdown during maturation probably results from the action of enzymes already present in the matrix rather than by a switchover of the maturation ameloblasts to proteolytic enzyme secretion. Uptake and transfer of the amelogenin fragments by the maturation-phase ameloblasts creates a gradient of concentration which will remove them from the deeper enamel. The removal of water probably occurs down osmotic gradients generated by the cells of the papillary layer secreting ions to the extracellular fluid. Movement of amelogenin fragments and water is almost certainly linked: either because the amelogenin fragments are osmotically active and water follows them, or because water movement itself can induce a streaming effect on the proteins. During maturation there is not only removal of water and protein but also addition of calcium and phosphate. Calcium has been detected in both maturation-phase ameloblasts and the papillary layer. Calmodulin is present in the polyribosomes, mitochondria, lysosomes and cytoplasm close to the cell membranes of ruffle-ended and smooth-ended ameloblasts and of papillary cells. Calbindin-D_{28K} is also present in all these cells and may function as a calcium buffer. Calcium-ATPase is not present in either ruffle- or smooth-ended ameloblasts and is found only in the papillary layer. This suggests that calcium ingress to the maturing enamel occurs via the intercellular spaces from the papillary layer and between the ameloblasts.

As maturation of the enamel is completed the papillary and ameloblast layers degenerate and form a thin cuticle over the erupting tooth.

The enamel matrix

Enamel matrix consists principally of amelogenins and enamelins. Amelogenins are low molecular weight proteins and protein fragments, rich in proline, glutamic acid, leucine and histidine The enamelins are of higher molecular weight and are rich in aspartic acid, serine, glutamic acid and glycine, but appear to be a mixture of proteins. There is evidence of *N*-acetylglucosamine and *N*-acetylgalactosamine and of chondroitin 1-sulphate and chondroitin 4-sulphate in maturing enamel. The presence of lipids is more difficult to establish. The lipids demonstrated thus far could all be cell membrane lipids, presumably derived from the process of exocytosis; early reports of sudanophilia are unhelpful as the enamel proteins themselves show some degree of sudanophilia.

In unfixed enamel matrix the protein appears as fibrils some 10 nm wide which are arranged in a helicoidal manner with four or five fibrils making a thicker fibre about 35 nm wide. The interior of the fibre tube is hydrophobic and may facilitate crystallisation by reducing the water content of the calcium-containing interstitial fluid. Certainly needle-like crystals appear within the fibres. Analysis of the matrix shows that during the secretory stage it contains around 28% calcium and 15% phosphate with a gradient to a slightly higher concentration at the amelodentinal junction, whilst during the maturation stage it seems to be more uniform with some 33% calcium and 16.6% phosphate (a molar ratio of 1.58 compared to the 1.66 of pure apatite). As the crystals grow and become smooth rectangular ribbons, the surrounding protein is removed, leaving only a thin coating of enamelins around the crystal. The initial crystal is possibly octacalcium phosphate which later tranforms into hydroxyapatite. However, it should be remembered that biological apatites almost invariably have other ions substituted into the crystal lattice. In enamel there is always a proportion of carbonate substitution for either phosphate or hydroxyl groups so that strictly it should be termed a carbonate apatite. A second anionic substitution is that of fluoride for a hydroxyl group. Fluoride accelerates hydroxyapatite formation and stabilises the crystals; in the calculated concentrations in the enamel organ one might still expect octacalcium phosphate to be formed but its transition to hydroxyapatite would be more rapid. There are also cationic substitutions, notably of sodium and magnesium. Magnesium substitutes for calcium and inhibits both precipitation and crystal growth. It reaches its maximum concentration in the forming enamel at the transition between the secretory stage and the maturation stage. It is suggested that magnesium may occupy vacant calcium sites at the crystal surface when the organic matrix is removed and before sufficient calcium is present to occupy them; calcium ions can displace the magnesium ions and so the magnesium concentration falls as maturation progresses. During maturation the crystals become progressively more stable as the calcium content increases and the acid phosphate and carbonate decrease, as shown by the increasing calcium molar ratio.

Calcification of cementum – cementogenesis

Cementum, like bone and dentine, is of mesodermal origin. In the process of dental development the tooth crown is formed first, and therefore cementum, as the outer layer of the tooth root, is the last of the three dental tissues to be laid down. The enamel organ and the dental papilla differentiate and begin to lay down their respective hard tissues before cementum formation begins.

Development of the tooth root

Extension away from the crown of an epithelial bilayer from the cervical loop triggers odontoblast differentiation and dentine formation in the tooth root

At the bell stage of the enamel organ the inner and outer enamel epithelial layers meet at the future neck of the tooth – forming the so-called cervical loop. The cells of the cervical loop begin to proliferate away from the crown of the tooth to form a bilayer (sometimes a trilayer) of epithelium which travels towards the future root apex and outlines the shape of the future root or roots (Fig. 3.13). In multi-rooted teeth the envelope of epithelium is first indented and then forms a tube for each root. This epithelial layer is termed the root sheath of Hertwig or the epithelial root sheath; it divides off the cells which form the pulp of the tooth from the surrounding cells which will ultimately form the periodontal ligament. There is formation of a basement membrane around inner and outer surfaces of the root sheath – presumably secreted by the epithelial cells themselves. The cells on the inner surface differentiate into pre-odontoblasts and then odontoblasts which begin to secrete collagen and other proteins of the dentinal matrix. The first randomly oriented fibres calcify as mantle dentine, as described earlier for those in the crown. The newly forming dentine extends inwards as circumpulpar dentine and away from the crown to elongate the root. In a human tooth the rate of extension of the root is about 6 μm/day. As the root extends apexwards the root sheath continues to extend in the same direction and the more coronal portion disintegrates. Remnants of the root sheath are thought to constitute the epithelial rests of Malassez later found in the periodontal ligament. At the growing tip of the root, then, there are the cells of the root sheath, odontoblasts, and newly formed predentine. This layer extends some 300 μm towards the crown. Mineralisation produces a core of dentine within the predentine extending to some 50–100 μm of the tip of the advancing predentine.

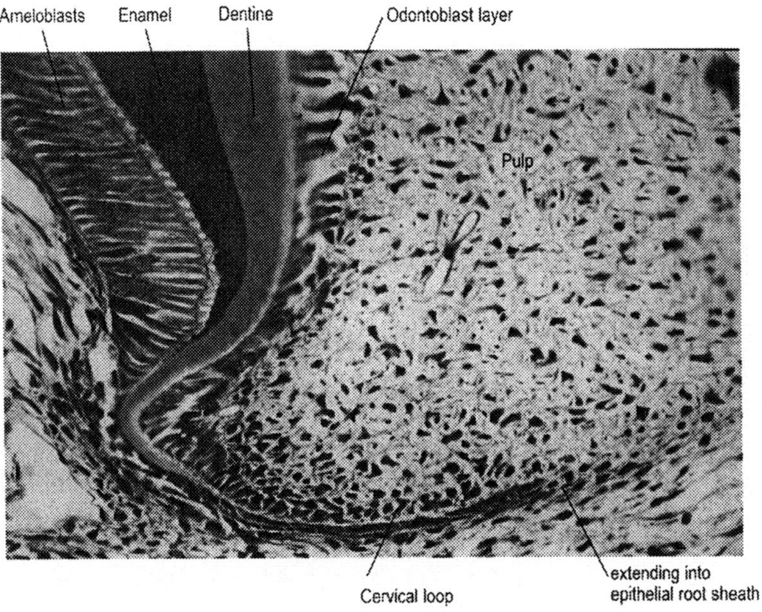

Fig. 3.13
The forming cervical margin of the tooth.

Cementoblast differentiation and cementum formation

Cementoblast differentiation occurs between the newly formed dentine and the epithelial root sheath

The inner layer of the root sheath is in contact with the predentine at the tip, but coronal to this the sheath appears to lose its inner layer and the outer layer separates from the forming root (Fig. 3.14). The cells which now appear between the dentine surface and this layer of epithelial cells are elongated fibroblast-like cells with an extensive rough endoplasmic reticulum and many desmosomal contacts. It is not clear whether these are ectomesenchymal cells migrating from the dental follicle in response to some signal from the epithelial cells, or whether they result from an unusual transformation of the epithelial root sheath cells into mesenchymal cells. They extend cytoplasmic processes towards the dentine which penetrate into the predentine and lay down collagen fibres which interdigitate with those of the predentine and project some 10–20 μm into the future periodontium as a fibre fringe. This layer of fibres later calcifies as the acellular extrinsic fibre cementum. The fibres are not connected with or related to the fibres of the future periodontal ligament, which at this stage lie parallel to the root surface in the dental follicle. The epithelial cells have been demonstrated to secrete proteins similar in structure to amelogenins. Although these might be involved in the formation of the initial layer of cementum, it seems more likely that they act as signal molecules which cause odontoblast differentiation. The predentine matrix calcifies after the meshing together of the predentine and cementoblast-derived collagen fibres. The cementum matrix laid down next to this contains collagen fibres, amelogenin-like proteins, osteopontin, bone sialoprotein,

The cementoblasts lay down a matrix of collagen and non-collagenous proteins

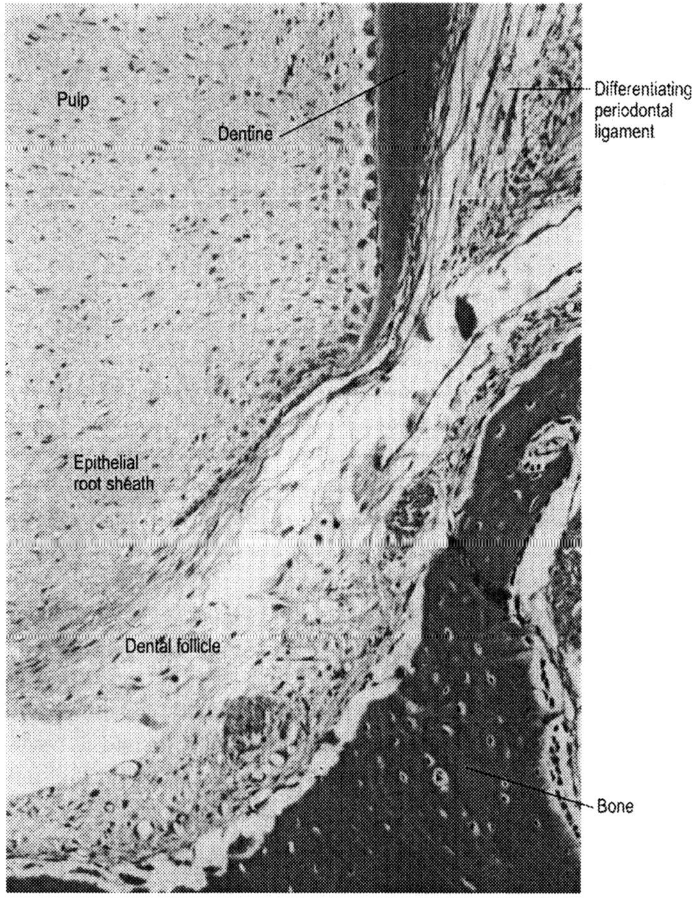

Fig. 3.14
Differentiation of the periodontal ligament and the site of cementoblast differentiation as the root develops.

The fibres of the periodontal ligament assume their final configuration some 5 years after root development has begun

osteocalcin and alpha-2 HS-glycoprotein. Bone acidic glycoprotein is not found in cementum matrix. Calcification begins in this matrix as discrete islands of crystals. The acellular extrinsic fibre cementum develops along the root surface and increases in thickness: the densely packed collagen fibres of the fringe increase in length as the cementum thickens. There is no apparent layer of cementoid analogous to osteoid: matrix calcification seems to occur as the matrix is laid down. The mature cementum is described as containing some non-calcified fibres. When the tooth follows its eruption pathway and reaches the oral epithelium the root is approximately two-thirds formed. At this stage the acellular extrinsic fibre cementum is about 7–9 μm thick at the cemento enamel junction. The root grows at about 6 μm/day and the cementum increases in thickness by just over 2 μm/year in a human premolar. Around 5 years after root development has begun the fibres of the periodontal ligament change direction from their initial parallelism with the long axis of the root and become either slightly oblique or perpendicular to the root surface. They now appear to interdigitate or even splice with the fringe fibres and further calcification causes them to become embedded in the cementum. They are then the principal fibres of the periodontal ligament (often called Sharpey's fibres) and they will adopt different alignments during tooth eruption until the so-called fibre groups can be identified. The final alignment of these fibres will be achieved as the tooth comes into occlusion.

Cementoblasts which form the cellular cementum and become embedded in it appear different from those which formed acellular cementum

At about the same time the formation of cementum on the final third of the root follows a new pattern. The cementoblasts which appear between the epithelial root sheath and the predentine begin as precementoblasts – small cells with long cytoplasmic processes penetrating the predentine. More coronally, the cementoblasts appear as large basophilic cells with large nuclei and extensive endoplasmic reticulum. These cells appear functionally different from those forming the acellular cementum but there is no evidence that they are different in origin – and, again, it is not clear whether they are derived from dental follicle cells or from the epithelial root sheath. The cementoblasts nearest the predentine send out long processes towards and into it. They begin to lay down matrix and the collagen fibres they produce interlock with the collagen fibres of the predentine. The cementum – cellular intrinsic fibre cementum – forms rapidly and cementoblasts become trapped in lacunae of the calcified material. These cementocytes are similar to the osteocytes in bone; communication may occur between them via long thin processes in the canaliculi which link the lacunae. The forming cementum incorporates extrinsic fibres which resemble the fringe fibres of the acellular extrinsic fibre cementum, but incorporation of the principal fibres of the periodontal ligament does not occur until these latter

Precipitation occurs when the ionic activity product exceeds the solubility product of the crystal

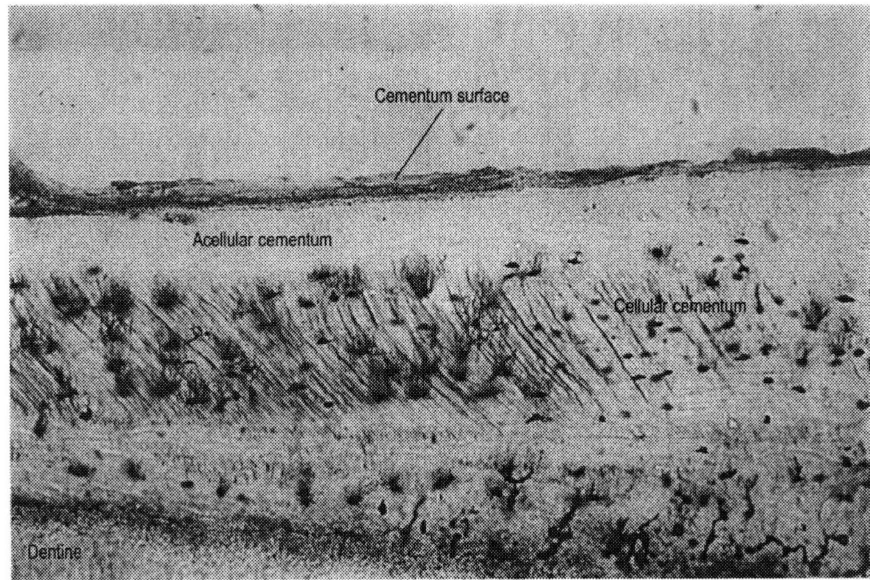

Fig. 3.15
Ground section of cementum showing layers of cellular and acellular cementum.

change direction as eruption proceeds. The cellular cementum is now termed cellular mixed stratified cementum. Formation of cementum continues throughout the life of the tooth as a result of cementoblast activity and the disposition of the different cementum types may be in any combination – cellular may overlay non-cellular or vice versa (Fig. 3.15).

Further Reading

Calcification in Biological Systems. Bonucci, E. (editor). CRC Press, Boca Raton, 1992

Mineral Aspects of Dentistry. Driessens, F.C.M. Monographs in Oral Science, Vol. 10. Karger, Basel, 1982

Calcium Phosphates in Biology and Medicine. LeGeros, R.Z. Monographs in Oral Science, Vol. 15. Karger, Basel, 1991

Symposium on Periodontal Ligament. Special issue of the Anatomical Record, 1996

4 The dental pulp

The dental pulp is the connective tissue inside the tooth which provides nutrition and sensation to the dentine and hence the tooth

The dental pulp is the connective tissue situated within the tooth, enclosed by dentine except at the apex of the root where it is continuous with the periodontal ligament. Each pulp is of small volume – estimated at about 0.02 ml in an adult tooth, giving a total volume of pulpal tissue in all the teeth of about 0.40 ml – and the apical foramen of the tooth, through which its nerve and blood supply pass, is reduced in adult life to a diameter barely large enough to allow access for the bundle of nerve fibres and vessels.

Although the pulp and dentine are described in different chapters, their functions are interlinked and they are sometimes referred to as the pulpodentinal complex (Fig. 4.1). The functions of the pulp are to maintain the health of the dentine by supplying nutrients, to provide a pathway for sensory impulses resulting from stimuli to dentine, and to initiate and govern repair of dentine when it is damaged. The layer of specialised cells immediately adjacent to the predentine or dentine – the odontoblasts – have processes which penetrate the dentine for varying distances, are responsible for the formation of dentinal matrix and its calcification, and may be involved in sensory perception from dentine. Although they are situated in the pulp and derive from pulpal cells, they will be considered in more detail in relation to dentine and to oral sensation.

Pulp matrix

Pulp consists of cells, fibres and a proteoglycan matrix penetrated by nerve fibres and blood vessels

Like all connective tissues, the pulp consists of fibres and cells situated in an apparently amorphous matrix, with nerves and the principal blood vessels arranged in bundles.

The matrix is made up of proteoglycans. The glycosaminoglycan parts of these molecules are long-chain carbohydrate polymers that retain water to form a gel. In many tissues the function of such a gel is to resist compression, but in the fully formed tooth where the pulpal cells and structures are protected by the surrounding dentine its role is more that of space filling. As the tooth ages there will be a progressive obliteration of the pulp by dentine; a more highly organised or cellular tissue would be replaced less easily. Such a role would be similar to that of the glycosaminoglycans in the stellate reticulum of the enamel organ during tooth development. The pulp contains

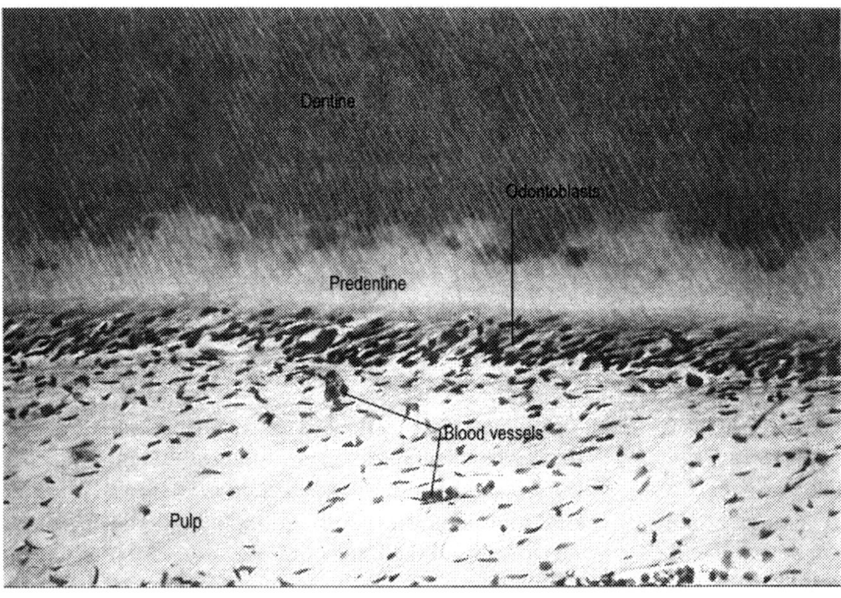

Fig. 4.1a
The pulpodentinal complex.

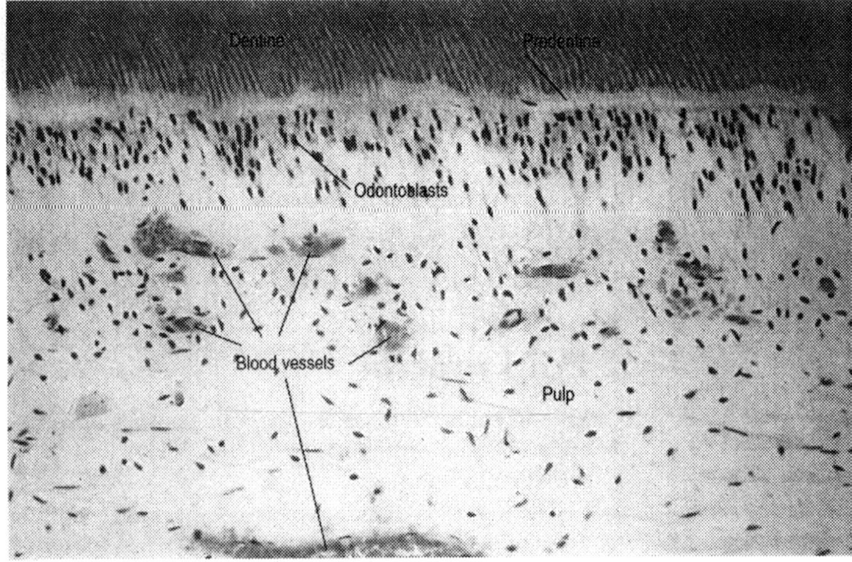

Fig. 4.1b
The dental pulp and dentine.

some 88% water, a proportion high in comparison with that of other tissues. The principal glycosaminoglycan of the pulp is chondroitin 4-sulphate (estimated at 55% of the total although the amount decreases in older pulps).

Table 4.1
Glycosaminoglycans of the dental pulp

Total amount 0.30±0.09 mg uronic acid/g wet weight of pulp	
Percentage of total glycosamines in human pulp tissue	
Hyaluronic acid	3.4
Keratan sulphate	28.0
Dermatan sulphate	13.0
Chondroitin 4-sulphate	55.7

Chondroitin 4-sulphate binds calcium readily; it helps to maintain a high calcium level in the pulp, providing a store of calcium to assist in the mineralisation of the dentine matrix. Next in concentration is keratin 1-sulphate (28%), most of which is linked to protein molecules. The only other glycosaminoglycan present in quantity is dermatan sulphate (13%), a substance which seems to be important in collagen fibrillogenesis. There is a small amount of hyaluronan, but virtually no heparan sulphate or chondroitin 6-sulphate (Table 4.1).

The fibres are collagen type III, with lesser amounts of type I and type VI

The fibrous component of the pulp is almost entirely collagen. Elastin is present only in the walls of the blood vessels. However, there are some glycoprotein fibrils present similar to those which surround elastin fibres; these constitute the oxytalan fibres. Collagen makes up about one-third of the dry weight of the pulp. The types normally present are types III, I and VI in order of their relative amounts. A very small amount of type V is also found. The normal function of these collagens is to confer some rigidity on a tissue; in the pulp that probably means the maintenance of position of the vessels, nerves and cells. Type III is usually associated with some degree of elasticity or extensibility of the tissue.

Other proteins demonstrated in the pulp include the glycoproteins fibronectin and tenascin. Fibronectin binds cells to collagen (particularly type III) and to the sulphated glycoproteins of the matrix; it is probably important in stabilising the spatial arrangement of pulp cells and fibres. It disappears from the mesenchyme when odontoblast differentiation begins and has therefore been suggested to play some role in this. However, a more likely candidate for an organiser molecule is tenascin, which is produced by the cells of the dental papilla but not by odontoblasts and has been shown to be widely distributed in dental pulps which retain the capacity to produce calcified tissue.

A number of enzymes have been detected and assayed in dental pulps. These include the enzymes of the glycolytic pathways. Alkaline phosphatase is associated with the odontoblasts and the predentine layer. A collagenase which has been detected is thought to be secreted by the odontoblasts. It is normally inactive because of the presence of inhibitors.

Pulp cells

If the cells making up the blood vessels and the nerve fibres are excluded, the cells of the pulp are the peripheral layer of highly differentiated odontoblasts

The cells of the dental pulp include immature mesenchymal cells, mature fibroblasts known as pulpocytes, and the layer of odontoblasts along the predentine surface

and the stellate cells with many processes which are usually termed fibroblasts. These latter, however, are of at least two types: the immature immature mesenchymal cells similar to those which originally made up the dental papilla, and the mature fibrocytes or pulpocytes. The mesenchymal cells of the dental papilla carry genetic information on the final size and shape of the tooth and they drive the differentiation of ectodermal cells into ameloblasts. In the pulp itself they synthesise collagen types I, III and V and they can develop into odontoblasts which retain the ability to synthesise collagen types I and V only. The committed fibroblasts of the pulp, or pulpocytes, are able to synthesise collagen types I, III, V and VI. The metabolism and functions of the odontoblasts will be described elsewhere.

In the healthy pulp the few blood cells found outside the blood vessels are mainly macrophages or histiocytes and the occasional lymphocyte.

Blood vessels

The pulp has an extensive blood supply

The pulp has a good blood supply derived from the appropriate alveolar artery. At the time of crown completion branches of the vessels curve towards the tooth germs and then split into two sets of branches, one supplying the coronal pulp and the other passing to the area around the reduced enamel epithelium which at this time covers the crown. This latter network gives rise to the dense capillary network beneath the epithelial attachment when the tooth erupts and also becomes the blood supply to the periodontal ligament as the tooth root forms. The main arterioles and venules lie along the longitudinal axis of the pulp and the arterioles pass up into the pulp horns (Fig. 4.2). They divide first into numerous small branches near the pulp surface and then into a capillary network on the surface – the terminal capillary network (Fig. 4.3). The venules are larger and less straight than the arterioles.

As the root reaches completion the distribution of the vessels changes. The larger arterioles lie centrally in the root canals whilst the venules travel along the walls. A few arterioles run along the walls towards the crown. The vascular bed itself is stratified into three layers: a terminal capillary network of flattened capillaries between the odontoblasts, a palisade of ascending precapillaries and descending postcapillaries, and reticulum of venules. In the floor of the pulp chamber only the terminal capillary network is present. As root development continues further and the pulp chamber narrows, the number of blood vessels passing through the root apex falls to seven or eight main arterioles and two or three main venules. The vessels of the network in the root canals and between the pulp horns narrow and the more superficial vessels appear coarse. The main venules now lie immediately below the superficial network, which appears as a single coarse layer. In some instances the terminal capillary layer forms short hairpin loops, particularly as secondary dentine formation proceeds. Some arteriovenous anastomoses are seen in the pulp but more unusually there are venovenous anastomoses between the networks supplied from different root canals and loops or coils are sometimes observed along the course of arterioles. It is possible that these could in some way serve as regulators of blood flow.

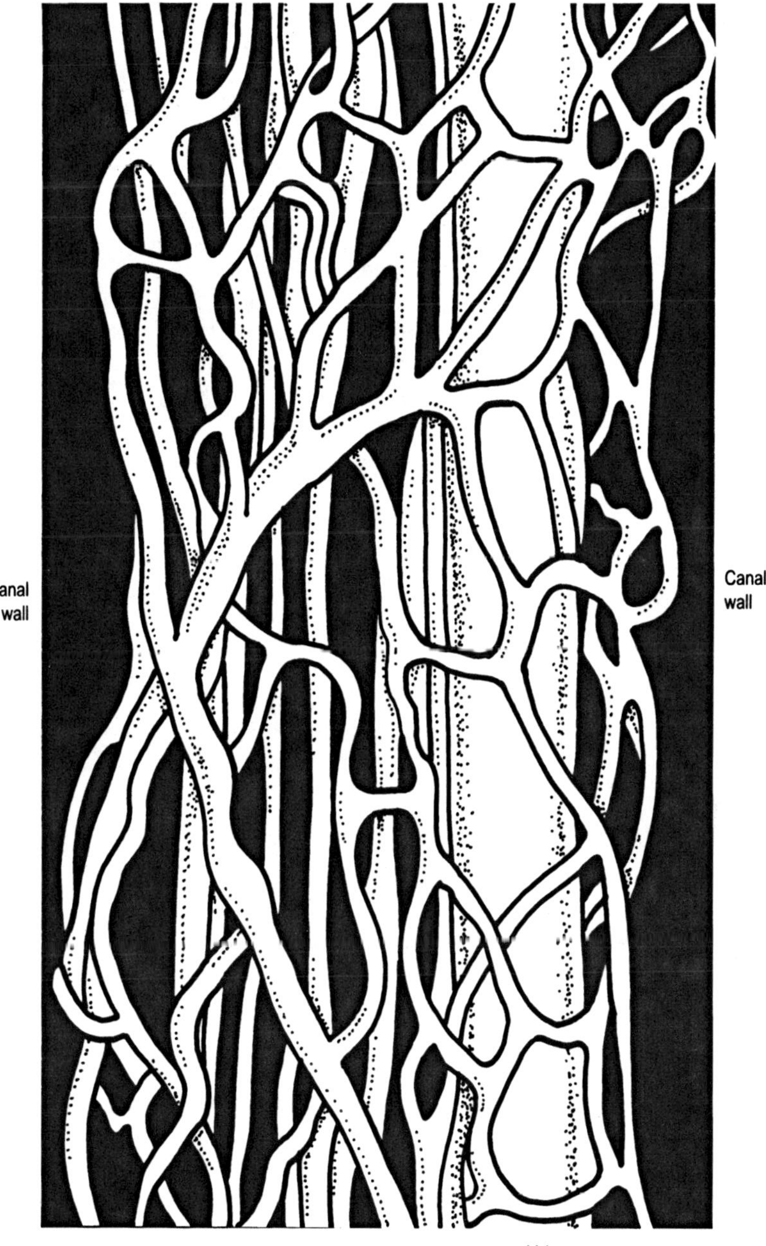

Fig. 4.2
Blood vessels in the root canal of a tooth. Note the large vein, the superficial plexus of capillaries and venules, and the straight parallel arteries passing up the centre of the root canal.

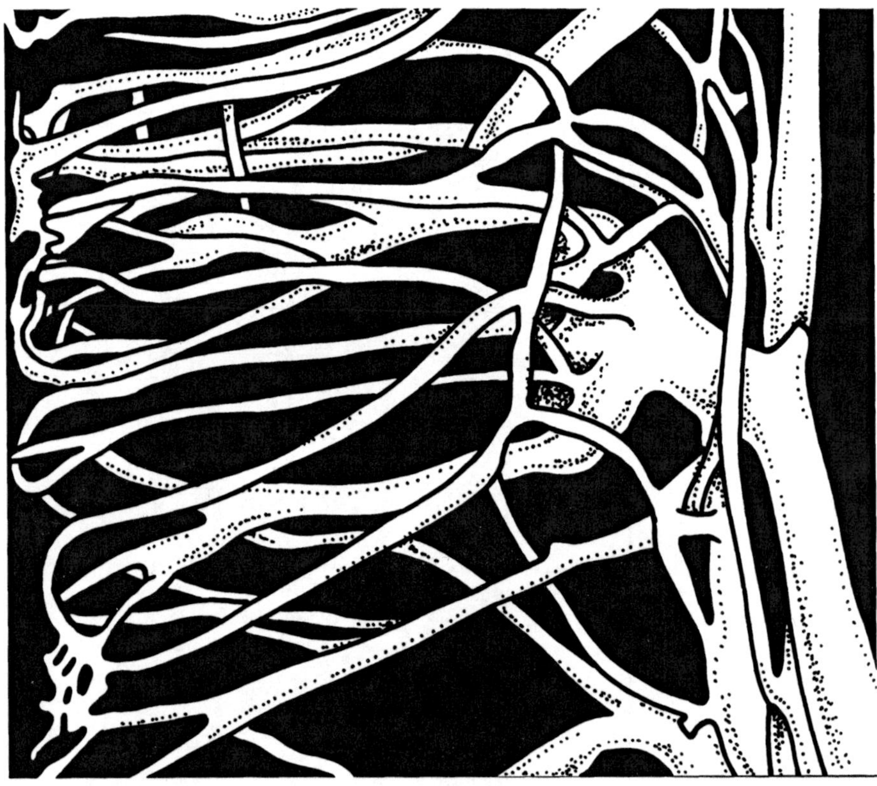

Blood vessels in the pulp chamber of a tooth. On the left is the capillary plexus around and below the odontoblasts; on the right is a vein draining these vessels.

Nerves

The nerve supply of the pulp is sensory with A delta and C fibres derived from the alveolar nerves, together with autonomic nerve fibres mainly concerned in the control of the blood vessels

The nerve fibres which have been observed by conventional optical microscopy in the dental pulp are sensory fibres of the A delta and C groups – fibre groups predominately associated with pain sensation. The use of enzyme histochemical techniques reveals cholinergic and adrenergic fibres and immunofluorescence studies enable peptidergic neurones to be visualised. Electron microscopy has shown three types of nerve terminals near blood vessels: large fibres, several micrometres in diameter, containing small vesicles, which resemble cholinergic endings; fibres up to 3 μm in diameter with numerous small dense-cored vesicles and a few large (60–150 nm) electron-dense vesicles, which are probably sympathetic fibres; and another group of small fibres with numerous large (80–200 nm) dense vesicles, which are probably purinergic or peptidergic endings. The second type are found mainly in the pulp horns and pulp chamber. The third type occur least frequently. In the adult the nerves enter at the apical foramen and pass, with relatively little branching, through the root canals to fan out in the crown and pass to the pulpodentinal border, forming a meshwork known as the plexus of Raschkow, or the subodontoblastic plexus. Individual axons divide into as many as eight terminal branches in this plexus.

In the earliest stages of tooth development branches of the alveolar nerve are seen close to the base of the dental papilla. During the early cap stage they form a local plexus and then pass first into the follicle and then the forming tooth. At the bell stage of development the fibres are unmyelinated. At eruption the number of nerve fibres increases markedly and continues to increase for a few years after eruption. Thus the first permanent molar has around 400 axons at eruption, whilst the premolar has less – 100 or more – but by 5 years after eruption has around 700. The distribution of fibre sizes remains fairly constant. The number of unmyelinated fibres also reaches a peak soon after eruption: typically at about 1800 axons. The average size of these fibres does seem to increase at eruption – possibly representing a transition towards myelination. As tooth development continues there is less grouping of non-myelinated fibres and the nerve plexuses decrease in size. This is probably related to the decreasing size of the pulp itself. In ageing pulps there is a decrease in the number of axons entering the pulp and an apparent reduction in fibre size of the myelinated nerves. The nerve fibres in the subodontoblastic plexus and the dentine–predentine area show little change with age.

The pattern of development of the innervation of the deciduous teeth is similar to that in the permanent dentition. The deciduous incisor after eruption has some 250 myelinated axons and between 1000 and 3000 unmyelinated axons: this is around two-thirds of the number in the permanent incisor. However, the deciduous canine has slightly more nerve fibres than the permanent canine or incisor although less than the premolar. There is therefore no adequate explanation of the lesser sensitivity of the deciduous teeth in terms of the number of nerve fibres supplying the teeth. When the deciduous teeth begin to resorb axon degeneration occurs and the number of nerve fibres progressively decreases until the tooth is shed.

Neurotrophic substances

Nerve growth substances are found in dental pulps

It is still unclear what determines the development and spread of nerve processes outside the central nervous system. Nerve growth factor has been studied extensively and it is known that, during the developmental stage of reduction in nerve cell numbers, nerve growth factor promotes the survival of the neural crest derived cells in the trigeminal ganglion. Again, nerve growth factor is produced in the maxillary process after it is reached by developing axons, and it appears to be important in maintaining their survival. It does not appear to have any role in directing the spread of fibres. The late invasion of the dental pulp tissue by nerve fibres suggests that the pulp may produce sprouting and trophic factors which can act on nearby nerves. Thus the permanent teeth are able to recruit some of their nerve supply from branches of axons previously supplying the deciduous teeth.

Reinnervation of implanted teeth occurs in a similar fashion. The extension of new nerve fibres into the odontoblast layer and dentine in reimplanted teeth may implicate the odontoblasts as possible sources of neurotrophic factors. Although nerve growth factor has not been demonstrated in the dental pulp, the evidence available shows that the properties of the neurotrophic factors in the pulp are distinct from those of nerve growth factor. None of the other defined survival or neurite growth-promoting factors described in other tissues have been demonstrated in, or shown to have effects on, nerves supplying the dental pulp.

Functions of the pulp nerves

Pulpal nerve fibres generate pain sensations when stimulated

The A delta fibres are myelinated, have diameters between 1 and 4 µm and are rapidly conducting (>2 m/s). In other tissues they are thought to mediate sharp, piercing pain sensations. In the tooth they are the nerves responsible for the sensitivity of dentine and they respond to any stimuli which cause fluid movement in the dentinal tubules – e.g. hydrodynamic stimuli such as drilling, drying and application of osmotically active solutions to dentine.

The C fibres are unmyelinated, less than 0.5 µm in diameter and conduct more slowly at <2m/s. They are polymodal and activated by thermal, mechanical and chemical stimuli. These last include histamine and bradykinin, which cause pain in the inflamed pulp. Such pain is dull, longer lasting and less well localised than that arising from impulses in the A delta nerves.

Neurotransmitter substances found in the pulp include CGRP, substance P and neurokinin A

A number of neurotransmitters have been identified in pulpal nerves. Of these, calcitonin gene-related peptide (CGRP), substance P and neurokinin A are present in fibres which arise from the alveolar nerves and are probably sensory. A large proportion of the pulpal nerves react with antibodies to calcitonin gene-related peptide. Substance P is detected only in fibres which also stain for calcitonin gene-related peptide, and neurokinin A only in fibres which contain both the other transmitters. Nerves fibres giving positive reactions for these peptides enter the pulp in bundles alongside the blood vessels in the apical foramen. Some narrow fibres with varicosities course along small blood vessels in the central portion of the pulp or form networks around the larger vessels. In human incisors and molars many fibres run directly into the pulp horns, turn to run parallel to the surface and then give off branches which pass between the odontoblasts and may enter the dentine. These peptide-containing fibres degenerate after section of the alveolar nerves but are unaffected by sympathectomy. The peptides are found in cells of the trigeminal ganglion: it is thought that they are synthesised there and pass by axonal flow to the terminals within the pulp. All three peptides are vasodilators, but it is possible that they are also in some way involved in modification of sensory inputs.

The autonomic nerve supply to the pulp includes both sympathetic and parasympathetic fibres. Of these, the majority are sympathetic; estimates of their numbers range from under 10% to over 50% of the nerve fibres entering the pulp. In the mouse about half of the sympathetic fibres are in the pulp horns, about a third in the pulp chamber, and the rest in the root canals. The main function of the sympathetic fibres is the control of pulp blood flow, but it has also been suggested that they may play some role in the regulation of odontogenesis and in the afferent transmission of impulses associated with

Sympathetic nerves are involved in the control of blood flow but may also affect dentine apposition

pain sensation. The evidence for these functions is partly anatomical: the majority of sympathetic nerve fibres are found in plexuses around blood vessels (usually arterioles) but some terminals are found close to the bases of odontoblasts and some pass into the predentine. Other evidence comes from observations after sympathectomy. After division of the sympathetic nerves vasodilatation occurs and there are changes in the rate of dentine apposition. Stimulation of the sympathetic nerves results in a decrease in pulpal pressure. The vascular effects of sympathetic stimulation are mediated mainly through alpha-1 adrenergic receptors. There are some beta-2 receptors: stimulation of these produces an immediate vasodilatation followed by a decrease in blood flow. Staining for neuropeptide Y has shown it to be present in some pulpal sympathetic nerves. Release of this peptide usually results in a more sustained vasoconstriction than is observed with noradrenaline alone.

Cholinergic fibres may modify sensation from dentine or have a possible indirect vasodilator effect

The functions of the cholinergic fibres detected in the dental pulp are less clear. As all neural crest derived cells are capable of acetylcholine synthesis, choline esterase has been identified in migrating neural crest cells as well as in developing nerves, and indeed is present in the enamel epithelium during tooth development. In cells other than nerve cells it usually disappears when morphogenetic movement is completed. The cholinergic fibres in the pulp include some sympathetic fibres, but the majority are thought to be parasympathetic. Thus removal of the superior cervical ganglion does cause some decrease in cholinesterase staining in the pulp whilst resection of the inferior alveolar nerve almost completely abolishes it. After resection of the inferior alveolar nerve in rats there is an increased rate of tooth eruption, a change usually associated with an increase in blood flow. Stimulation of the cut end of the nerve causes vasoconstriction in the extrapulpal branches of the mandibular artery but an increase in intrapulpal pressure. Some of the nerve fibres in the dentinal tubules and in the subodontoblastic layer have been identified as cholinergic. It is thought that they, like the sympathetic fibres in the odontogenic region, may modify the sensory output resulting from stimulation of dentine. Observations on nerve fibres in the dental pulp of cat teeth have identified vasoactive intestinal peptide (VIP) in association with acetylcholine in the parasympathetic nerve terminals. It is possible that this may be responsible for any vasodilator activity of the these nerves.

Blood supply to the dental pulp

Blood pressure in dental pulps is typical of that close to capillaries in other peripheral tissues, but the enclosed nature of the pulp renders the blood supply of low compliance

There have been few measurements of blood pressure in human tooth pulps. Arterial pressure has been recorded as 4.3 kPa systolic and 3.5 kPa diastolic with a mean pressure of 3.7 kPa. The intersitial fluid pressure has been measured in dogs with results varying between 0 and 8 kPa and in cats with values around 2.4 kPa, but the most reliable methods give figures of around 0.8 kPa and values in humans are unlikely to be very different. The enclosure of the pulp tissue and vessels within the rigid dentine walls of the pulp cavity gives the pulpal circulation a low compliance: small changes in volume result in major changes in pressure. Thus formation of interstitial fluid is a self-limiting process – factors tending to increase interstitial fluid formation will rapidly increase interstitial fluid pressure to equalise the transcapillary pressures or even compress the blood vessels and reduce blood flow. There is now evidence of a lymphatic drainage from the tooth pulp. As lymph vessels must also pass through the narrow apical foramen, they too are liable to compression if tissue pressures increase.

Pulpal blood flow has been more extensively studied than has pulpal blood pressure – partly because it is a more informative measurement and partly because it is technically easier to measure. Nevertheless, few data exist for human teeth and most measurements have been carried out on dogs. Similarly, studies of the factors affecting pulp blood flow have also been carried out in dogs. It is probable, however, that the conclusions are equally valid in humans. The normal pulp blood flow in humans is of the same order as that in the dog: 40–50 ml/min/100 g of tissue. This is a relatively high figure – the highest recorded in oral tissues – and it is not immediately obvious why a tissue with no apparent special metabolic needs should have a high blood flow. A possible function of the rapid rate of flow may be the need for rapid removal of potentially toxic substances which had penetrated dentine or been released from the pulpal tissue itself.

Pulpal blood flow is high

Flow is not uniform throughout the pulp, being highest in the tips of the pulp horns and least in the root canals. These differences are due to the distribution of the blood vessels. The effect of mastication on pulpal blood flow has not been explored, but it is likely that the compression of the periodontal ligament during the biting stroke will compress the supply vessels, momentarily and rhythmically interrupting blood flow.

Pulp blood flow depends more upon nervous control than on local metabolic products, but the effects of the various vasoactive stimuli are modified by the low compliance of the pulpal circulation and the higher compliances of the parallel circulations such as those in the periodontal ligament and gingivae. Three types of response have been described. The response to most vasoconstrictor stimuli is a simple reduction in blood flow. Thus stimulation of the superior cervical ganglion or the cervical sympathetic chain causes vasoconstriction and reduction in blood flow. Infusion of adrenaline or noradrenaline, or application of noradrenaline to a cavity cut in dentine has similar effects. Pulpal pressure is decreased. All these actions can be blocked by alpha adrenoceptor blocking agents such as phentolamine. In contrast, adrenaline applied directly to the pulp increases blood flow. Vasoconstrictors other than sympathomimetic agents, including serotonin (5-hydroxytryptamine) and prostaglandin F_{2alpha}, also reduce blood flow.

Most vasodilator agents give a biphasic response, with a brief increase in blood flow being followed by a longer-lasting decrease. Such a response is seen with close arterial injection of acetylcholine, histamine, isoproterenol, bradykinin, vasoactive intestinal peptide, substance P, calcitonin gene-related peptide and prostaglandin E_2. This response may be due to a simultaneous vasodilatation in parallel circulations, which because of their higher compliance effectively shift the blood away from the higher resistance pathway. Further, the rise in tissue pressure as a result of the volume increase in the pulp compresses the venules leaving the pulp chamber so that blood flow decreases until the tissue pressure falls sufficiently to allow outflow. The simultaneous compression of the lymphatic vessels means that pressure may remain high for some time. It is also possible that vasodilators may open

The vasodilator response of pulpal blood vessels is complicated by the low compliance

arteriovenous shunts and thus decrease tissue perfusion, but there is no evidence of this. Topical application of vasodilator substances either directly to the pulp or to cavities cut in dentine increases blood flow. Stimulation of the inferior alveolar nerve also produces a vasodilator response. This response is not inhibited by atropine or by propranolol, suggesting that it is not a cholinergic response. Substance P is known to be released in the pulp after stimulation of this nerve, and is also known to increase pulpal blood flow and pulpal pressure. This response is abolished by somatostatin.

The third type of blood flow response is a slow decrease in blood flow which occurs when substances increasing capillary permeability and tissue fluid formation are either injected into vessels or applied to the pulp. This is again a response caused by the enclosed nature of the pulp.

Metabolic stimuli are ineffective in the pulp. The pulpal circulation does not demonstrate any response similar to reactive hyperaemia and it does not respond rapidly to local hypoxia.

Systemic factors acting on the circulation do, however, produce similar results in the dental pulp to those elsewhere. Baroreceptor, respiratory chemoreceptor and blood volume reflexes all include the pulpal blood vessels.

Nociceptive response

The axon response described in skin subjected to painful stimuli is readily identified in the dental pulp

The dental pulp reacts initially to electrical, mechanical or chemical stimulation of dentine via an axon reflex. The sensory C fibres are stimulated and a retrograde impulse in their branches results in the release of substance P at their terminals. Substance P acts on the blood vessels to cause vasodilatation. In young teeth with relatively wide apical canals there is an increase in blood flow to the coronal pulp and the terminal capillaries in the subodontoblastic layer. The response in older teeth is more variable. Although blood flow may be increased in some teeth, in others there is a decreased flow in the capillary network as a result of vasodilatation in a low compliance circulation. Where vasodilatation occurs it is followed by increased fluid transfer across the capillary walls and tissue oedema. Substance P also causes the release of histamine from mast cells, increasing capillary permeability and fluid extravasation. Noxious stimulation of the pulp is associated with bradykinin formation. This too may be stimulated by substance P. Bradykinin contributes further to the vasodilatation, but may also stimulate the release of encephalins, particularly met-encephalin, from pulpal cells. The encephalins are anti-inflammatory and in turn inhibit bradykinin release – a protective negative feedback reaction. Both met-encephalin and its precursor, met-encephalin-arg-phe, have been demonstrated in pulp cells and their concentration increases after noxious stimulation.

Another group of substances associated with responses to noxious stimuli and inflammatory responses in tissues in general is the eicosanoid group – metabolites of arachidonic acid which include the prostaglandins and the leucotrienes. The dental pulp phospholipids are high in arachidonic acid content and pathways are present for synthesis of both prostaglandins and leucotrienes. Prostaglandin I_2 is produced by endothelial cells and inhibits platelet aggregation as well as being vasodilator; thromboxane A_2, produced by platelets and other cells such as fibroblasts, stimulates platelet aggregation. Both of these are present normally in the pulp, with prostaglandin I_2 being in the higher concentration. Prostaglandins F_{2alpha} and E_2 are also present in human dental pulps with F_{2alpha} in the higer concentration. Of the leucotrienes, 12-HETE and LTC_4 have been identified in human pulps.

Inflammation of the pulp resulting from bacterial, mechanical or chemical irritation causes an increase in prostaglandin E_2 and F_{2alpha}, and both these compounds are found in much higher concentration in painful pulps. These increased concentrations do not seem to be related to the increases in histamine and bradykinin concentrations seen in inflammation, although serotonin, another contributor to the inflammatory process, stimulates prostaglandin I_2 release. The role of the prostaglandins in pulpal inflammation is probably mainly in relation to vasodilatation, but they do also increase the pain-producing properties of the other characteristic molecules of inflammation: histamine, bradykinin and serotonin. Relief of pain from an inflamed pulp may be achieved by the administration of aspirin, an inhibitor of cyclo-oxygenase and therefore of prostaglandin synthesis. Medicaments used in root canal treatment such as phenol, *p*-chlorophenol, cresol, thymol and guaiacol, in addition to their antibacterial effect, have an analgesic action which is partly due to their ability to inhibit synthesis of prostaglandins and leucotrienes. Eugenol, used both on dentine and in root canals, is even more effective than these other phenols in inhibiting prostaglandin synthesis. Evaluation of these phenolic substances has been made difficult by the observation that in low concentrations they may stimulate production of prostaglandins, whilst having the reverse effect at high concentrations.

Pulpitis and pulp necrosis

Injury to dentine, including cavity preparation, usually results in nerve fibres and odontoblast cell bodies being pulled by hydrodynamic forces into the dentinal tubules and separated from the underlying pulpal tissue. This is discussed in relation to pain in dentine on page 234. Nerve fibres may be damaged and odontoblast cells actually killed by this. Small areas of damage may be sealed off by new reparative dentine formation. This will block reinnervation, but the innervation of neighbouring areas may be increased. If damage to the odontoblast layer in the crown is slight, there is sprouting of new fibres from the CGRP (calcitonin gene-related peptide) reactive axons and even root dentine may become innervated by these sprouts.

Inflammation of the pulp frequently leads to necrosis. There is some possibility of reparative dentine formation and of reinnervation

As the lesion heals these new fibres disappear. If the cavity reaches the pulp, and the odontoblast layer is destroyed, inflammation occurs locally. With small lesions a dentine bridge may be formed, the inflammation resolve, and the pulp heal. In these circumstances the area of inflammation is often demarcated by a zone of fibrous tissue, and outside this there is sprouting of CGRP nerve fibres. With more severe pulpal exposures necrosis occurs, and again the zone is usually bounded by fibrous tissue and beyond that CGRP nerve sprouting is observed. Extension of the lesion to the root apex is associated with nerve sprouting in the periapical tissues. The role of these CGRP nerve fibres is complex: they seem to be associated with pain sensation from the damaged areas, but, in addition, the neurotransmitters seem to interact with inflammatory products and cells in the total reaction. It is thought that the increase in number of nerve fibres may explain hypersensitivity in early pulpitis, whilst the separation of the fibres from the area of inflammation by fibrous tissue may explain the lack of pain at a later stage. The increase in number of nerve fibres may also contribute to the difficulty of achieving local anaesthesia in and around a tooth with an inflamed pulp.

Further reading

Dynamic Aspects of Dental Pulp. Inoki, R., Kudo, T., Olgart, L.M. Chapman & Hall, London, 1990

The Biology of Dental Tissues. Nanci, A., McKee, M.D., Smith, C.E. (editors). Anatomical Record 245: 127–592; 1996

5 The periodontal ligament

The periodontium

The periodontal ligament is a thin (0.2 mm wide) layer of fibrous connective tissue between the tooth and the bony alveolus

The periodontal ligament is a narrow band of dense connective tissue interposed between the tooth and its bony socket. It is continuous with the gingival tissue which covers the surface of the alveolar bone and is situated between the teeth (Figs 5.1 and 5.2). Its function has been described as to support the tooth in its socket, although this can also be regarded as permitting tooth movement inside the relatively rigid bony socket in response to axial or lateral stresses. Additionally the fibroblasts and collagen fibres of the ligament have been proposed as agents in the continued eruption of the tooth within the oral cavity, and in the transmission of stresses to the bone which initiate resorption and deposition of bone mineral.

The term ligament is used here in a somewhat different way from the more normal usage in relation to bands of tissue connecting one bone with another and limiting joint movement.

The width of the periodontal ligament is of the order of 0.2 mm around the permanent teeth and slightly more than this around the deciduous teeth; it is narrower around non-functional teeth and wider when the teeth are involved in more vigorous masticatory usage. The width of the ligament varies along the root of the tooth, being greatest at the alveolar crest and the root apex, and narrowest at a level about one-third of the length of the root from the apex. This level is identified as the axis of rotation of the tooth in response to lateral displacing forces. This width of periodontal ligament of the same order as the thickness of cementum, so that the volume of the two tissues is very similar – ranging from as little as 150 mm^3 around a small single root up to as much as 450 mm^3 around a molar.

The fibres are mainly type I collagen with about 20% of type III

The periodontal ligament is made up largely of bundles of collagen fibres in a proteoglycan matrix. The organic matrix which surrounds them also contains other fibres, blood vessels, nerve fibres and cells. It is usually described as dense connective tissue because the cells and fibres make up between one-half and three-quarters of its volume. The ligament becomes less dense with age. Some 20% of the collagen fibres are of type III – a fibre type often associated with tissues which are subject to compressive stresses; the remainder are of the collagen type I typical of bone. The fibres are arranged in bundles described according to their orientation or situation. Thus most of the bundles run

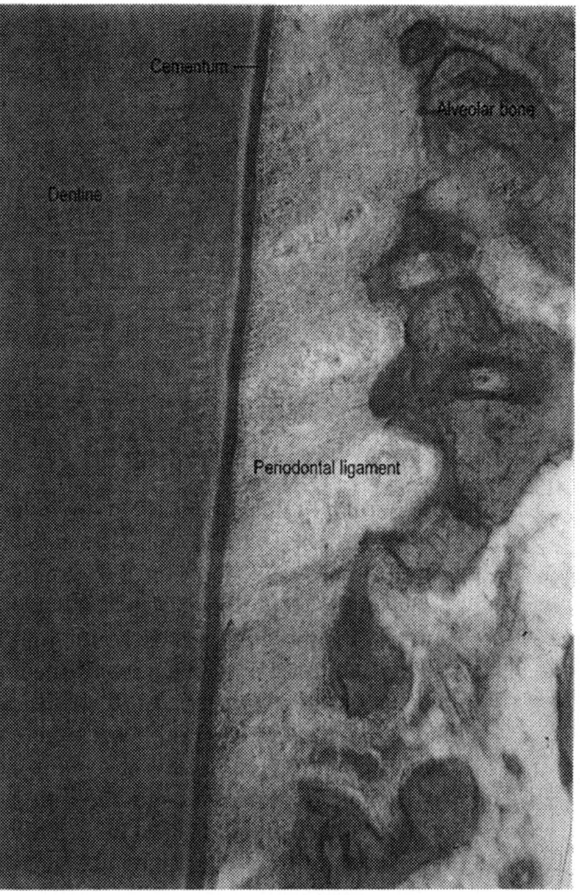

Fig. 5.1
The periodontal ligament. The fibres run obliquely from the alveolar bone to the cementum, suspending the tooth in its socket.

obliquely downward from the bony wall of the socket to the root of the tooth and are termed oblique fibres; others are identified by histologists as free fibres terminating in gingival tissue, horizontal fibres, apical fibres, interradicular fibres and crestal or interdental fibres. Fibres may pass into bone or cementum and be embedded in calcified material: they are then termed Sharpey's fibres. There has been some discussion as to whether fibres can bridge the full distance between bone and cementum or whether they terminate in an intermediate plexus. The intermediate plexus is now thought to be a sectioning artefact and it is thought that the fibres branch, with fibrils joining neighbouring fibres as they cross the ligament. However, the density of collagen fibre bundles appears greater at the periphery and less in the midline of the ligament. Each fibre bundle attached to a functioning tooth is about 4 μm in diameter, and it has been estimated that each square millimetre of cementum has around 50 000 bundles inserted into it. The actual surface of

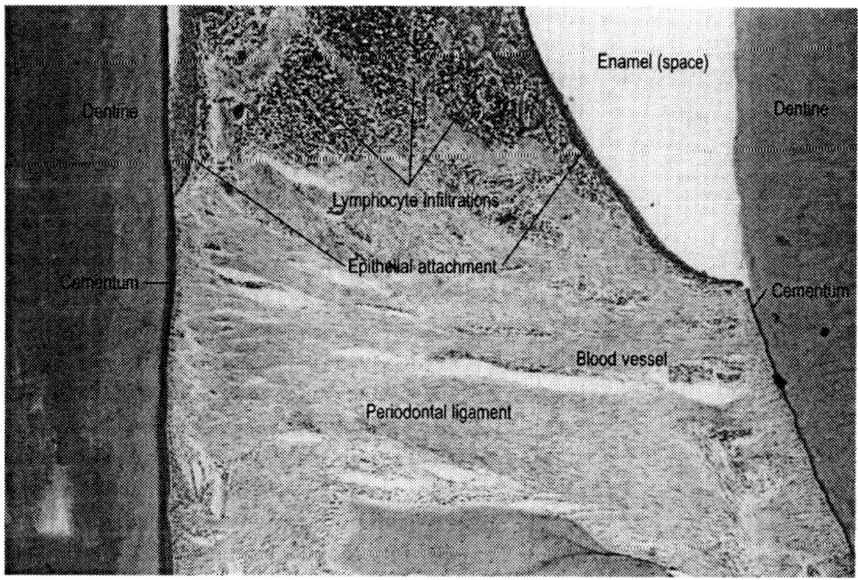

Fig. 5.2
The marginal periodontium. The arrangement of the periodontal fibres above the interdental septum can be seen. The epithelial attachment is on enamel on the right tooth but has extended down on to cementum on the left tooth.

bone available for insertion of collagen bundles is thought to be less than that of cementum because the bone is pierced by many fine foramina through which blood vessels and nerves enter the periodontal ligament. These constitute some 5–10% of the surface of the bone – hence the description of the socket boundary as a cribriform plate. The presence of many small fibres inserting into the cementum and the smaller number of larger bundles inserting into bone may explain why cementoclasts find it more difficult to approach the cementum surface than do osteoclasts to approach bone. Thus when tooth movements occur it is bone rather than cementum that is remodelled. Regularly applied pressure to the tooth causes the bundles of fibres to increase in size and number. Further increases in pressure result in the remodelling of bone and cementum and tooth movement. There is continual turnover of periodontal ligament fibres: the fibroblasts both synthesise and break down collagen fibrils at a rate twice as great as that in gingival tissue and four times as great as that in skin. Thus the half-life of collagen in the periodontal ligament is about one-fifth that in gingiva and about one-fifteenth that in skin. Turnover slows with ageing. In vitamin C deficiency, production of new collagen fibres may cease completely and there is no replacement of the fibres which are removed by the fibroblasts.

There is relatively rapid turnover of periodontal ligament fibres

The only elastic fibres in the ligament are those around blood vessels, but there are coarser fibres present which stain like elastin and are known as oxytalan fibres. These are anchored in cementum but they terminate within the ligament, usually close to blood vessels. This suggests that they may play some role in the control of blood flow in the ligament. Although their actual function is still unknown, oxytalan fibres are found more often, and appear thicker, in the periodontal ligaments of teeth subject to heavier masticatory loads or subject to orthodontic forces.

Most ligaments associated with joints have a poor blood supply as it is the mechanical properties of their fibres which are important, but the periodontal ligament is generously supplied with blood vessels. The blood vessels in the alveolar bone send branches to perforate the compact cortical bone lining the socket and these then run in bundles of nerves and vessels in grooves along the walls of the alveolus or between the collagen fibre bundles. The larger vessels are found close to the alveolar wall and run parallel to the long axis of the roots whilst the main capillary plexus forms a basket-like mesh around the teeth. The coiled portions of arterioles seen in some histological sections used to be described as glomerular structures and were thought to be arteriovenous shunts, but they are not evident in corrosion preparations – preparations in which the blood vessels are filled with a plastic which polymerises to a solid and remains to show the structure when the rest of the tissue is dissolved away. The pressure of mastication is sufficient to stop the flow of blood through the vessels and this can cause the appearance of swellings on some vessels. These are described as small aneurysm-like swellings. They increase the elasticity of the ligament. The increased pressure in these vessels causes more transudation of tissue fluid and increases the effective fluid cushion. Tissue pressure in the periodontal ligament has been calculated at 0.3 kPa. Both veins and lymphatic vessels run alongside the arterioles. The nerve fibres which also travel together with the blood vessels are large, rapidly conducting A alpha and A beta fibres which terminate in Ruffini-type endings, and the A delta and C fibres which are the more slowly conducting pain fibres with typical bare endings. The Ruffini-type end-organs respond to pressure in the ligament: their function is rather like that of a conventional muscle tendon organ – to limit the load applied by the muscles and protect the teeth and jaws from excess masticatory pressure. As such they are important moderating influences on the process of mastication (see p. 259). Unmyelinated sympathetic nerves form networks around the blood vessels.

The ligament has a good supply of vessels and nerves. The nerves detect pressure and their their input is important in the control of mastication

The cells of the periodontal ligament vary according to site. At the bony boundary of the tooth socket there are osteoblasts and osteoclasts; in the body of the ligament there are fibroblasts and uncommitted mesodermal cells; and at the cemental edge there are cementocytes. Unusually there may be cementoclasts at points along this edge. In addition, there are epithelial cells derived from the root sheath of Hertwig, and leucocytes which have migrated from the blood vessels. The fibroblasts are spindle-shaped or flat discs with ovoid nuclei and long processes which form a dense network around and in the fibre bundles. They contain acid phosphatase and proteolytic enzymes as well as the enzymes necessary for collagen synthesis. The presence of short lengths of collagen fibrils within them indicates that they phagocytose and destroy collagen as well as synthesising it. Some of the apparently inactive fibroblasts at the periphery are actually the progenitor cells for the forming and resorbing cells of bone and cementum. The differentiated cementoblasts are cuboidal or ovoid in shape and are seen when cementum is being laid down; the osteoblasts form a continuous layer over the osteoid when bone is being formed. Multinucleated osteoclasts lie in the lacunae which result as they resorb bone during remodelling. The epithelial cells of the periodontal ligament are remnants of the epithelial root sheath which form a net-like layer close to and around the root. This slowly disappears with age so that the continuous mesh which can be seen around newly erupted teeth is reduced to isolated cell clusters or strands in older individuals. The cells are small and show no distinctive features. In a healthy periodontal ligament there will always be some lymphocytes and macrophages dispersed among the fibre bundles.

The marginal periodontium

The marginal periodontium is the tissue around the neck of the tooth above the crest of the alveolar bone

The term marginal periodontium is applied to the tissues surrounding the neck of the tooth above the crest of the alveolar bone. It includes the marginal or free gingiva with its collagen fibres and epithelial covering, and the epithelial attachment to the tooth surface (Figs 5.2 and 5.3). The space bounded by the tooth surface, the epithelial attachment and the free gingiva is termed the gingival crevice or sulcus and is normally less than 0.5 mm deep when the gingiva is healthy. Inflammation causes swelling of the gingival crest and then increased rate of loss of the most superficial cells of the epithelial attachment with a consequent deepening of the sulcus.

It includes the free gingiva with its parakeratinised oral epithelial covering, and the marginal periodontium

The free gingiva is so termed because it can be readily separated from the tooth, as the epithelial attachment itself can be split by very small lateral forces. It is between 1 and 2 mm in extent, increasing with age. It contains collagen fibre bundles inserted into the cementum (coronal and horizontal dentogingival fibres) and the crest of the alveolar bone (alveologingival fibres), as well as the circular and intercircular fibres that surround the neck of the tooth and link to their counterparts around adjacent teeth. Between the level of the apical end of the epithelial attachment and the crest of the alveolar bone is another 0.5 mm of gingiva (the part of the so-called attached gingiva nearest the crown of the tooth), which is also made up of collagen fibres inserted into cementum (the apical dentogingival fibres) and the alveolar crest (alveologingival fibres) together with the dentoperiostal fibres from cementum to the alveolar crest and the periosteogingival fibres which bind down the gingiva to the outer surface of the alveolar bone. The circular and intergingival fibres encircle the tooth and pass along the vestibular and lingual aspects.

The gingival tissue of the marginal periodontium is covered by the typical oral epithelium of the gingiva. It has a basal lamina separating it from the underlying connective tissue, and an actively dividing basal layer of cells. The basal lamina is a structure produced by epithelial cells where they come into contact with non-epithelial surfaces – i.e. connective tissue, enamel, cementum, or inert implant materials. It is made up of laminin, heparan sulphate and type IV collagen. The epithelial cells are attached to it by hemidesmosomes, whilst connective tissue attaches to it by secreting fibrils which form loops anchored at each end in the basal lamina and projecting about 100 μm into the connective tissue. Through these loops pass collagen and reticulin fibres from the connective tissue.

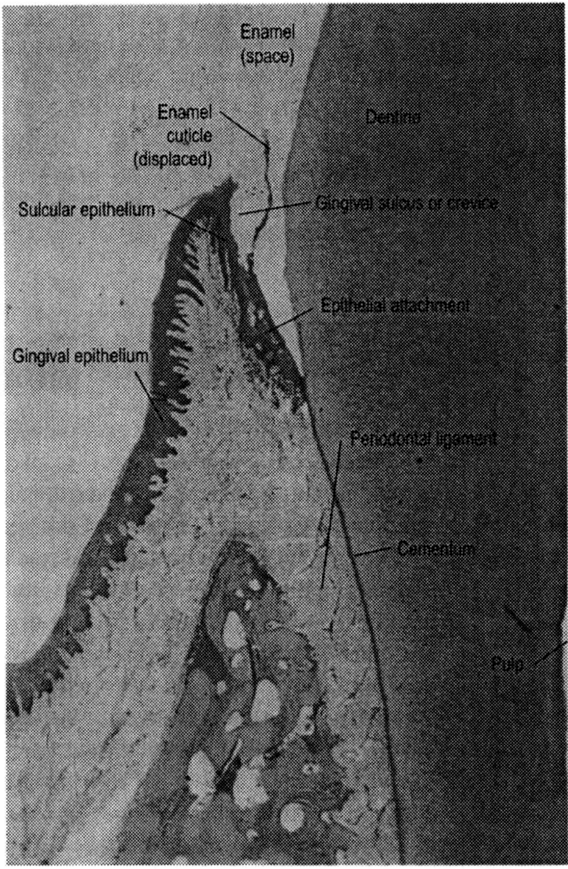

Fig. 5.3
The marginal periodontium. The gingival margin and the epithelial attachment can be seen.

The basal cell layer is folded so that it projects down into the connective tissue, increasing its effective length and strengthening the bond between it and the connective tissue. As the cells divide, the daughter cells pass towards the gingival surface, becoming less cuboidal as the flattened cells of the spinous layer, and synthesising tonofilaments and keratohyalin granules. By the time the cells reach the granular layer the keratohyalin granules have become the dominant cytological feature. Keratin fibres are the typical product of epithelial cells. A number of different keratins have now been identified, and immunological staining of the gingival epithelium shows that most of the normally occurring keratins are present. The gingival epithelium is described as parakeratinised; the outermost cornified layer consists of cells which have keratinised but still retain some remnants of their nuclei and cytoplasmic organelles. The process of keratinisation appears to occur relatively rapidly; in response to some chemical signal, the cells from the granular layer lose their granules to form an impermeable barrier in the cell spaces, and they themselves become filled with keratin filaments as their nuclei and organelles disintegrate. The gingival epithelium in a theoretically perfect and healthy state abuts the tooth surface, where it is continuous with a modified epithelium, the junctional epithelium, which extends some 2 mm down the tooth surface (Figs 5.3 and 5.4). Trauma or inflammation causes accelerated loss of the desquamating cells of the junctional epithelium and a narrow space develops between tooth and gingiva. This is termed the gingival crevice or sulcus. A gingival sulcus depth of up to 0.5 mm, as measured with gentle insertion of a blunt probe into the crevice, is considered as being within the range accepted as clinically healthy.

The junctional epithelium adjoins the tooth surface and is linked to it by hemidesmosomes and a basal lamina

The junctional epithelium secretes a basal lamina on its basal, or gingival, side and also on the side next to the tooth surface. The two are continuous at the apical tip of the junctional epithelium (Fig. 5.4), although that next to the tooth surface is given the title 'epithelial attachment' to describe its situation between tooth and epithelium. It represents the final seal separating the oral fluids from the periodontal tissues and closing the potential gap in the epithelial layer separating body tissues from the external environment. The seal, however, is mechanically weak: even slight pressure from a sharp probe causes cleavage between epithelial attachment and the tooth surface. The cells of the junctional epithelium are separated less readily by such mechanical means.

The junctional epithelium is made up of only two cell zones: a basal zone and a suprabasal zone. The basal cells are actively dividing cuboidal cells; the suprabasal cells are the daughter cells which are more flattened and elongated. They remain this shape as they are displaced towards the tooth surface and the base of the gingival sulcus, and do not undergo the changes seen in cells in the outer zones of the gingival and sulcular epithelium. At the base of the gingival sulcus they are desquamated. There are relatively few desmosomes or other intercellular junctions and the lack of keratohyaline granule products render this epithelium very permeable. It is through this epithelial layer that blood proteins present in the extracellular fluid and water can diffuse to form the gingival crevicular fluid (Ch. 7). Although no data are available for rates of cell turnover in the epithelia of the human marginal periodontium, data from monkeys suggests a turnover rate of 8–10 days for the gingival epithelium and 4–6 days for the junctional epithelium. The junctional epithelium of a newly erupted tooth is derived from the reduced enamel epithelium – the collapsed remains of the enamel organ – but if the marginal periodontium is removed by gingivectomy the junctional epithelium regenerates from the basal layer of the gingival epithelium.

Gingival crevicular fluid is formed across the marginal and junctional epithelium

The gingival epithelium contains other non-epithelial cell types. In the basal layer are found melanocytes and also Merkel cells, which have short processes, link to the epithelial cells by desmosomes and to nerve axons by synapse-like junctions. Neuropeptides have been detected in these cells. They are thought to be involved in touch and pressure sensation. In the spinous layer are found Langerhans cells, antigen-presenting cells with OK1a and OKT6 antigens and Fc-IgG and complement receptors on their surfaces. They are derived from monocytes. Small lymphocytes, predominantly T helper cells, are also found in the gingival epithelium. The only non-epithelial cells found in the junctional epithelium are leucocytes – mainly neutrophil

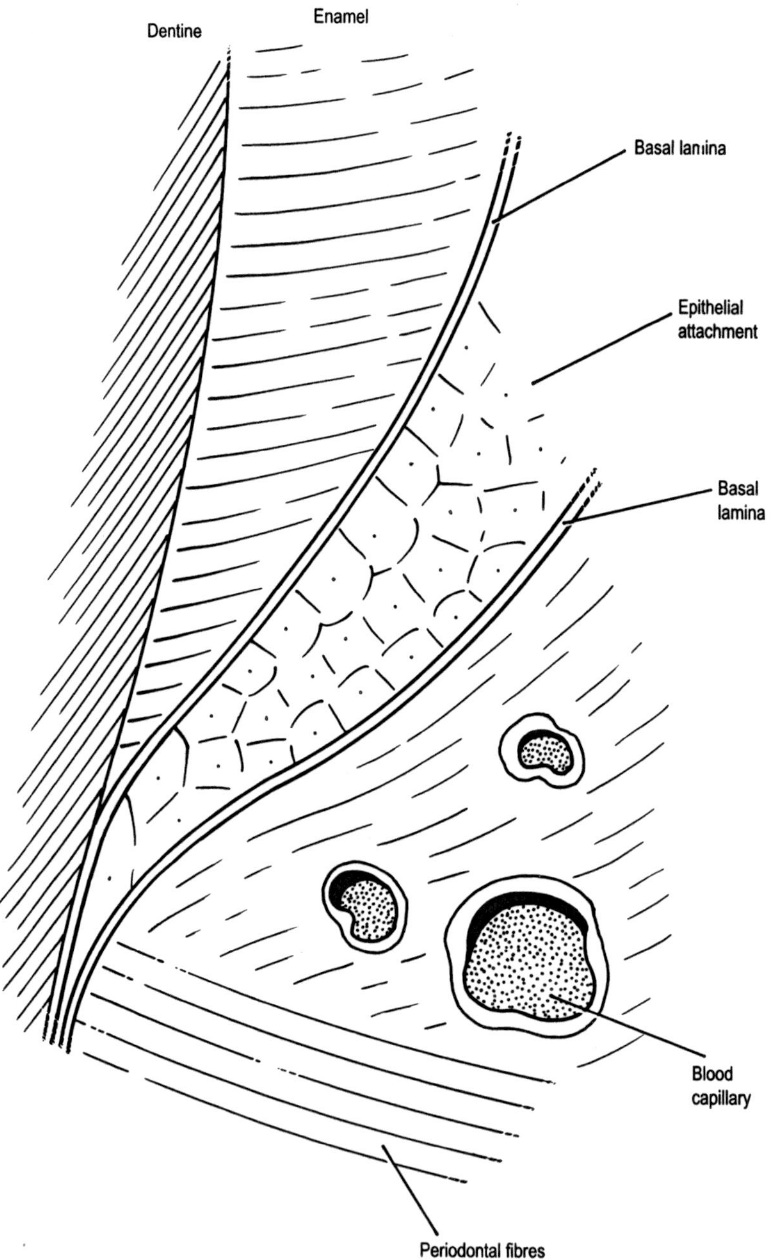

Fig. 5.4
The epithelial attachment. The diagram illustrates the thinning down to a unicellular layer towards the root of the tooth, and the situation of the basal lamina between epithelial attachment and the tooth as well as between the attachment and the underlying connective tissue.

granulocytes. These migrate through the junctional epithelium, perhaps chemotactically attracted by products of dental plaque, and reach the oral fluids by this route. Their numbers increase in proportion to the degree of inflammation and when sufficient are present in the epithelium they cause separation of the epithelial cells and more rapid exfoliation with consequent deepening of the sulcus. As permeability of the junctional epithelium increases, the rate of transudation of gingival crevical fluid increases and so measurement of crevicular fluid production can be used to assess semiquantitatively the degree of gingival inflammation present. Even normal junctional epithelium is highly permeable in both directions. Serum albumin has been shown to pass through readily. Products of bacterial dental plaque such as bacterial antigens and endotoxins, and even the plaque dextrans, can diffuse across this epithelial layer. This apparently weak link in the epithelial defensive barrier is defended by leucocytes. There is a continuous flow of neutrophil polymorphonuclear leucocytes from the capillary plexus close to the junctional epithelium, across the intercellular spaces and out into the sulcus between the epithelial cells (Fig. 5.5). It is these leucocytes which are found in the oral fluid in a dead or dying state, although in the sulcus they are phagocytically active. In the basal layer of the epithelium and the subjacent connective tissue there are lymphocytes and macrophages: the lymphocytes give a second line of defence by triggering immune responses to foreign antigens. Accumulation of dental plaque and increasing exposure to bacterial toxins increases neutrophil migration and initiates the outward flow of gingival crevicular fluid.

More severe inflammation of the gingiva increases cell loss further and the sulcus deepens. It is then termed a pocket. Accumulation of bacteria in the pocket can then lead to a chronic inflammation (Fig. 5.6) with possible destruction of the epithelium and the underlying collagen fibres. Once the collagen fibres inserted into cementum have been destroyed the connective tissue attachment to that part of the tooth cannot be renewed unless the periodontal ligament is protected from epithelial invasion and bacterial plaque. This can be achieved by the so-called guided tissue regeneration – the insertion of a plastic filter barrier over the surgical wound. Collagen barriers have also been used, and the incorporation of fibronectin and heparan sulphate into the membranes is said to enhance periodontal repair. New bone formation on the alveolar crest is claimed to result from guided tissue regeneration: certainly several bone morphogenetic proteins and other growth factors are present in the healing tissue. The epithelial attachment readily reforms from the basal cells of the marginal gingiva and, in the absence of a guided tissue regeneration membrane, a new attachment is generated more apically on the tooth root if the pocket is cleaned and its depth reduced surgically.

Eruption

The process of tooth eruption has been the subject of intensive study over many years. The use of rodent incisors as a model system has been customary but is open to several objections in relation to the eruption of teeth of limited

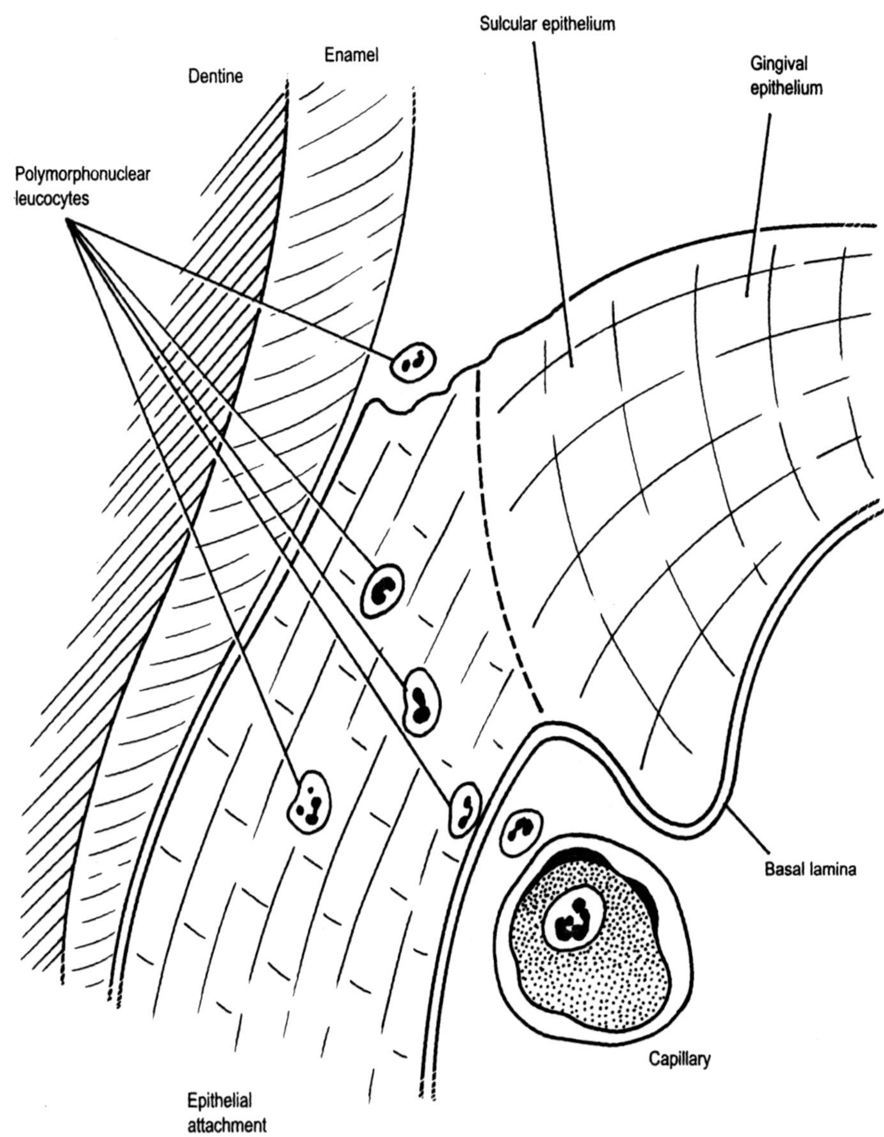

Fig. 5.5
Polymorphonuclear leucocytes pass through the epithelial attachment.

The process of tooth eruption is a result of many possible interacting mechanisms: growth factors play an important part in preparing the eruption pathway

growth such as those of the human. Rodent incisors erupt continuously in order to compensate for the wear of their tips. Although this is the normal situation, the rodent incisor continues to erupt when unimpeded – i.e. when the opposing incisor is shortened or extracted. The anatomical structure of the rodent incisor differs from that of the human tooth as the pulp chamber remains widely open and the direction of eruption at the apex of the root is parallel to the long axis of the jaw rather than at right-angles to it. The tissues

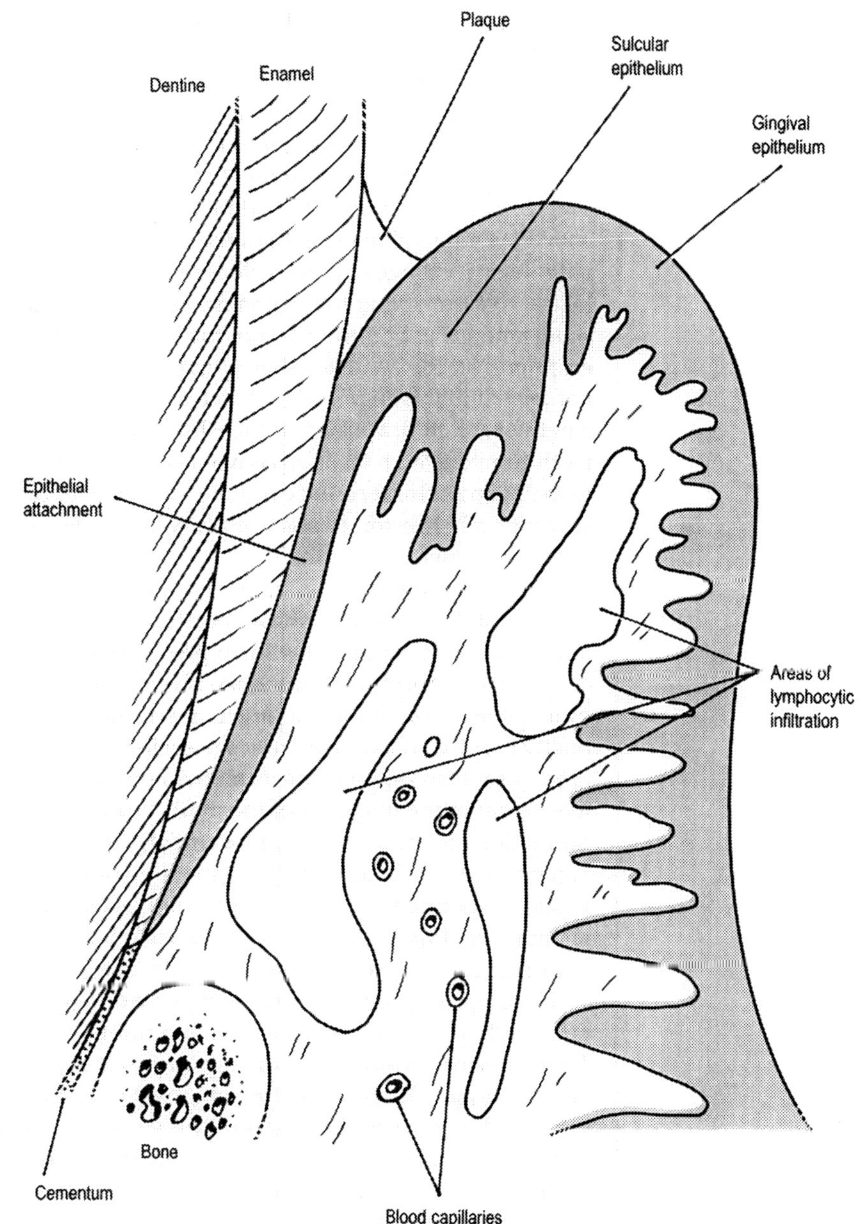

Fig. 5.6
The gingival sulcus develops, plaque extends downwards and a chronic inflammatory reaction is seen in the marginal gingiva.

of the tooth are differently arranged and hence the relationship of the tissues to the direction of eruption is different.

In the human tooth there is a period of eruption during the development of the tooth during which the pulp chamber is also open at the apex of the root

(Fig. 2.1). However, eruption continues after the tooth root is more completely defined and the apical foramen is reduced to a narrow canal. Little evidence is available as to the continuance of eruption after the teeth have come into occlusion with those in the other jaw: statements that eruption continues in the vertical plane (i.e. at right-angles to the long axis of the jaw) throughout life are based upon the observation of the movement of the tooth attachment progressively more apically and the elongation of the visible tooth crown above the gingival margin. Both these effects could be explained by minor pathological changes in the periodontal, alveolar and gingival tissues. It is logical to assume that the maintenance of tooth contact after the relatively small amount of occlusal wear of the human tooth is due to continued eruption, but the evidence shows that the movement of the tooth attachment is not related to the degree of occlusal wear. Such wear should maintain the length of the clinical crown rather than increasing it. However, extraction of a tooth from one arch leads to compensatory eruption of teeth in the other arch to maintain occlusal contact and the replacement of the occlusal surface by a crown or other restoration is rapidly followed by restoration of functional occlusal contact.

Tooth eruption has been defined as the movement of a tooth from its position of development within the alveolar process to its functional position in the oral cavity. It includes small pre-eruptive movements of the forming crown, active eruption through the alveolar bone when the root begins to form, penetration of the oral mucosa, eruption up to the occlusal position, and finally eruptive movement after the establishment of occlusal position, a process said to continue slowly throughout life. Although primarily a movement in the long axis of the tooth, eruption may also include lateral translation and even rotating movements. Thus, while a deciduous incisor appears to erupt axially, the permanent incisors also move in a facial direction, whilst the permanent molars move from a stepped arrangement to a linear relationship. Rates of eruption are variable but specific to the stage of eruption. The final tooth position is subject to genetic control.

The eruptive process has to be explained in terms of the forces available, or potentially available, to move the tooth through the tissues into the oral cavity. These may be considered as arising from soft tissue forces or from the growth of hard tissues. Thus tissue pressure exerted by the interstitial fluid and perhaps due to changes in blood supply is one possibility. Multiplication of soft tissue cells could force a tooth in the direction of least resistance. The arrangement of collagen fibres which sling the tooth in its socket is designed to resist the axial forces of occlusion which tend to drive the tooth into its socket. If such forces were absent it is conceivable that the elasticity of these fibres could move the tooth towards the oral cavity. Finally, there are forces generated by the apposition of hard tissues – perhaps dentine during the early phases of eruption, cementum later, or alveolar bone throughout life. There is experimental evidence which eliminates any one of these as the sole force contributing to eruption. The current view is that eruption depends upon a combination of factors: root elongation, alveolar bone remodelling and periodontal ligament formation. All these processes are products of the activity of the dental follicle and most recent work assigns a crucial role to this tissue. Even when the tooth has penetrated the oral epithelium and the dental follicle itself has disappeared, tissues and activities derived from it can continue to govern the later stages of eruption. Root formation by itself is not essential for eruption: teeth without roots and those in dentine dysplasia type I can still erupt. Equally, bone formation is not sufficient to maintain eruption. In osteopetrosis, eruption fails because bone resorption does not occur. It is therefore bone remodelling – both appropriate formation and resorption – which is necessary. The periodontal ligament appears to be essential for the continuous eruption of rodent incisors, but its role is more questionable in teeth of limited growth. Its presence in relation to teeth which fail to erupt in cases of osteopetrosis, and its absence from rootless teeth which do erupt suggest that it is not a major factor in human tooth eruption. In the pre-eruptive stage of tooth development there are small apparently random changes in position of the tooth crown for most teeth. The premolar teeth, however, are initiated lingual to the deciduous molars, and when these erupt the premolar crowns move facially to develop in the tissues between the roots of the deciduous molars.

Eruption proper begins with an infiltration of mononuclear cells into the dental follicle coronal to the developing tooth and a proliferation of follicle cells apically. The mononuclear cells appear to be precursors of osteoclasts which now proceed to open up a pathway for eruption through the bony covering of the tooth crypt. Collagen synthesis ceases in this area. The infiltration of mononuclear cells is triggered by release of transforming growth factor beta. Epidermal growth factor is known to stimulate early eruption of rat incisors: it is found in the follicle when eruption begins and the follicle cells have specific receptors for this factor at an earlier stage. Cells from the enamel organ produce transforming growth factor beta in response to epidermal growth factor and this may be the source of the transforming growth factor. Further, the cells of the enamel organ can synthesise interleukin 1-alpha in response to epidermal growth factor. Interleukin 1-alpha is a powerful promoter of bone resorption by itself, but it also stimulates the follicle cells to produce colony-stimulating factor-1 which attracts monocytes into the follicle and osteoclasts to the bony surfaces of the crypt. Animal experiments have shown that colony-stimulating factor-1 stimulates eruption only if present during a short time period specific to a particular tooth. The apical follicle cells also bind epidermal growth factor; after a short period in which root formation begins and bone resorption occurs so that the tooth crown does not move axially, bone formation occurs at the forming root apex. These simultaneous forces move the tooth towards and into the bony channel already forming. There is also evidence that the follicle and the enamel epithelium have some cells containing granules of two large proteins (167 and 200 kDa, respectively) which can inhibit eruption. This suggests that the process is very precisely controlled by the interaction of a number of factors. The highly hydrated connective tissue of the follicle increases in weight and volume by synthesis of collagen and proteoglycans as eruption commences, although in the part of the follicle immediately below the future eruption pathway the cessation of collagen formation moves the balance of collagen turnover towards fibre breakdown, easing the eruption route. At the onset of eruption, follicular tissue (which cannot be separated from the reduced enamel epithelium for analysis) undergoes a change in protein composition: a sialoprotein of 95 kDa, termed DF-95, is broken down to yield three small proteins each of around 20–25 kDa. The sialoprotein is probably an enamel organ protein. The follicular content of the metalloproteinases collagenase and stromelysin is reduced during eruption.

The processes outlined above proceed at different rates, and the passage of the erupting tooth varies from time to time: at first, the root grows into an area where bone has been resorbed, but when the eruption pathway is created the varying speeds of pathway creation and root growth will be accompanied by apical bone growth, stasis or even resorption. It is possible that in human teeth the increased rate of production and turnover of periodontal ligament fibres is related more to stabilising the position of the erupting tooth than to any role in the eruptive movement itself. The rate of eruption through the alveolus varies between 1 and 10 μm/day.

As soon as the tooth cusps reach the surface epithelium the enamel epithelium fuses with it. This process is accompanied by proliferation of the outer enamel epithelium and local proteolytic activity. It forms the junctional epithelium which can then proliferate basally and be shed superficially in a controlled manner so that it moves down the crown of the tooth as it erupts. The rate of eruption increases at this stage and reaches a maximum of around 75 μm/day as the tooth moves into occlusion. The eruptive movement is achieved by root growth and bony apposition in the basal or apical end of the tooth socket. Simultaneously the walls of the alveolus are increasing in height.

The systemic health upsets experienced by most children at the time of tooth eruption are difficult to explain. The area of mucosa immediately overlying the unworn and therefore sharp cusps of the erupting tooth will be particularly sensitive to the pressures of mastication, and minute lesions of the surface epithelium will be readily infected by the oral bacteria. The protective mechanism of the junctional epithelium and gingival fluid generation is not yet developed and inflammation can easily occur. Some workers have postulated that the proteins of the enamel epithelium may themselves generate a local hypersensitivity reaction; this would explain the local erythema, the rhinitis and fever described as teething pains.

Once in occlusion the tooth continues to erupt at a very slow rate for the next 40 years or so. The final stage of root growth may require some resorption of bone at the tooth apex but after this point further eruption depends upon cementum apposition on the root and bone growth in the socket. As the tooth becomes subject to occlusal forces the periodontal ligament adopts a mature distribution of fibres and the alveolar bone remodels to give support to the teeth.

Tooth movement

Teeth move in response to external forces, and the alveolar bone around them is resorbed and deposited to maintain the width of the periodontal ligament

The process of tooth eruption is clearly one of tooth movement, but the term is more usually applied to lateral movement of the tooth within the alveolar bone. It therefore includes physiological mesial drift, the movement of teeth which occurs after extraction of neighbouring teeth, lateral movement in response to occlusal forces, and the movement of teeth produced by orthodontically applied forces.

In general, the position of a tooth within the dental arch is that at which opposing forces cancel out each other. With the teeth of the two jaws slightly separated in the normal rest position of the mandible, the pressures will be those exerted by the lips and cheeks on the outer face of the arch and by the tongue on the inner face. When the teeth in the two arches are brought together, the forces exerted by the masticatory muscles can be translated into vertical and horizontal vectors at each point of contact. The teeth will be moved into positions which minimise the horizontal force vectors. This is possible because of the small degree of elasticity afforded by the periodontal ligament, but more importantly by the possibility of altering the position of the tooth in the alveolar bone by the synchronised removal of bone on the side of the socket where the periodontal ligament is compressed, deposition of bone on the side of periodontal ligament stretching, remodelling of periodontal ligament fibres, and deposition of new cementum on the root surface.

Although wear of dental enamel might be expected to occur only on the occlusal surfaces of teeth which are subjected to the abrasive action of food particles between the occluding surfaces, the small degree of movement of the teeth in their sockets causes the approximal surfaces of the teeth to rub and wear against each other. This can be observed in the difference between the small area of a contact point in newly erupted teeth and the broad contact area observed in teeth from older subjects. The loss of mesiodistal length in the teeth of primitive people eating a tougher, more fibrous and abrasive diet can reduce the length of the dental arch by as much as 8 mm. Even in modern European subjects, the distance between the mesial surface of the first premolar and the distal surface of the third molar decreases by some 0.3 mm over a period of 9 years. Thus between 1 and 10 µm of enamel thickness is lost from each contact area over a year. Experimental evidence demonstrates that the mesial movement of the teeth which maintains the teeth in contact with their neighbours despite the loss of enamel at the contact area is a result of the tension in the collagen fibre bundles which pass over the interdental bony septum from the cementum of one tooth to that of the next – the transseptal fibres. The very small forces involved in this physiological mesial drift maintain a slow turnover of the precursor cell compartment of the periodontal ligament with the maturation of osteoblasts and cementoblasts on the distal tension side of the ligament, osteoclasts on the mesial compression side, and fibroblasts to break down and renew the collagen fibre apparatus (Fig. 5.7).

Orthodontic movement with small forces is similar to the physiological movement

The ability of the periodontal tissues to accommodate tooth movement makes possible, and is exploited in, the process of orthodontic adjustment of tooth position. The forces produced by orthodontic appliances are of much greater magnitude and exerted over shorter time periods. The critical factor in the progress of orthodontic tooth movement is thought to be the blood supply to the ligament: if the force exerted is sufficient to occlude the capillary network on the compression side local necrosis will take place. The pressure in the capillaries of the periodontal ligament should be expected to be around 3.3 kPa (or kN/m^2) and experimental observations suggest that forces around 25 g are sufficient to occlude the capillaries. Application of unilateral forces perpendicular to the long axis of the tooth results in cellular proliferation, with fibroblast and osteoblast production appearing after about 12 h and reaching a peak at about 24 h. At this point osteoclasts begin to appear on the surface of the alveolar bone on the compression side; some 12 h later new

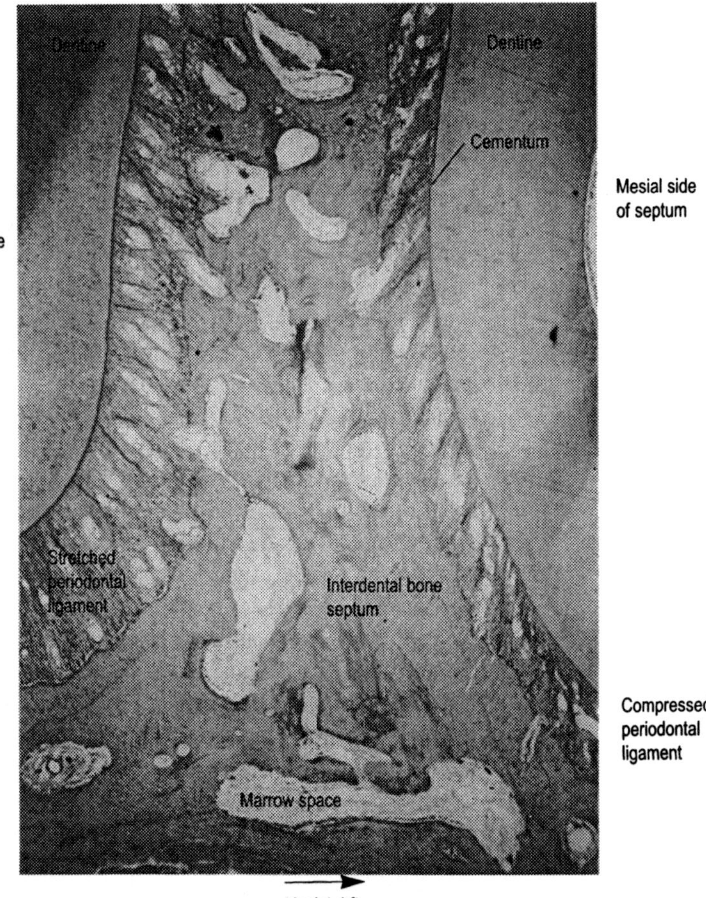

Fig. 5.7
Two adjacent teeth and the tissues between them. The mesial drift of the teeth results in compression of the periodontal ligament on the mesial side with resorption of the bone lining the socket, and stretching of the ligament on the distal side with the deposition of new bone.

Prostaglandin E_2 is secreted by stretched fibroblasts

osteoblasts line the surface of the alveolar bone on the tension side (Fig. 5.7). Over the next 48 h these cells lay down a layer of osteoid and the stretched fibres of the periodontal ligament are embedded in forming bundle bone. The cellular mechanisms involved in these processes are not fully understood. It is possible that the tension exerted by the stretched fibres on the alveolar bone may cause deformation and the movement of bone crystals then generate minute electrical currents (a piezo-electric effect) which in turn stimulate osteoblastic activity. However, disruption of collagen fibres by certain types of drug does not seem to affect the osteoblast activation. Such observations would also rule out any direct effect of the stretched fibres on bone cells. Experiments in which layers of fibroblasts have been stretched show that the fibroblasts respond by secreting prostaglandin E_2. The cells show increased levels of intracellular messengers, both cAMP and inositol trisphosphate being raised. Intracellular ionic calcium concentrations increase, either because of the opening of stretch-activated calcium channels or as a result of the increase in cAMP and inositol trisphosphate. On the compression side it seems more likely that the newly developed osteoblasts in some way transduce the pressure signal by secreting prostanoids and cytokines which attract, localise and then activate the osteoclasts. Prostaglandin E_1 has been implicated in this process but other larger molecules have also been detected. If the osteoblasts themselves are not the transducing cells, then some other cellular component such as the fibroblasts or even blood cells must be able to stimulate the osteoblasts, probably by one of the recognised pathways of production of interleukin 1-alpha and -beta, tumour necrosis factors alpha and beta, and/or transforming growth factors.

When the movement is completed, there has usually been a greater resorption of bone in the resorption lacunae than is necessary, and bone deposition occurs, smoothing out the irregularities in the resorbed surface. The first matrix laid down in this process contains chondroitin sulphate, followed by osteopontin which is thought to mediate osteoblast adhesion to the surface, and then bone sialoprotein which precedes nucleation. Fibronectin is involved only in cell–cell adhesion of the osteoblasts. It is probable that decorin and biglycan are present. Calcification of this initial layer forms a resting line (sometimes confusingly known as a cement line) which stains with basophilic dyes. New bundle bone formation continues on the resting line and later this may be converted into new lamellated bone.

It has been shown that orthodontic movement can be enhanced by injections of prostaglandin E_1 and slowed by administration of indomethacin, which blocks prostaglandin synthesis. There is some evidence to show that intermittent application of force is more effective than continuous loading, although it is difficult to see how the rates of force application tried experimentally could be used in orthodontic practice.

On the tooth itself the cementoblasts lay down cementum on the compression side and there is a continuous process of remodelling of the periodontal fibre to cementum linkages.

Larger orthodontic forces cause necrosis in the periodontal ligament and adjacent bone. Movement of the tooth occurs when the necrotic tissue resorbs

Orthodontic forces sufficiently large to occlude the smaller blood vessels cause local necrosis of the periodontal ligament and the alveolar bone on the compression side. Within 48 h the fibroblasts of the ligament and the endothelial cells of the capillaries show changes in the cell organelles: swelling of the mitochondria and the rough endoplasmic reticulum The nuclei then become pyknotic and break up. Vacuoles appear in the cytoplasm and the cell membranes rupture. After this the necrosis cannot be reversed and the tissue is effectively dead. The vessel walls break up and the remains of the nuclei can be seen outside the remaining cells. Collagen fibres appear intact but are slowly broken down over the next 10–20 days by lysosomal enzymes released from the dead cells. Osteoclasts cannot develop in this necrotic tissue, and the bone lining the socket, having been deprived of its blood supply, is also dead. The products of tissue destruction, however, can stimulate the osteoblasts in the marrow spaces which still retain their blood supply. The osteoblasts in turn secrete the factors which attract the blood cell precursors of the osteoclasts, stimulate them to develop, and initiate resorption of the dead bone from within the bone itself. Blood-borne macrophages digest the dead tissue and when this is completed new bone and periodontal ligament are laid down. Clinically there is a pattern of little or no tooth movement until the necrotic tissue is removed and then a sudden movement of the tooth occurs, to be followed by a more gradual steady movement. On the tension side of the ligament the blood supply is unaffected and so there is no necrosis: the cell proliferation seen on this side with lower orthodontic forces is greatly increased and the alveolar bone surface is rapidly covered by a layer of osteoblasts.

Where necrosis of the periodontal ligament occurs there may be resorption of the tooth root. Resorption lacunae develop and fuse as a result of the appearance of cells best termed odontoclasts, since they are capable of resorbing dentine as well as cementum. Normally this resorption ceases as orthodontic movement is completed and first acellular intrinsic fibre cementum is laid down in the resorption lacunae and then new periodontal ligament fibres attach to new extrinsic fibre cementum. In some instances resorption occurs at the root apex and permanent shortening of the root results.

Dental implants

Reimplantation of avulsed teeth

Avulsed teeth can be reimplanted if the periodontal ligament remains vital

A tooth which has been extracted or lost by accidental trauma may be replaced in its socket and become functional again if the periodontal ligament remaining attached to the cementum can be kept viable. The evidence is that if the tooth can be kept moist with a suitable fluid the ligament can survive up to about 30 min and the periodontal cells can participate in a reattachment. The pulp usually dies immediately, although in incompletely formed roots it may be replaced by granulation tissue and new odontoblasts may develop. The replanted tooth is usually, therefore, non-vital and hence it may be useful to treat it endodontically before reimplantation. Clearly there would be advantages if teeth could be transplanted – a third molar into a first molar socket, or even a tooth from one individual into another – to restore a dentition. This can be successful if the transplanted tooth still has incomplete root formation and there are no immunological reactions.

If teeth are replanted after the periodontal remnants have been removed from the root surface, a bony union with the alveolar bone follows, the root is resorbed and the crown is exfoliated.

Prosthetic dental implants

Metal implants can be inserted into predrilled holes in bone and attain a functional union

Since there is little possibility of replacement of teeth which have been extracted, their replacement with synthetic structures has been explored and developed. Such structures do not normally aim to replace the teeth themselves but to provide support from the bone of the jaw for prosthetic units. When a biologically inert post of titanium is inserted into a hole drilled into bone so that it fits tightly, the repair process, if successful, will provide a functional union. Two types of union have been described, although neither of these emulates the periodontal ligament attachment of the teeth. Implants are not covered by cementum, so that there is no possibility of attachment of collagen fibres to the implant or an attachment to the bone of the implant socket by these. Implants are described as osseointegrated when the implant surface is covered by a thin layer of calcified material similar to that in resorption or cement lines, or as fibro-osteal integrated when a fibrous capsule surrounds the implant and separates it from direct contact with the alveolar bone. In either case the union lacks the mobility conferred by a periodontal ligament and there is no possibility of implant movement in the bone when the precursor cell population of the periodontal ligament is absent. Implants can therefore be used as stable points for anchorage of orthodontic appliances. Osseointegration can be achieved with implants made of titanium or zirconium, and also from hydroxyapatite ceramic materials or hydroxyapatite-coated materials. The latter have the useful property of encouraging bone growth along their surfaces – a particularly useful property when the implant is situated in cancellous bone.

When the implant is inserted into the accurately matched hole drilled into bone, it displaces the blood in the hole. Single-stage implants are inserted to be level with the mucosal surface but two-stage implants are left below the surface with their internally screwed hole sealed by a plastic screw cover and the mucosa is allowed to heal over them. The two-stage implant is subsequently exposed through the mucosal surface for attachment of the supramucosal part of the implant. The blood clot around the implant and in the marrow spaces is invaded by leucocytes and then by endosteal cells and undifferentiated mesenchymal cells, both of which cell types can become osteogenic. In cortical bone with a less good blood supply, or in the screw threads of a screwed implant, some osteonecrosis may occur and the dead bone should later be replaced by new bone. The osteoblast cells in the clot area lay down a non-collagenous matrix against the implant surface. This first layer of matrix is similar to that of the reversal lines observed when osteoclast activity gives way to bone deposition. Subsequently bone is laid down in a collagenous matrix. Bone production is usually seen next to the existing bone of the alveolus: thus in cancellous bone it does not usually form to seal the marrow spaces unless an osteoconductive material such as hydroxyapatite is on the implant surface. At the mucosal surface the basal layer of the gingival epithelium proliferates down the side of the implant for a short distance and develops a hemidesmosome type of attachment to a basal lamina secreted onto the implant surface. This appears to be identical with the epithelial attachment on the natural tooth surface. In the absence of bacterial attack or inflammation a junctional epithelium will remain limited in extent. A sulcus may develop later, but only if infection penetrates the junctional epithelium will proliferation occur and the equivalent of a periodontal lesion develop. The implant may then be lost.

Fibro-osteal integration occurs if the bone is overheated during preparation of the implant socket and bone necrosis is more extensive. The use of membranes, as in the guided tissue regeneration methods of periodontal treatment, has helped to provide conditions in which osseointegration and a healthy mucosal junction can be obtained.

Further reading

The Biology of Dental Tissues. Nanci, A., McKee, M.D., Smith, C.E. (editors). Anatomical Record 245 (2): 127–592; 1996

The Periodontium. Schroeder, H.E. Handbook of Microscopic Anatomy, Vol. V/5. Springer-Verlag, Berlin, 1986

The Periodontal Ligament in Health and Disease. Berkovitz, B.K., Moxham, B.J., Newman, H.N. Pergamon, London, 1982

SECTION TWO

Oral fluids, deposits and nutrients

6 The salivary glands and their secretions

The salivary glands produce secretions which lubricate the oral soft tissues, protect the teeth by their calcium and phosphate content and by buffering acid, and begin the digestion of starch. Saliva also has antimicrobial components

The mouth is the entrance to the digestive tract and its main function is to take in food, begin its processing – both mechanical and chemical – and to pass it on via the oesophagus to the next processing organ, the stomach. Mechanical processing, the process of mastication, is dealt with in Ch. 12. Sufficient here to say that it involves the teeth, tongue, cheeks and palate, and all these need to be maintained and protected in order to continue to carry out their functions. Soft tissues throughout the digestive tract are protected by a lubricating layer of mucin – a solution of complex long-chain carbohydrate molecules attached to protein cores – secreted by single cells or by aggregations of cells to form glands. The teeth themselves require protection, less against physical damage than against chemical damage, as the hard enamel surface is slightly soluble in water and very soluble in acid. The glands of the mouth are termed salivary glands, and the composite of their secretions, saliva. The functions of saliva are to protect the oral tissues by keeping them moist and by providing a lubricating mucoid secretion, by maintaining a fluid environment with high calcium and phosphate concentrations and the power of buffering acids, and to initiate the digestion of starch, one of the principal dietary components. Saliva also contains antibacterial substances, giving some protection against the bacteria which inevitably gain access to the digestive tube by this external orifice.

The salivary glands

The salivary glands include the paired parotid, submandibular and sublingual glands, together with several hundred minor glands throughout the oral mucosa

The glands which produce saliva include three major paired glands – the parotid glands, the submandibular glands and the sublingual glands (Fig. 6.1) – together with several hundred smaller glands scattered on the inner surface of the lips and cheeks (Fig. 6.2), over the hard and soft palates and on the surface of the tongue. The small glands are often referred to collectively as the accessory, or minor, salivary glands. Their secretion, with the exception of those on the tongue around the circumvallate papillae, is predominately mucous – i.e. rich in mucoproteins – and their main function is lubrication, although they also secrete immunoglobulins and other proteins. Those around the circumvallate papillae are known as glands of von Ebner, and they secrete a watery secretion whose purpose is to solubilise substances to give them the

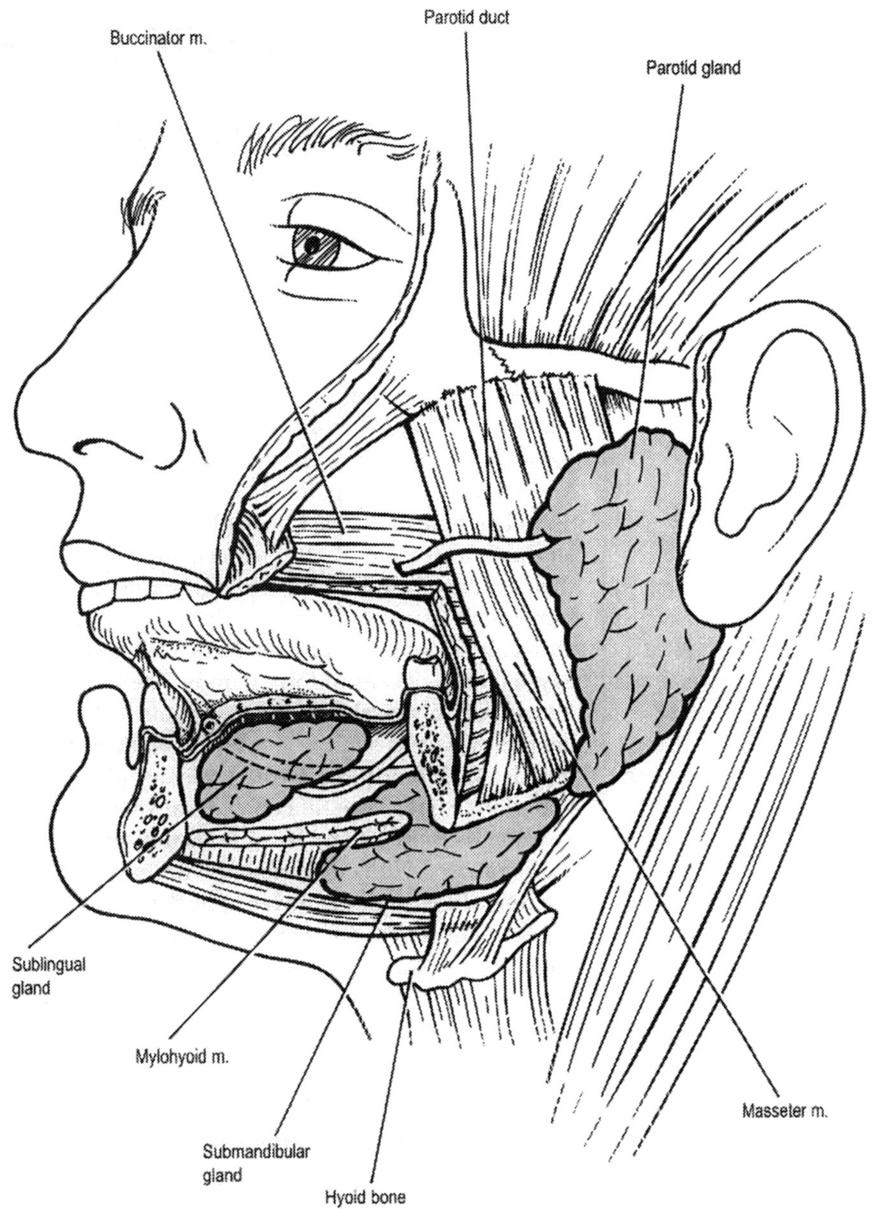

The major salivary glands. The left cheek and the part of the body of the mandible have been removed, and the mylohyoid muscle cut and reflected to show the positions of the major salivary glands on the left side. The duct of the submandibular gland passes between the sublingual gland and the genioglossus muscle to reach its opening at the side of the frenum of the tongue. The ducts of the sublingual gland pierce the floor of the mouth lateral to the side of the tongue.

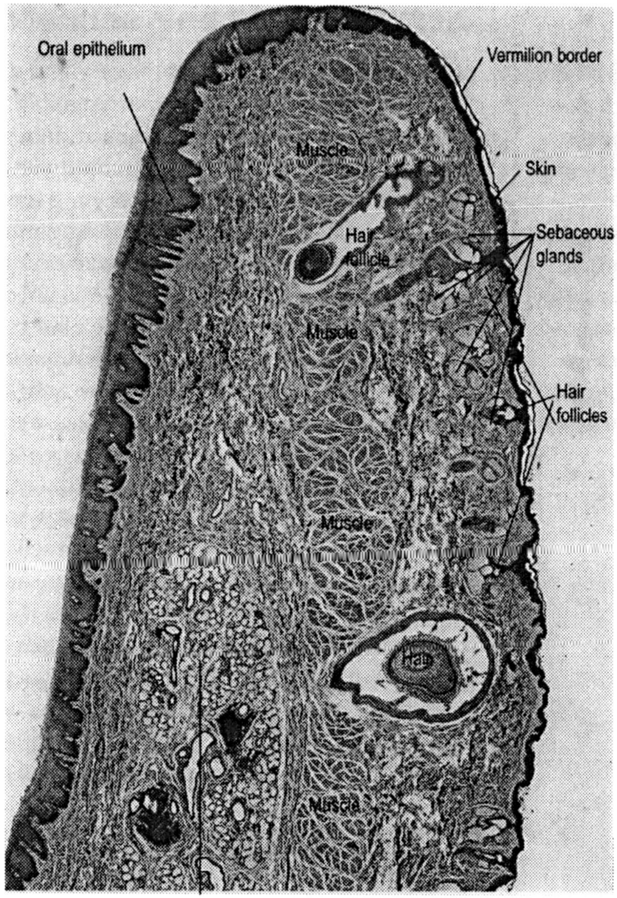

Fig. 6.2
Section through the lip showing labial salivary glands.

possibility of stimulating the taste cells around the papillae. It is likely that the minor glands are continuously active, and there is evidence that the usual stimuli to secretion which affect the major glands have little effect on the minor glands. The submandibular and sublingual glands also secrete continuously at a low level, but can increase this 10–20 times when stimulated appropriately. The parotid glands have no measurable unstimulated secretion in most individuals but become the major source of saliva when stimulated. The composition of the saliva collected by dribbling or spitting – variously termed whole or mixed saliva, or perhaps more precisely, oral fluid – therefore varies according to the particular mixture of secretions from the different glands elicited by the degree of stimulation. Thus, an unstimulated whole saliva is dominated by the submandibular components, whilst an acid-stimulated saliva has a composition much closer to that of parotid saliva.

Structure of the secretory unit

The secretory unit of a salivary gland is the acinus, which passes secretion into a sequence of ducts which progressively join together to become the final excretory duct. Draining directly from the acinus is a short intercalated duct and then, in many glands, a striated duct

A section through a typical salivary gland (Fig. 6.3) shows a bewildering mixture of cells, some clearly arranged in a circle with a central space, others apparently forming small islands and, in some glands, still others capping the islands of cells (Fig. 6.4). If one could view such a section in three dimensions, one would see epithelial cells forming the walls of ducts, arranged as spherical aggregations in the acini, and forming minor components on the surface of these spherical structures. The excretory duct of a salivary glands is in continuity with the oral mucosa: it is lined with a stratified squamous epithelium. As one passes into the gland this duct divides into main branches, the lobular ducts, lined with a columnar epithelium (Fig. 6.5), and these in turn continue to divide into smaller and smaller branches. The epithelium remains columnar as the ducts decrease in size but becomes striated in appearance because of extensive invaginations in the base of the cells. These striated ducts give way to the cuboidal cell walled intercalated ducts and finally reach a blind end in the acinus with its surrounding secretory cells. In glands such as the submandibular which contain both mucous and serous cells, the mucous cells usually form the acinus and the flattened (semilunar) serous cells surround the mucous cells (Fig. 6.4). The striated ducts are present in the parotid and submandibular glands but absent from the sublingual and many of the minor salivary glands. Myoepithelial cells with a central nucleus and long processes extending round the acinus or sometimes the duct are termed basket cells because of this morphological appearance. The acinar cells are of two types when stained for optical microscopy: the basophilic serous

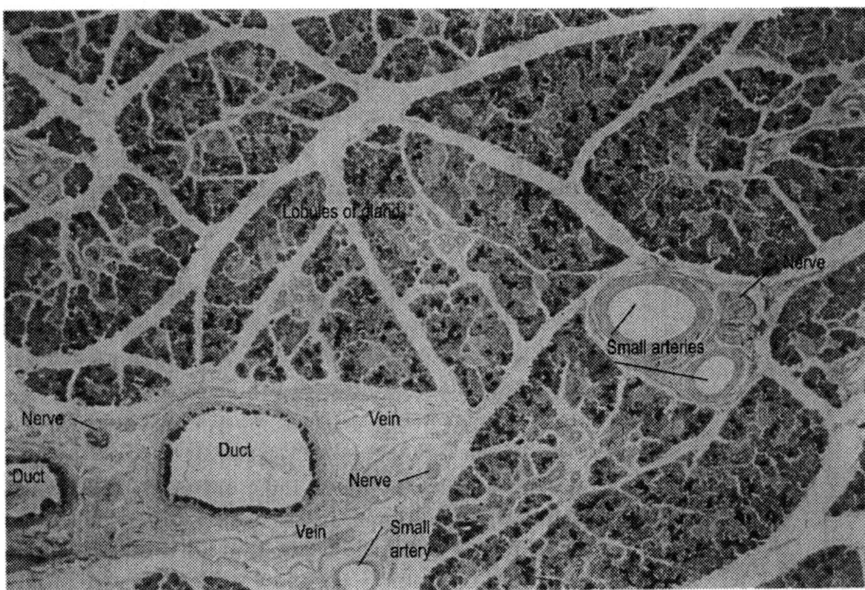

Fig. 6.3
Low power view of a section of a parotid salivary gland showing the lobular structure.

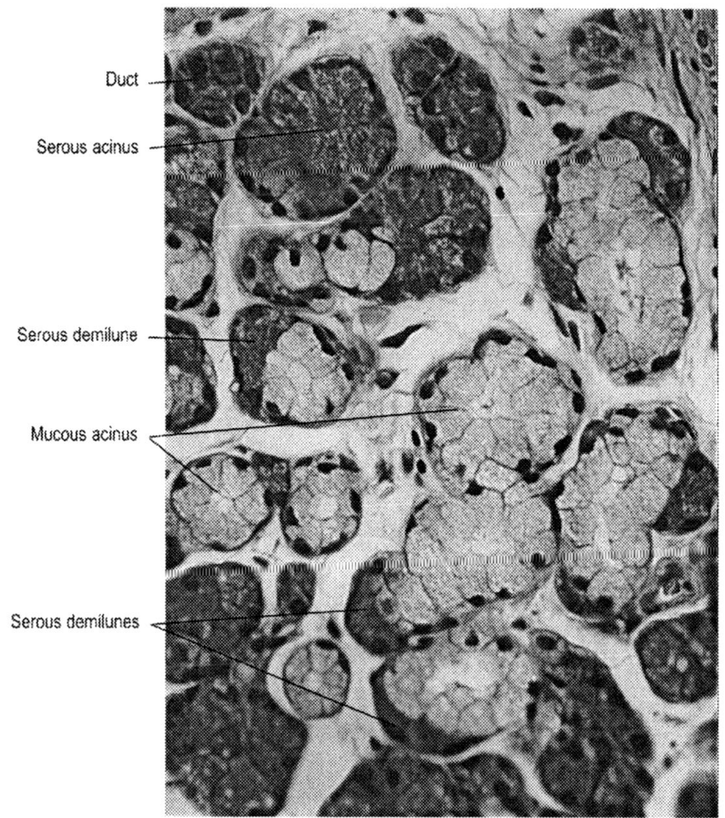

Fig. 6.4
Higher power view of a section of submandibular gland showing serous and mucous acini, serous demilunes and a duct. Note that the ductal cells have centrally situated nuclei, in contrast to the basal situation of the nuclei of the secretory cells.

cells with their secretory granules and the eosinophilic mucous cells with their pale-staining vacuoles containing mucoproteins. Electron microscopy confirms these differences. The serous cell has a basally situated nucleus, an extensive endoplasmic reticulum, well-developed Golgi apparatus and numerous granules passing to the acinar surface for exocytosis. The mucous cell is almost filled with vacuoles of secretory material; the nucleus is crushed towards the base of the cell, the Golgi apparatus lies more apically and the rough endoplasmic reticulum is basal and between the vacuoles. The intercalated duct is short and its cells appear relatively unspecialised. One of the functions of these cells may be to act as progenitors for the acinar cells but they do also seem to have some secretory functions.

Cells of the intercalated ducts may be secretory or may be precursors of the acinar cells. The striated ducts modify the ion content of the acinar secretions

The cells of the striated ducts are concerned with the modification of the saliva initially formed in the acini. They have extensively infolded basal membranes, many mitochondria and intense sodium–potassium-ATPase activity basally. These features are typical of cells engaged in unidirectional transport of ions.

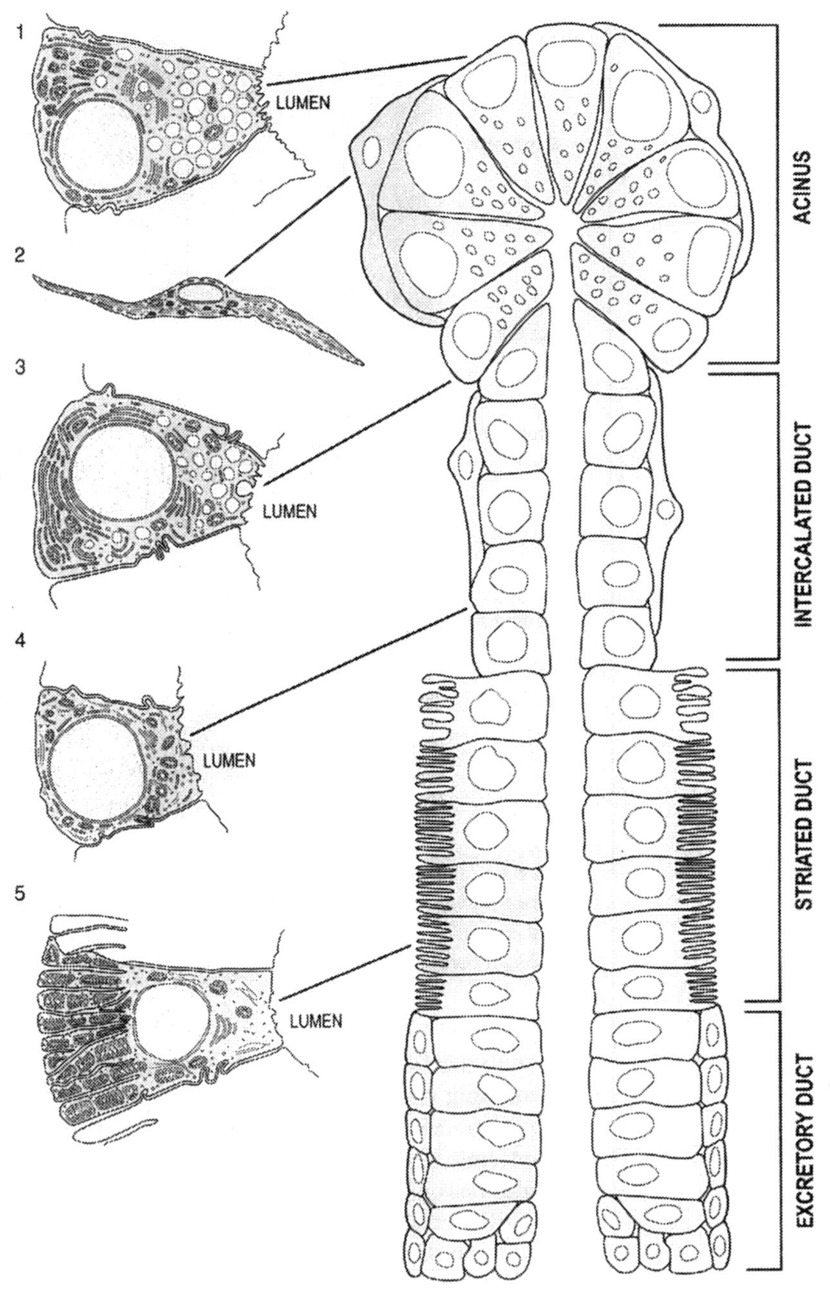

Diagram of the parts of the secretory unit of salivary glands. The component cells are shown to the left: 1, acinar serous cell; 2, myoepithelial cell; 3, acinar mucous cell; 4, intercalated duct cell; 5, striated duct cell. Mucous and serous cells do not normally appear side by side in the same acinus as shown diagrammatically here, but in mixed acini the serous cells are arranged in a demilune on the acinar surface as shown in Fig. 6.4.

The blood supply to the major salivary glands

Local circulation in a salivary gland may be a portal system

The blood circulation to the glands is obviously important in saliva production. There is some interesting research which suggests that the pressure produced by the secretion of saliva – the pressure driving saliva along the ducts and out into the mouth – depends upon the arterial blood pressure within the gland. Earlier suggestions of a filtration process in saliva formation cannot be fitted into current theories of saliva formation and so these observations remain unexplained. Stimulation of the parasympathetic supply to the salivary glands results in an increased blood flow to them. The blood supply, like that of the kidney, is thought to be a portal one – that is to say, one where two capillary systems are in series. The arterioles break up into a capillary bed around the ducts, the capillaries recombine and then a second set of capillaries are formed around the acini. Thus the reabsorption of ions around the ducts is balanced by the transfer of ions to the secretory epithelium of the acini. It is equally possible that the two capillary systems are arranged the other way round, with the acinar capillaries first and the ductal second. However, the histological appearance of the glands makes it difficult to tell which of these arrangements is correct and the lack of separation of ductal and acinar portions of the gland may mean that such a dual system is unnecessary – a single capillary bed could serve both acini and ducts.

The nerve supply to the major salivary glands

Parasympathetic nerves carry the main secretomotor supply to salivary glands

The main control of the salivary glands is through the parasympathetic nerves. Although these originate in the salivatory nuclei they synapse in ganglia near or in the glands and the final efferent fibres are short. The neurotransmitter in the ganglia is acetylcholine and the receptors are nicotinic; the neurotransmitter at the cells of the gland is also acetylcholine but the receptors on the acinar cells are muscarinic. It is possible that other transmitters in addition to acetylcholine can be released from the varicosities of the parasympathetic nerve fibres (parasympathetic nerves usually provide an en passant innervation rather than a multitude of nerve terminals) and experiments in animals have demonstrated receptors for a number of neuropeptides such as substance P. It is not clear how important these are in humans although some of the atropine resistant effects of parasympathetic stimulation may be due to these. The parasympathetic fibres to the submandibular and sublingual glands pass in the facial nerve to the inner ear and then in its chorda tympani branch to the submandibular ganglion (Fig. 11.6). The efferent supply to the parotid gland travels in the glossopharyngeal nerve to the otic ganglion and thence to the gland. The sympathetic fibres pass from the second thoracic segment of the spinal cord to the superior cervical ganglion on each side and the postganglionic fibres travel with blood vessels to the gland. The neurotransmitter in the ganglion is acetylcholine, whilst that at the acinar cells is noradrenaline: the adrenoreceptors there are both alpha-1 and beta-2 in their responses. The glands do not solely consist of acini: they have ductal systems which modify the initial secretion, myoepithelial cells which may assist in the expulsion of saliva from the gland, and blood vessels which supply nutrients, metabolic subtrates, water and ions necessary for secretion to occur. Even the secretory cells are of two types, one type described as mucous and secreting mucoproteins, and the other, described as serous, producing a less viscous secretion with amylase and proline-rich proteins as the main organic constituents. There is no direct evidence to suggest that the innervation of the serous and mucous cells is different, but it is possible that the distribution and sensitivity of receptors on the cells may differ and provide selective responses. Cholinesterase activity has been demonstrated in or close to ductal cells, suggesting that they may have a parasympathetic innervation. The innervation of the myoepithelial cells is uncertain; in animal experiments they have been shown to respond to neurotransmitters of both the sympathetic and parasympathetic systems and also to bradykinin. There is continuing debate as to the role and importance of these cells. The blood vessels of the salivary glands are, like blood vessels elsewhere in the body, subject to parasympathetic control and stimulation of the parasympathetic supply leads to activation of alpha receptors and a vasoconstriction. However, these blood vessels also have a parasympathetic nerve supply and respond to stimulation with vasodilatation – one of the very few instances of parasympathetic induced vasodilatation in the human body. The neurotransmitter involved is almost certainly not acetylcholine but is probably vasoactive intestinal peptide (VIP). Nitric oxide (NO) is another likely candidate, but this possibility has not as yet been explored. The difficulty of explaining how sympathetic stimulation can result in secretion when it simultaneously causes vasoconstriction has been overcome by the suggestion that kallikrein is one of the secretory products of the ductal cells and this can diffuse back into the extracellular space and generate bradykinin in the local circulation: bradykinin is a vasodilator associated with secretion in other glands in the body.

Salivary ducts are innervated by the parasympathetic system

Parasympathetic nerves are vasodilator to the salivary glands, possibly using VIP as a neurotransmitter

The process of secretion

Stimuli to secretion

Saliva secretion may be stimulated by psychic stimuli, by taste and smell, or by irritation of the oesophagus

It is often convenient to think of stimuli to digestive organs as occurring in three phases: cephalic, intraorgan and interorgan. As the mouth is a cephalic organ the first phase has to be considered in a slightly different way: it includes a psychological phase – the thought of food – and the related visual phase – the sight of food – as well as the more direct olfactory stage – the smell of food. It has even been suggested that the sound of cooking of some foods may stimulate salivary flow. These stimuli are conditioned stimuli because they represent an association of the stimulus with actual food intake rather than the direct oral stimulus of food intake. There is still debate as to how far they increase salivary secretion: their effect, if any, is very small, and it may be that these stimuli lead to an enhanced awareness of saliva in the mouth rather than an actual increase in secretion. Experimentally, it is impossible to demonstrate anything as dramatic as the description 'mouth-watering' suggests.

The within-organ stimuli are the most important for salivary secretion. They include the mechanical stimuli – those involving touch or pressure on oral structures and movements of the masticatory muscles and mandible – and those involving chemical substances which stimulate the taste receptors. The stimuli vary in their effects, with mechanical stimuli being least effective in producing a flow of saliva and acid-tasting substances being most effective. As the nasal cavity is continuous with the oral cavity, smell does affect the flavour of foods (see Ch. 11) and so there is a possibility of a direct olfactory stimulus to secretion, but there is no evidence to support this. However, olfactory irritants can increase salivary flow, presumably by a direct rather than a conditioned reflex. Stimulation of taste, touch and muscle and joint proprioceptive receptors unilaterally stimulates secretion on the ipsilateral side of the mouth.

Stimuli to taste receptors innervated by the lingual nerve and chorda tympani result in a greater stimulation of the sublingual and submandibular glands which are innervated by efferent fibres in the same nerve, whilst stimuli to taste receptors innervated by the glossopharyngeal nerve are more effective in stimulated the glossopharyngeal–innervated parotid gland.

The final group of controls in the digestive system are the interorgan controls. The only interorgan control for the salivary glands is the stimulatory effect on secretion of irritation to the oesophagus; there is, however, a secretory response as part of the vomiting reflex.

The output pathways of all the salivary reflexes are via nerves.

Hormones do not stimulate secretion but can modify it

Hormones are not involved in the control of salivary secretion, although circulating aldosterone can affect the composition. The major glands have a dual nerve supply from the sympathetic and parasympathetic divisions of the autonomic nervous system. The cell bodies of the secretomotor neurones in the parasympathetic system are in the peripheral ganglia close to the glands, but the preganglionic fibres have cell bodies grouped together in the reticular formation to form two salivatory centres, the superior related to the nucleus of the facial nerve and controlling the submandibular and sublingual glands, the inferior related to the nucleus of the glossopharyngeal nerve and controlling the parotid glands. Stimulation of these centres induces salivation on the ipsilateral side. The preganglionic cell bodies in the sympathetic nervous system are located at the level of the second thoracic nerve. Cells in either system may receive inputs from the various receptors either directly or via interneurones and may also be excited or inhibited by impulses from higher centres. These latter may form parts of the patterned reflexes in which certain stimuli generate stereotyped patterns of response integrated across several effector systems. Vomiting, with its preparatory stimulation of salivary flow, is an example of this. Stimulation of the cerebral cortex at the lower end of the fissure of Rolando and the junction of the frontal and anterior sigmoidal gyri, or stimulation of the rhinencephalon near the amygdaloid nucleus, can provoke a feeding reaction which includes increased flow of saliva. The hypothalamus exerts an overriding control as a higher centre: in addition to its

There are salivatory centres in the pons

The hypothalamus modulates the activity of lower centres

direct connections with the sympathetic system it mediates the primitive reactions of fear, rage and excitement, which include both dryness of mouth and excess salivation in different circumstances. Salivation is normally inhibited or reduced during sleep – another central control. The progressive reduction in the unstimulated salivary flow rates of infants between birth and 5 years of age – a period when maturation of the brain and nervous responses is occurring – demonstrates the progressive increase in inhibitory signals from higher centres.

The formation of the initial acinar fluid

Parasympathetic stimuli act on secretory cells via G-proteins and the IP_3/Ca secondary messenger system

Parasympathetic stimulation results in the binding of acetylcholine to the muscarinic receptors on the acinar cells. This activates a G-protein pathway (Figs 6.6 and 6.7), causing the activation of phospholipase C and the splitting of phosphatidylinositol 4,5-diphosphate to give inositol trisphosphate and diacylglycerol. Inositol trisphosphate (IP_3) stimulates calcium release from the calcium stores within the cell and this free ionised calcium passes through the cell to give three effects. It causes the opening of basal potassium channels, the opening of apical chloride channels, and the movement of secretory granules or vesicles towards the apical membrane and their fusion with the membrane to begin the process of exocytosis. The opening of potassium channels results in outward diffusion of potassium ions. This can sometimes be detected as a very high concentration of potassium in the first few drops of saliva collected after stimulation. Basally it raises the concentration of potassium in the extracellular fluid and this activates a sodium–potassium–chloride transporter in the basal and basolateral cell membranes, carrying the three ions into the cell. The energy for this transport is derived from the sodium ion concentration gradient maintained by the basolateral and lateral sodium–potassium-ATPase pumps. The ions are carried as two potassiums and three chlorides for every sodium ion transported. The potassium replaces that lost through the potassium channels and the sodium is excreted from the cell by the sodium–potassium pumps. The increasing concentration of chloride ions results in their diffusion out through the apical, or acinar, cell membrane into the acinar space. Increasing concentrations of chloride in the acinar fluid drag sodium ions to balance the charge and water down an osmotic gradient, probably between the acinar cells despite their tight apical junctions. Protein and mucoprotein are exocytosed into the acinar space where the tight junctions prevent their diffusion away from the acinar fluid.

Sympathetic stimulation acts via alpha receptors on the same second messenger system but via beta-2 receptors on the cAMP system. This latter causes protein rather than fluid secretion

Sympathetic stimulation at alpha receptors activates the same pathway as acetylcholine, but at the beta-2 receptors a different second messenger system is invoked. Activation of the excitatory G-protein (Figs 6.8 and 6.9) results in adenylyl cyclase activation and the production of cyclic adenosine monophosphate (cAMP). This in turn activates protein kinase A and also causes mobilisation of calcium ions. At least a proportion of the increase in ionic calcium concentration results from opening of calcium channels permitting calcium to flow into the cells. There is a rapid opening of potassium channels and the process of fluid secretion is initiated. However, this is on a much smaller scale than that induced by the inositol trisphosphate

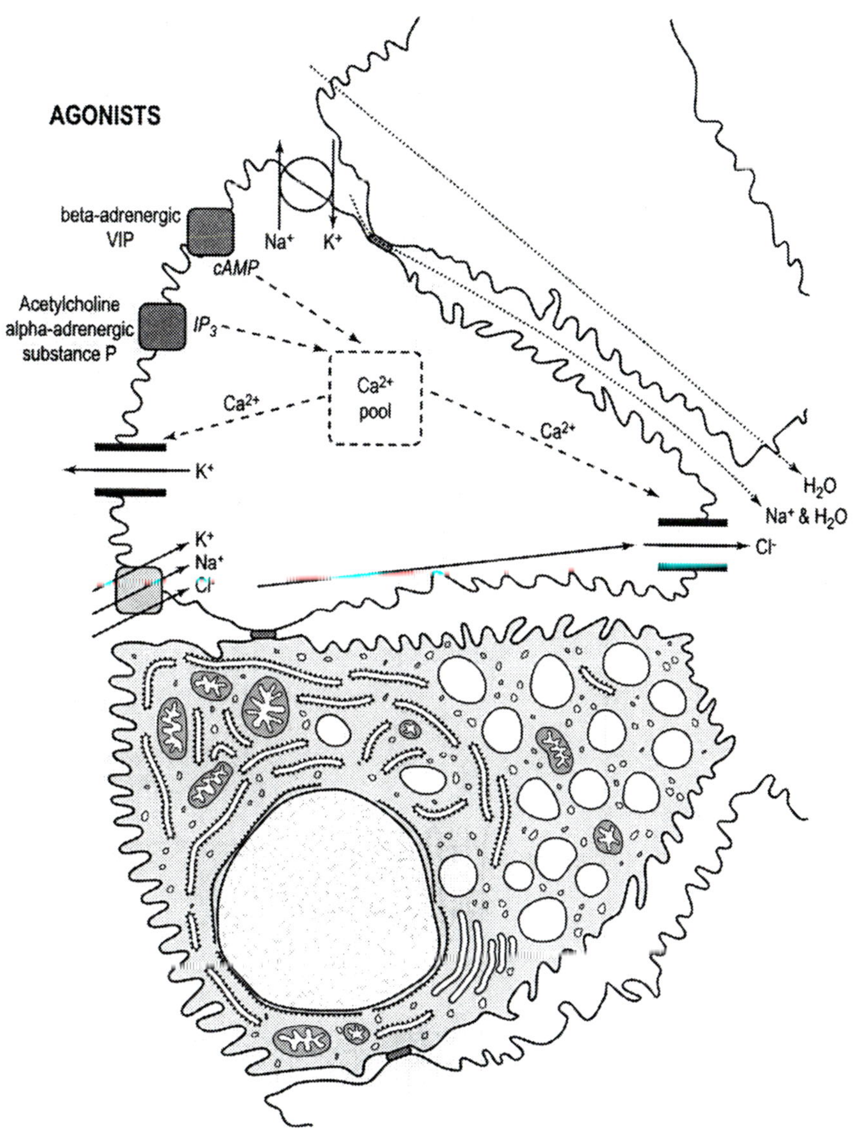

The process of secretion of ions by acinar cells. Chloride ions are secreted as a result of their increased intracellular concentration produced by the sodium–potassium–chloride transporter. Sodium ions follow down a gradient of charge and water down the resultant osmotic gradient. Sodium ions are thought to pass by an intercellular route. Water may pass by an intercellular route, but aquaporins may permit it also to pass transcellularly.

pathway, and the major result of sympathetic stimulation is the secretion of protein and mucoprotein, giving a thick viscous saliva.

Both neurotransmitters, acetylcholine and noradrenaline, are broken down rapidly: acetylcholinesterase is present in the acinar cell membranes

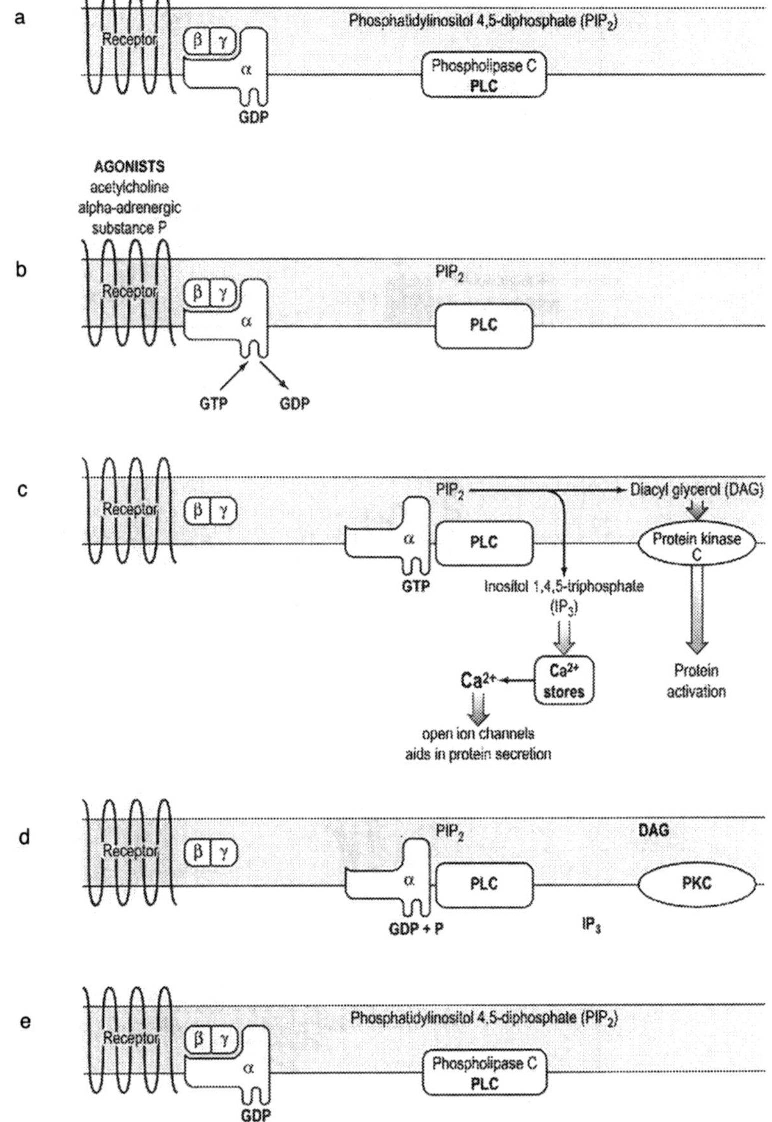

Activation of stimulatory G-proteins (**a**) by binding of agonists to receptors, resulting in the secretion of ions. (**b**) Binding of an agonist to the receptor causes the alpha subunit of the stimulatory G-protein complex to bind GTP instead of GDP. As a result (**c**) the alpha subunit separates from the beta and gamma subunits and activates phospholipase C. This splits phosphatidylinositol 4,5-diphosphate (PIP_2) to yield diacylglycerol and inositol 1,4,5-trisphosphate (IP_3). IP_3 in turn causes release of calcium ions from intracellular stores. The calcium ions cause opening of potassium ion channels basally and chloride ion channels apically. The diacylglycerol activates phosphokinase C which activates cellular proteins and enzymes. The alpha subunit itself splits off the third phosphate ion from GTP (**d**) and returns to its binding with the other two subunits and the receptor (**e**).

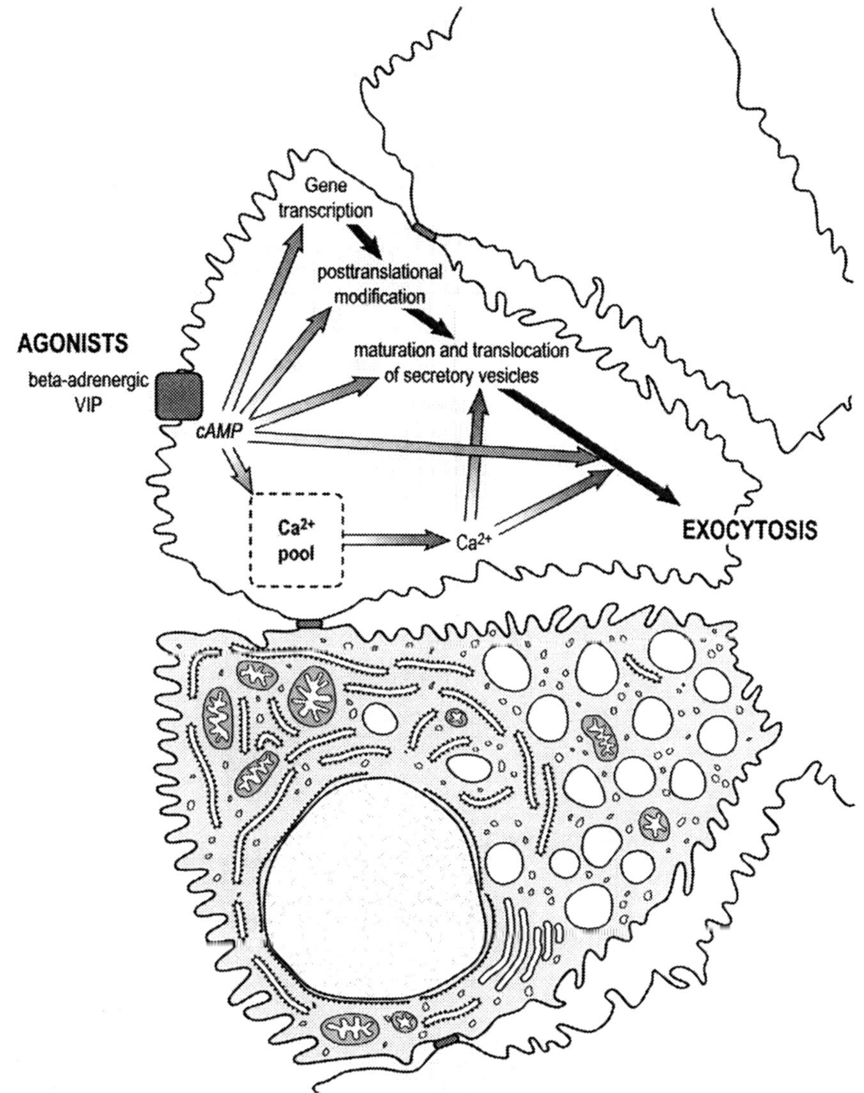

Fig. 6.8
The process of secretion of proteins and mucins by acinar cells.

and the salivary glands contain high concentrations of monoamine oxidases.

There are other effects of stimulation on the acinar cells: the net inward movement of chloride brings in water down an osmotic gradient and the cells tend to swell, whilst the increased cell activity increases the cell acidity. The former activates stretch-sensitive calcium channels in the cell membrane and outward movement of calcium reduces the ionic excess in the cells. Cell buffering is achieved by outward pumping of hydrogen ions or by exchange of hydrogen carbonate and chloride ions.

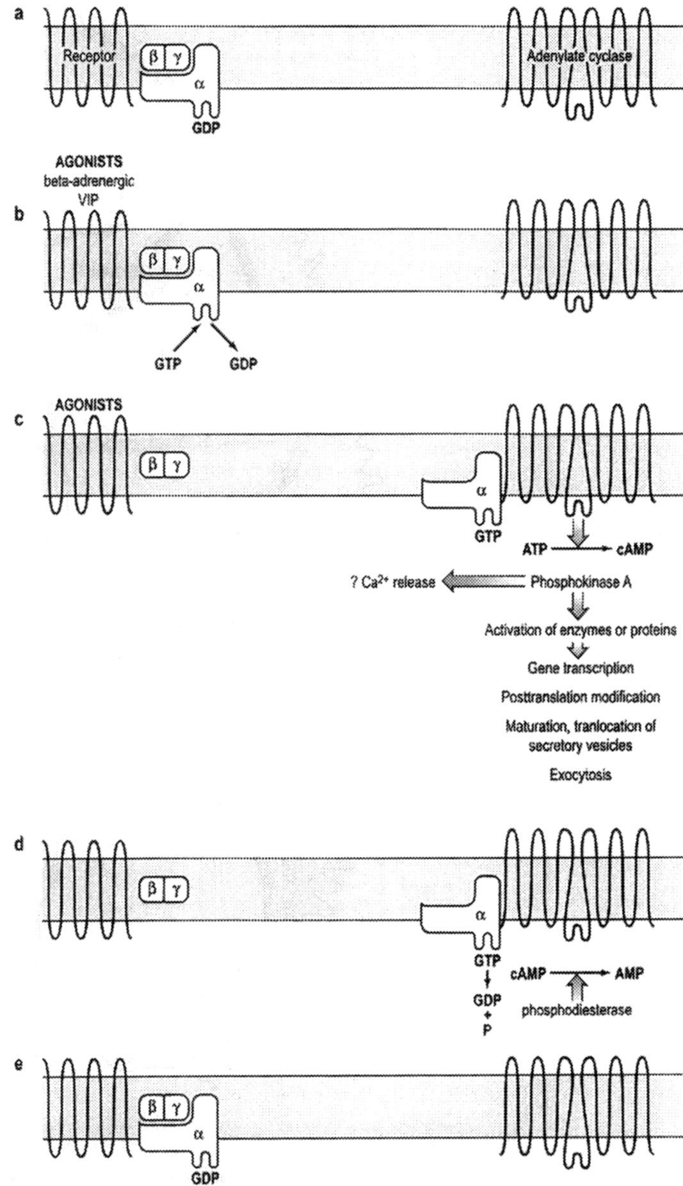

Activation of stimulatory G-proteins by binding of agonists to receptors, resulting in the secretion of proteins and mucins. The initial steps in activation of the alpha subunit of the stimulatory G-protein are similar to those in Fig. 6.7 (**a** and **b** in each figure). The alpha subunit after exchanging GDP for GTP now separates from the beta and gamma subunits and activates the enzyme adenylyl cyclase. This splits ATP to yield cyclic adenosine monophosphate (cAMP) (**c**) which activates phosphokinase A, and this activates all stages of protein synthesis and modification leading to final exocytosis of the salivary proteins or mucoproteins. Calcium ion release is also stimulated and these ions assist in exocytosis. The alpha subunit splits off a phosphate ion from the attached GTP and reverts to its former state (**d**, **e**) whilst the cAMP is converted to AMP by cellular phosphodiesterase.

It is not known whether stimulation by either pathway can cause synthesis of new protein for export or whether replenishment of protein stores is simply an ongoing process. Prolonged stimulation of the parotid gland results in a diminution in protein concentration of the secretion but in the short term – say half an hour – the protein concentration remains remarkably steady at a given level of stimulation. The net result of these processes is the formation of an acinar, or initial, secretion which is roughly similar in ionic composition to interstitial fluid in sodium and chloride concentrations, but with slightly higher potassium and calcium concentrations. It also contains the exocytosed proteins, but large molecules such as these have little effect on the osmotic activity of the solution and so the initial saliva is virtually isotonic with plasma.

Acinar fluid is similar to interstitial fluid in its ionic concentrations

Ductal modification of the acinar secretion

Saliva as secreted into the oral cavity is a hypotonic solution which varies in sodium concentrations from less than 10 mmol/l up to around 100 mmol/l. Chloride concentrations are similarly variable and below those in extracellular fluids generally, whilst hydrogen carbonate concentrations are usually in excess of those in extracellular fluids (Table 6.1). These changes are accomplished within the ducts and, more particularly, in the striated ducts.

The intercalated ducts are short in humans and no specific functions have been identified for them. Nevertheless, it has been suggested that they can secrete proteins similar to those from the acinar cells. They do not contain any significant number organelles which would normally be seen in secreting cells. In rodents there is another type of cell in this part of the ductal system: it contains many granules and hence the duct is described as the granular duct. It secretes kallikrein and a number of other proteolytic enzymes. It is possible that the human intercalated duct is the site of kallikrein secretion. A number of other proteins found in human saliva are secreted in the ductal system but the exact site of secretion has not been identified. In the case of secretory IgA this is not too suprising as the immunoglobulin is synthesised in the lymphoid follicles dispersed throughout the glands and probably passes between the relatively loosely connected ductal cells. Lysozyme and lactoferrin are proteins of ductal origin, as is carbonic anhydrase (Fig. 6.10). Serum albumin also

Lysozyme, lactoferrin and carbonic anhydrase are secreted by ductal cells. It is not known whether these functions are localised to any part of the ducts

Table 6.1
Composition of primary acinar fluid (mmol/l)

Component	Acinar fluid	Plasma	Saliva	
			Slow flow	Fast flow
Sodium	136	152	<10	80
Potassium	8	4	21	22
Calcium		2.5	1.2	1.8
Magnesium	0.75	1.5	0.15	0.12
Chloride	112	112	10	40
Hydrogen carbonate	30	24	4	35

reaches saliva by intercellular diffusion in very small amounts, although the higher concentrations observed in whole saliva result from the mixing in the mouth with gingival fluid. The salivary amylase found in plasma passes across the ductal epithelium in the opposite direction: when a salivary duct is obstructed, the intraluminal pressure rises and the ductal epithelium becomes

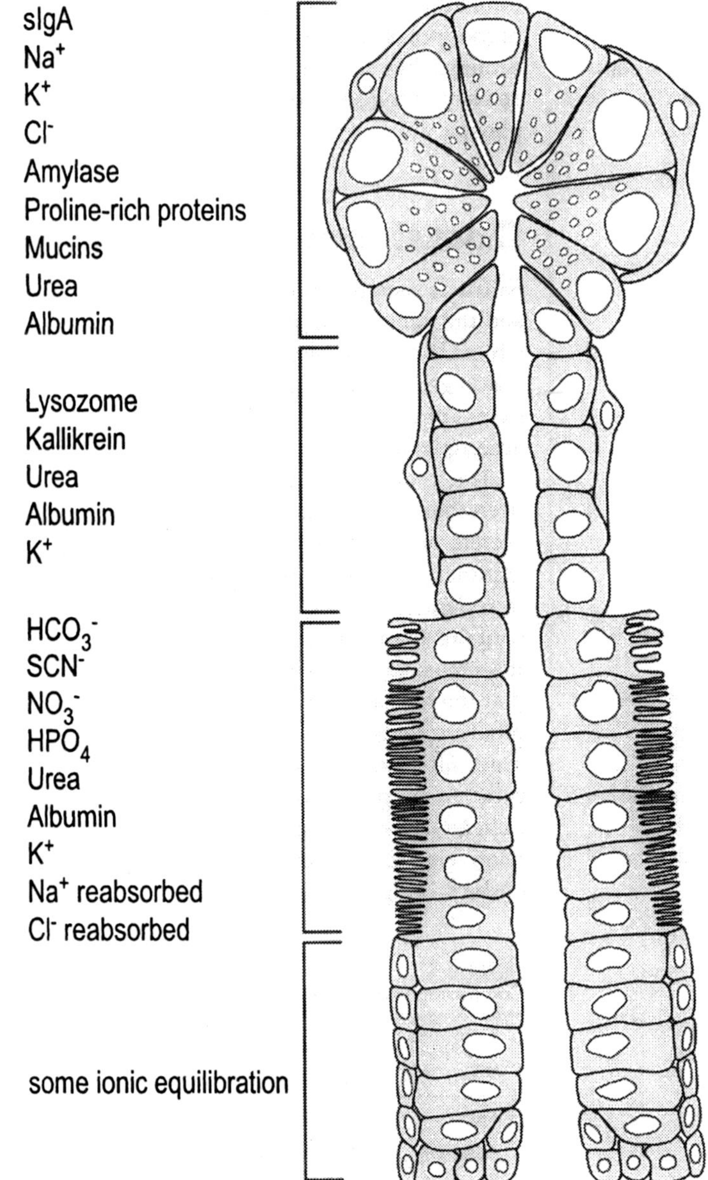

Areas of the secretory unit involved in the secretion of different proteins and ions.

very 'leaky'; plasma salivary amylase concentrations rise markedly when this happens.

The striated ducts which are found in the parotid and submandibular glands are the main sites of modification of ionic composition. They are said to be absent in the sublingual and minor glands, but there is evidence that some labial glands may be able to produce a hypotonic saliva. Sodium–potassium pumps in the intercalated duct cells are found mainly on the infolded basal surface where the infoldings result in a greatly increased surface area. Activation of these pumps generates a concentration gradient across the cells and sodium passes from the luminal fluid into the cells and out across the basal membrane (Fig. 6.11) – a process very similar to that in the proximal tubules of the kidney. These cells differ from those of the kidney proximal tubule, however, in being relatively impermeable to water, so that the fluid in the proximal tubule remains isotonic and that in the striated duct becomes hypotonic. The duct is capable of reducing the sodium concentration almost to zero if the saliva stays in it for a sufficiently long period: in very slow flowing saliva the sodium concentrations are less than 10 mmol/l. The process of reabsorption is time-dependent and hence sodium concentrations rise as saliva flow rate increases. Damage to the ductal cells, such as may occur as a result of radiation, will increase the sodium concentrations in the saliva reaching the oral cavity.

The striated ducts remove sodium and chloride from the saliva to leave a fluid hypotonic to interstitial fluid. Their activity is time-limited and so they are less effective at fast secretion rates

Throughout the ductal system there is addition of potassium ions to the ductal fluid but, as in the kidney, the removal of sodium in the striated duct does not have a major role in this, probably because the accompanying movement of chloride ions balances the charge difference. Chloride ions are reabsorbed in the striated duct by two mechanisms: the transport gives a charge gradient for anions, and the presence of chloride–hydrogen-carbonate exchange proteins in the apical cell membranes allows chloride to pass into the cells and hydrogen carbonate to pass out. It is in this part of the duct, therefore, that chloride concentrations fall and hydrogen carbonate concentrations rise.

In the remainder of the ductal system there may be some addition of potassium ions to the ductal fluid; whether any of the ductal-derived proteins mentioned above reach the fluid in these later parts of the system is unknown.

The movements of water and ions take place across the salivary gland epithelium by the various processes outlined above; the ultimate source of water and ions in saliva is the blood plasma and the interstitial fluid derived from it.

Composition of saliva

The composition of saliva from different glands varies, and it is difficult to define the composition of fluid in contact with either the teeth or the oral mucosa

The fluid which is normally present in the mouth, forming a thin layer between the surfaces of the cheeks and lips, the teeth, the tongue and the palate, is a mixture of secretions with a substantial component from the minor glands. Mixing of secretions takes place, but fluids near the orifices of the ducts of the major glands will obviously be nearer in composition to the appropriate secretion. During mastication when there is increased flow and the effective volume of the mouth which is available for saliva is increased by

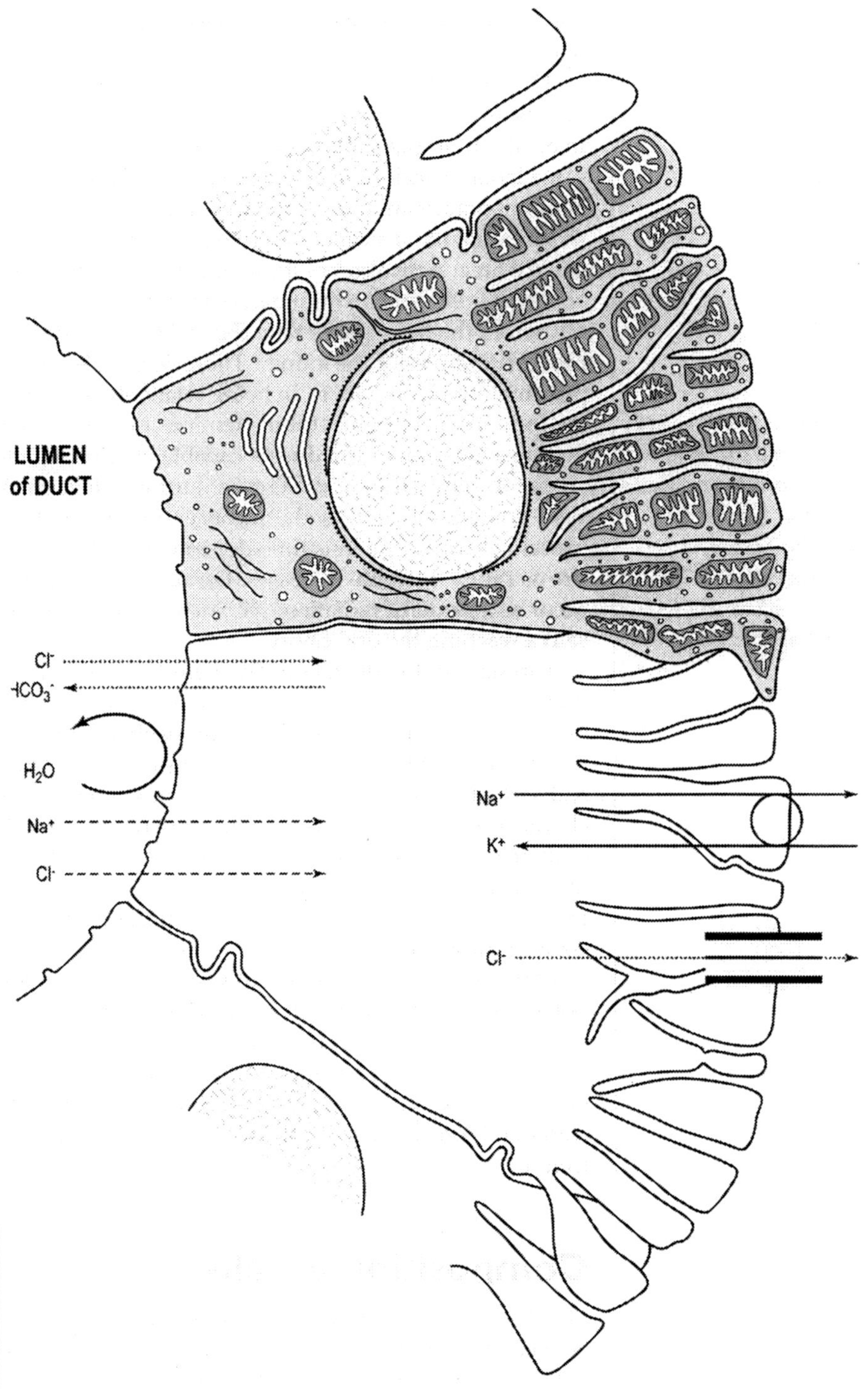

Fig. 6.11
The reabsorption of sodium and chloride across the cells of the striated duct. Water is not reabsorbed here, resulting in a final hypotonic saliva.

the presence of food: the saliva in the mouth is mixed with the food. It is difficult therefore to define the resting environment of the teeth, with their covering of dental plaque, and that of the oral soft tissues, in terms of the different salivary secretions. The mixed secretions which are collected by expectoration (spitting) are termed whole saliva or mixed saliva by different writers; neither of these terms is entirely satisfactory and the term 'oral fluid' sometimes used in USA is a better alternative. Such terminology also avoids the implication that the expectorated fluid contains only the secretions of salivary glands. In fact (Table 6.2), the fluid contains a contribution from gingival crevicular fluid (Ch. 12), bacteria and white blood cells. It is rare for it contain food particles except during and immediately after food intake.

There is a much greater amount of information available in relation to parotid saliva than to the other secretions, largely because there is an effective method in the Lashley (Carlson-Crittenden) cannula or cup for the easy collection of large volumes of a pure secretion. A superficial judgement suggests that whole saliva (oral fluid) should give the best assessment of the nature of the oral environment, but if the calculations on the volume of saliva normally in the mouth are valid the possibility exists of major differences in different parts of the mouth. It would seem appropriate therefore to describe the composition of saliva principally in terms of whole saliva (oral fluid) (Table 6.3), but such information as is available for the different glandular secretions is given separately in Tables 6.4–6.7.

Ionic composition

Calcium and phosphate concentrations are important both in relation to acid dissolution of tooth enamel and to the precipitation of dental calculus

Calcium and phosphate

In terms of ionic composition the three ions in saliva which concern the dentist most are calcium, phosphate and hydrogen carbonate – the first two because they will help to prevent dissolution of dental enamel and the last because of its buffering power. There are two other ions which play a part in the protection of the enamel surface: fluoride because of its ability to

Table 6.2
The components of oral fluid

Cells	
Bacteria	$60–70 \times 10^6$/l
Leucocytes	$25–650 \times 10^3$/l
Buccal squames	$6–600 \times 10^3$/l
Secretions from:	
2 parotid glands	Varying proportions according to the degree of stimulation
2 submandibular glands	
2 sublingual glands	
>600 minor salivary glands	
Gingival crevicular fluid	Varying in amount according to degree of gingival inflammation

Table 6.3
Composition of oral fluid (whole saliva, mixed saliva)

	Unstimulated		Stimulated	
Flow rate (ml/min)	0.25–0.35		1.0–3.0	
pH	6.0	5.7–6.2		up to 8.0
	Mean ± SD	Range	Mean ± SD	Range
Inorganic				
Sodium	7.7 ± 3.0	2 – 26	32 ± 20	13 – 80
Potassium	21 ± 4	13 – 40	22 ± 12	13 – 38
Calcium	1.35 ± 0.45	0.5 – 2.8	1.70 ± 1.0	0.2 – 4.7
Magnesium	0.31 ± 0.22	0.15 – 0.6	0.18 ± 0.15	0.2 – 0.6
Chloride	24 ± 8	8 – 40	25 ± 18	10 – 56
Hydrogen carbonate	2.9 ± 2.4	0.1 – 8.0	20 ± 8	4 – 40
Phosphate	5.5	2 – 22	10	1.5 – 25
Thiocyanate	2.5	0.4 – 5.0	1.2	0.4 – 3.0
Iodide (μmol/l)	5.5 ± 4.2	2 – 22	10 ± 7	2 – 30
Fluoride (μmol/l)	1.5	0.2 – 2.8	5.0	0.8 – 6.3
Organic				
Protein (g/l)			1.75	1.0 – 6.4
Serum albumin (mg/l)			25	
Gamma globulins (mg/l)			50	
Mucoproteins (g/l)			0.45	
MG1				
MG2				
Amylase (g/l)			0.42	
Lysozyme (g/l)			0.14	
Proline-rich proteins (mg/l)		0 – 80		
Histidine-rich proteins				
Lactoferrin				
Carbonic anhydrase				
Fibronectin (mg/l)		0.2 – 2.0		
Statherin (mg/l)		16 – 147		
Carbohydrate (g/l)				0.27 – 0.40
Blood group substances (mg/l)				10 – 20
Glucose				0.02 – 0.17
Lipids (mg/l)			20	
Cortisol (nmol/l)				2 – 20
Amino acids (mg/l)			40	
Urea				2.0 – 4.20
Ammonia				0.6 – 7.0

All concentrations are given in mmol/l unless otherwise designated. Components present in saliva but for which no quantitative data have been found are listed without such data.

Table 6.4
Composition of individual gland secretions: parotid

	Unstimulated		Stimulated	
Flow rate (ml/min)	0–0.11		1.40–3.00	
	Mean ± SD	Range	Mean ± SD	Range
Inorganic				
Sodium	1.3 ± 1.4	0.5 – 6.0	36 ± 12	8 – 80
Potassium	24 ± 6.5	30 – 80	21 ± 5	8 – 44
Calcium	1.05 ± 0.35	0.5 – 2.1	1.6 ± 0.8	0.2 – 2.7
Magnesium	0.16 ± 0.07	0.07 – 0.50	0.12 ± 0.15	0.01 – 0.4
Chloride	22 ± 6	17 – 40	28 ± 15	4 – 56
Hydrogen carbonate	1.1 ± 0.1	0.5 – 5.0	30 ± 9.6	5 – 60
Phosphate	9 ± 3.5	3.9 – 20	3.7 ± 1.0	2.3 – 9.3
Fluoride (μmol/l)	1.5		1.0 ± 0.3	4.0 – 13
Organic				
Protein (g/l)			2.3	
Serum albumin (mg/l)			100	
Gamma globulins (mg/l)				96 – 102 (sIgA)
Mucoproteins (g/l)			0.8	
MG1				
MG2				
Amylase (mg/l)				650 – 800
Lysozyme (g/l)			0.2	
Proline-rich proteins (mg/l)				100 – 900
Histidine-rich proteins				
Lactoferrin (mg/l)				1 – 2
Carbonic anhydrase				
Peroxidase (mg/l)				5 – 6
Fibronectin (mg/l)				2 – 6
Carbohydrate (g/l)			0.45	
Blood group substances			0	
Glucose			0.03	
Lipids (mg/l)			20	
Cortisol (nmol/l)				2 – 20
Amino acids (mg/l)			10	
Urea				2.0 – 4.2
Ammonia				0.6 – 7.0

All concentrations are given in mmol/l unless otherwise designated. Components present in saliva but for which no quantitative data have been found are listed without such data.

Table 6.5
Composition of individual gland secretions: submandibular

Flow rate (ml/min)	Unstimulated		Stimulated	
	0–0.28			
	Mean ± SD	Range	Mean ± SD	Range
Inorganic				
Sodium	3.3 ± 3.9		45 ± 23	10 – 60
Potassium	14.4 ± 2.2	10 – 22	17 ± 4	10 – 22
Calcium	1.56 ± 0.45	0.5 – 5.0	2.4 ± 0.6	0.7 – 3.7
Magnesium	0.07 ± 0.03		0.04 ± 0.01	0.01 – 0.5
Chloride	12 ± 4.6	3 – 24	25 ± 11	10 – 42
Hydrogen carbonate	4.0		18	3 – 36
Phosphate	5.6 ± 1.9	3 – 12	5.5 ± 4.0	0.2 – 7.4
Organic				
Protein (g/l)			1.1	
Serum albumin (mg/l)			11	
Gamma globulins (mg/l)			60	
Mucoproteins (g/l)			0.8	
MG1				
MG2 (mg/l)				14 – 203
Amylase (g/l)			0.3	
Lysozyme				
Proline-rich proteins (mg/l)			430	
Histidine-rich proteins				
Lactoferrin (mg/l)				1 – 2
Carbonic anhydrase				
Fibronectin (mg/l)				0.2 – 2.0
Carbohydrate (g/l)			0.3	
Blood group substances (mg/l)				10 – 20
Glucose			0.03	
Lipids (mg/l)			20	
Cortisol				
Amino acids			20	
Urea				0.7 – 1.7
Ammonia				0.2 – 7.0

All concentrations are given in mmol/l unless otherwise designated. Components present in saliva but for which no quantitative data have been found are listed without such data.

substitute into the hydroxyapatite lattice, and thiocyanate because of its antibacterial activity when converted to hypothiocyanate by salivary lactoperoxidase. Calcium and phosphate are present in whole saliva typically at 1.4 mmol/l and 6 mmol/l, respectively, in unstimulated saliva and 1.7 and 4

Table 6.6
Composition of individual gland secretions: sublingual

Flow rate (ml/min)	Stimulated	
	Mean ± SD	Range
Inorganic		
Sodium	32.7 ± 10.4	22 – 55
Potassium	13 ± 2	10 – 17
Calcium	2.1 ± 0.4	1.7 – 2.95
Chloride	26 ± 10	12 – 37
Hydrogen carbonate	11 ± 4	5 – 17
Phosphate	4.1 ± 0.8	2.5 – 5.0
Organic		
Protein		
Serum albumin		
Gamma globulins		
Mucoproteins		
MG1		
MG2 (mg/l)		14 – 203
Amylase (g/l)	0.25 ± 0.06	
Lysozyme		
Proline-rich proteins		
Histidine-rich proteins		
Lactoferrin (mg/l)		1 – 2
Carbonic anhydrase		
Fibronectin (mg/l)		0.2 – 2.0
Carbohydrate		
Blood group substances (mg/l)		80 – 150
Glucose		
Lipids		
Cortisol		
Amino acids		
Urea		
Ammonia		

All concentrations are given in mmol/l unless otherwise designated. Components present in saliva but for which no quantitative data have been found are listed without such data.

mmol/l in stimulated saliva. The values for calcium are misleading because they are for total calcium and only around 50% of calcium in saliva is present in an ionic form – about 40% is complexed with other ions and about 10% bound by salivary protein. Phosphate, on the other hand, is almost all in the ionic form – perhaps 10% being organic phosphate and in some subjects a

Table 6.7
Composition of individual gland secretions: labial glands

Flow rate	Unstimulated		Stimulated	
	Mean ± SD	Range	Mean ± SD	Range
Inorganic				
Sodium	14 ± 12	3 – 37	37 ± 22	11 – 98
Potassium	19 ± 5	10 – 29	17 ± 4	11 – 25
Calcium	2.29 ± 0.47	1.6 – 3.2	2.03 ± 0.38	1.64 – 2.48
Magnesium	0.65 ± 0.25	0.41 – 1.22	0.54 ± 0.14	0.38 – 0.8
Chloride	31 ± 14	16 – 54	56 ± 30	19 – 109
Hydrogen carbonate	Virtually zero		Virtually zero	
Phosphate	0.62 ± 0.23	0.25 – 1.07	0.45 ± 0.11	0.2 – 0.6
Organic				
Protein (g/l)	2.96 ± 1.02	1.45 – 5.60	2.58 ± 0.72	1.45 – 3.55
Serum albumin				
Gamma globulins				
Mucoproteins				
MG1				
MG2				
Amylase				
Lysozyme				
Proline-rich proteins				
Histidine-rich proteins				
Lactoferrin				
Carbonic anhydrase				
Carbohydrate				
Blood group substances (mg/l)				60 – 350
Glucose				
Lipids				
Cortisol				
Amino acids				
Urea			280	170 – 350
Ammonia				

All concentrations are given in mmol/l unless otherwise designated. Components present in saliva but for which no quantitative data have been found are listed without such data.

small amount of pyrophosphate is present. If these values are substituted into the equation for the solubility product of hydroxyapatite, it is apparent that hydroxyapatite is unlikely to dissolve in saliva at a pH around 6.0 – the pH of resting saliva. However, increases in pH or in calcium or phosphate concentration could result in precipitation of calcium salts as in the formation of dental calculus. It is difficult to predict how calcium concentrations in whole saliva will vary at different flow rates because, although in individual secretions calcium concentrations increase with flow rate (Fig. 6.12), whole saliva will have a smaller proportion of submandibular saliva and a greater proportion of parotid saliva at high flow rates and parotid saliva has only about half the calcium concentration of submandibular saliva. Phosphate concentrations in saliva tend to decrease at higher rates of flow (Fig. 6.12). This may be because phosphate is probably secreted into saliva in the ducts and more rapidly secreted saliva traverses the ducts more quickly. If this explanation is correct the output of phosphate in unit time should be roughly constant. Phosphate concentrations are particularly low in minor gland saliva. The higher calcium concentration in submandibular saliva helps to explain why calculus is particularly likely to form on the lingual side of the lower incisors. Calculus formation on the buccal surface of the upper first molar – another common site – is more difficult to explain. Whilst calcium and phosphate concentrations in saliva have not been shown to relate to overall calculus formation, individuals with more pyrophosphate in their saliva form less calculus. This is not surprising as pyrophosphate is a well-known inhibitor of calcification and is now used as the active ingredient of anti-tartar toothpastes.

Hydrogen carbonate

Hydrogen carbonate is an important buffer

Hydrogen carbonate concentrations are low in unstimulated saliva from all the glands but increase markedly at fast flow rates (Fig. 6.12). Hydrogen carbonate is the major buffer in saliva: it pushes the pH of stimulated saliva up towards pH 8.0 and is active as a buffer around the so-called critical pH of 5.6 in dental plaque – the pH at which enamel begins to dissolve in saliva. It can easily be shown that the pH fall in dental plaque exposed to sugar solutions can be greatly reduced by saliva collected at fast flow rates and that the pH fall in dental plaque on a tooth surface from which saliva is excluded is greater than that in the presence of saliva. Thus hydrogen carbonate is an effective defence against the acid produced by cariogenic bacteria. The lower caries experience of subjects with faster saliva flow rates may be due to this factor. A paper strip test is available (formerly known as Dentobuff©, but now Vivacult BC©) which measures salivary buffer capacity as a means of assessing susceptibility to dental caries. The hydrogen carbonate is ultimately derived from the carbon dioxide generated by metabolic activity in the salivary glands, which contain much carbonic anhydrase and can readily hydrate the carbon dioxide. This explains the increased concentration at higher flow rates. The ion is in equilibrium with dissolved carbon dioxide in saliva, but loss of carbon dioxide from saliva increases its alkalinity and so calcium salts may precipitate out from saliva on standing.

Fluoride

Fluoride is present in saliva

Fluoride concentrations in saliva are low and very similar to those in plasma and extracellular fluids in general. Intake of fluoride increases plasma levels

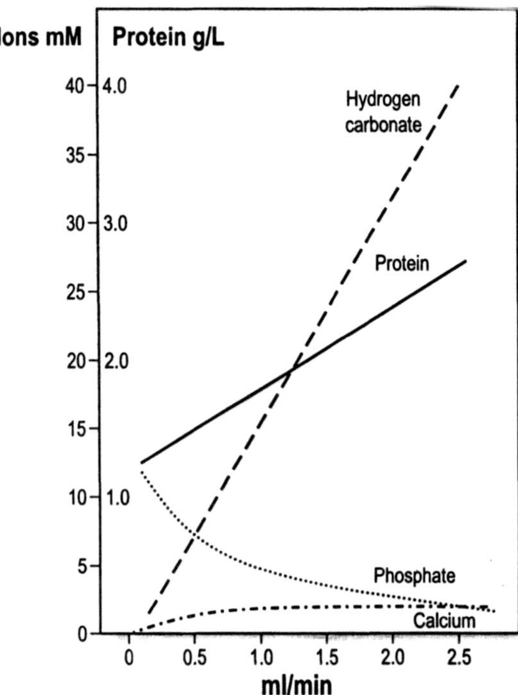

Variation in concentrations of some salivary components at different rates of flow.

transiently and that increase is also observed in saliva. Although flouride concentrations in unstimulated saliva are slightly higher, there is little variation with rates of saliva flow.

Thiocyanate

Thiocyanate is a component of an antibacterial system in saliva

Thiocyanate in saliva has been found to be associated with a lower incidence of dental caries. The mechanism by which this is achieved is the oxidation of thiocyanate to hypothiocyanite by the active oxygen resulting from bacterial peroxides being broken down by salivary lactoperoxidase. Hypothiocyanite is a powerful antibacterial agent. Thiocyanate reaches saliva by transport in the ducts and so decreases in concentration as flow rate increases. It is particularly high in concentration in saliva from cigarette smokers and can be used to identify children who smoke, although people subjected to high levels of atmospheric cigarette smoke also have high concentrations of the ion in saliva.

Sodium, potassium and chloride

Sodium and chloride concentrations vary at different flow rates

The other ions in saliva are of interest more for their role in the secretion of saliva than for their activity in the oral cavity. Thus the concentrations of sodium, potassium and chloride and effects of flow on these have already been dealt with above.

Lead, cadmium, copper

Saliva may reflect systemic concentrations of some ions

Apart from those already mentioned, data exist on a number of other ions whose concentrations might be expected to reflect plasma concentrations and hence might be useful in diagnosis and treatment. Thus lead, cadmium and copper indicate pollution of various kinds and lithium concentrations reflect the use of lithium in the treatment of depression.

Iodine

Iodine is secreted into saliva

Iodine is stored by the salivary glands and secreted into saliva: there is some dental interest in iodine handling by the glands because radio-iodine can be used to visualise them in the same way as it is used to visualise the thyroid gland.

Major organic components of saliva

The main organic components of saliva are the proteins and mucoproteins

Proteins with lubricating properties

Mucins

Glycoproteins with more than 40% carbohydrate in the molecule are termed mucins; they act as lubricants on epithelial surfaces throughout the digestive tract

If the main function of saliva is lubrication, the most important organic constituents are the mucins or mucoproteins. These are usually defined as glycoproteins containing more than 40% carbohydrate. They have protein cores with many oligosaccharide side-chains attached by *O*-glycosidic linkages. The two principal mucins of submandibular saliva have been isolated and characterised. They are known as MG1 and MG2. The smaller of these, MG2, has a molecular size of 200–250 kDa whilst that of the larger, MG1, is over 1000 kDa. The protein core of MG2 is a single peptide chain with threonine, proline, serine and alanine as the major amino acids. This peptide chain accounts for about 30% of the molecule and the remainder is largely carbohydrate with some 170 short (2–7 residues) oligosaccharide chains attached like the bristles of a bottlebrush. In solution the molecules probably exist as random coils and therefore contribute to the viscosity of the solution. The larger mucin has a protein core with the same general composition as that of MG2 but this accounts for only some 15% of the total weight. The oligosaccharide chains are larger than those of MG2, varying between 4 and 16 sugar residues. In both mucoproteins the carbohydrate residues include fucose and large amounts of both *N*-acetylglucosamine and *N*-acetylgalactosamine. The long molecules of MG1 contribute to the lubricating properties of saliva.

Proline-rich proteins

Both parotid and submandibular saliva contain glycoproteins rich in proline; these also have around 40% carbohydrate in their molecules. These proline-rich glycoproteins have a single peptide chain with six oligosaccharide units attached. Their role in lubrication is probably small.

Digestive proteins

Amylase is the main digestive enzyme in saliva, but its action is limited by the short time available in the mouth and its inactivation by gastric acid

The second function of saliva mentioned above is that of digestion. This is accomplished by the enzyme amylase which breaks down starch at O-glycosidic linkages to give maltase and longer chain polysaccharides. The enzyme is active above pH 6 and is therefore inactivated in the stomach, except in the centre of a food bolus. Its time of action in the mouth is short although it may break down starchy foods remaining on the teeth after a meal. This could have a cleansing effect but would also provide disaccharide substrate for acid production by oral bacteria. The enzyme is secreted mainly from the parotid glands, making up about 30% of the total protein in parotid saliva. The remainder is largely made up by the proline-rich proteins, with the acidic ones contributing twice as much as the basic ones. Amylase has a molecular mass of between 55 and 60 kDa and exists in a glycosylated and a non-glycosylated form. Both forms are produced by the same gene, which is closely related to the genes responsible for amylase production in the pancreas and situated at chromosome 1p21. Amylase can cross the walls of the salivary ducts to increase the serum amylase concentrations, particularly if there is any obstruction in the ducts. It binds to apatite and selectively to some bacteria.

Parotid lipase is important only when pancreatic lipase secretion is reduced

There are a very large number of enzymes present in whole saliva but most of these are bacterial in origin and in very low concentrations. A lipase in saliva is secreted by the parotid and some of the lingual glands; it is thought to be of little importance in healthy subjects but may have significant activity in patients unable to secrete pancreatic lipase.

Proteins with antimicrobial properties

Sialoperoxidase, lysozyme, lactoferrin and sIgA are antibacterial; the histatins are anti-candidal

The third group of proteins are those having antibacterial activity. They include the sialoperoxidase already mentioned, lysozyme, IgA and lactoferrin. Lysozyme is found in most exocrine secretions. It is also termed muramidase, since its function is to break down muramic acid in bacterial cell walls. IgA is synthesised as a monomer by plasma cells in the lymphatic tissue present in the glands. These cells also synthesise a small protein termed the J-protein, which links two molecules of IgA to form a dimer. In the ductal epithelium, it binds to a cell membrane receptor and is then transported through the cell. At the luminal surface it is released into the saliva, still bound to a part of the receptor molecule. This latter is termed the secretory piece, and the dimeric IgA with the secretory piece protects the antibody from breakdown in the oral fluids. The concentration of sIgA in saliva is greater than that of other immunoglobulins and its association with lower levels of dental caries suggests that it is active against cariogenic bacteria. Lactoferrin is an iron-binding protein which deprives bacteria of the trace amounts of iron in the environment and hence inhibits their metabolic processes. The histatins are a group of some six histidine-rich peptides. They have been demonstrated to have anti-candidal properties. The presence of a protein known as salivary leucocyte proteinase inhibitor (SLPI) in saliva is thought to account for the inability of the human immunodeficiency virus (HIV) to be transferred via saliva.

Proteins binding calcium

Statherin and the acidic proline-rich proteins bind calcium and reduce calculus formation

The proline-rich proteins constitute the major protein fraction of parotid saliva

Another protein with protective functions is statherin: this small protein binds calcium and prevents precipitation of calcium phosphates in the ducts of the glands as well as reducing the possibility of dental calculus formation.

The major protein fraction in parotid saliva is the proline-rich protein component. The group of proteins are found in secretions of the trachea and pharynx as well as in the mouth. They have been found in saliva in many animal species. Their function is unclear. Like statherin, the acidic proline-rich proteins bind calcium and reduce the possibility of precipitation of calcium phosphates. All the proline-rich proteins have the property of binding tannins, and feeding of high tannin diets to rats results in greater synthesis of proline-rich proteins. Chronic administration of physostigmine has a similar effect, although then coupled with hyperplasia of the glands. Whilst tannins are harmful to epithelial tissues, this scarcely justifies a response on the scale suggested by the proline-rich protein content of human saliva. The proteins result from the activity of a group of genes on chromosome 12, and the large number of proteins is due to their splitting by proteolytic enzymes such as kallikrein in the glands. They contain some 40% of proline residues; other amino acids are present in much lower proportions (Fig. 6.13). They are coded by a group of genes which form the salivary protein complex on the short arm of chromosome 12.

Proline-rich proteins are usually subdivided into three groups on the basis of their amino acid and carbohydrate content, the acidic group making up around 45%, the basis group making up 30%, and the glycosylated group making up 25%. The proportion of proline rich proteins in other salivary secretions is lower, and in whole saliva many of the larger ones are broken down by proteolytic activity.

P P Q G $^{K}_{R}$ P Q G P P Q Q G G H Q G Q P P P

P Q G P P P Q G G

P P P G K P Q G P P P Q G G N K P Q G P P

Three different aminoacid sequences which have been identified as repeating sequences in the proline-rich proteins. The preponderance of proline, glutamine and glycine is obvious.

Fig. 6.13
Three different amino acid sequences which have been identified as repeating sequences in the proline-rich proteins. The upper one is repeated five times in the acidic proline-rich protein PRP3 which has an additional 51 amino acid sequence at the N-terminal and a six amino acid sequence at the C-terminal. The middle sequence is also found in acidic proline-rich proteins, whilst the lower sequence is characteristic of the basic proline-rich proteins such as IB6.

Other organic components

Blood group substances

ABO blood group substances in saliva have been identified in criminal cases involving bitemarks

Some 80% of people in Western communities secrete blood group substances of the ABO blood groups into their saliva. Other blood group antigens, with the exception of Lewis A and Lewis B, are not secreted, although Lewis A is also secreted by subjects of otherwise non-secretor status. Parotid saliva does not contain blood group substances. The blood group antigens are predominantly carbohydrate in nature with a small amount of protein; they include the H substance produced by people in group O as well as A and B substances. This property of saliva is of some importance forensically.

Sugars

A number of small sugars are found in saliva; concentrations of glucose follow those of plasma glucose but are some 100 times lower.

Lipids

Steroid hormones are found in saliva in proportion to their free concentration in plasma

The lipid content of saliva is very low but it does include steroid hormones. These are important for two reasons: there is evidence that oestrogen and testosterone affect the oral bacterial population, and the fact that only non-protein-bound forms of the steroids can gain access to saliva means that salivary steroids can be assayed to give a measure of free steroid concentrations in plasma. This means that the non-invasive collection of whole saliva can be used to monitor plasma hormone levels.

Amino acids, ammonia, urea, sialin

A number of nitrogen-containing compounds in saliva can be converted to ammonia by plaque bacteria

Among the other components of saliva are amino acids, a tetrapeptide named sialin with the composition GGKR (gly-gly-lys-arg), urea, uric acid, ammonia and creatinine. Urea is readily broken down by plaque ureases to yield ammonia, sialin is also converted into ammonia in plaque, and ammonia is itself present. The pH of dental plaque is raised by ammonia from these three sources: this provides a means of combating plaque acid production and maintains a more alkaline plaque during fasting periods.

Normal variations in salivary composition

Variations in the flow rate and composition of oral fluid will depend upon the activity of the individual salivary glands

It will be apparent from the tables summarising the composition of saliva that there are wide variations in both the flow rate and composition of saliva. Oral fluid, or whole saliva, is a mixture of the secretions from all the salivary glands and hence its flow rate will be the sum of the individual gland flow rates, and its composition will be dependent upon the particular mixture of secretions at the time. By measuring the flow rates produced by the individual major glands and comparing this with the total flow rate of oral fluid, an estimate of the contribution of the minor glands can be derived. However, whilst a non-stimulated total flow can be measured, the use of collecting devices over the major glands introduces some degree of oral stimulation and it is impossible to obtain comparable flow values for them. The available data estimates suggest that at low flow rates during sleep the oral fluid is predominantly from the submandibular glands (72%), with no measurable secretion from the parotid glands and roughly equal proportions from the sublingual glands and all the minor glands (14% each). If, as may well be the case, the minor glands continue to secrete at the same rate as during waking hours, they would have a total flow rate equivalent to that from the submandibular glands and the above figures would have to be revised.

Unstimulated oral fluid has more submandibular saliva and hence more calcium; stimulated oral fluid has more parotid saliva and hence more amylase

Unstimulated flow of oral fluid is thought to be largely from the submandibular glands (70%), with the parotid glands providing around 20% and the accessory glands around 7%. The contribution of the sublingual glands is less than 2% of either unstimulated or stimulated oral fluid. With acid stimulation parotid and submandibular contributions become roughly equal at around 45%, and the stimulus of chewing evokes nearly twice as much parotid saliva as submandibular. These changes in proportion of the individual secretions affect the composition of oral fluid. A secretion rich in parotid saliva has a greatly increased amylase content, while a secretion rich in submandibular saliva will have higher calcium concentrations.

Sodium, chloride and hydrogen carbonate concentrations increase with flow rate as does protein. Phosphate and immunoglobulin concentrations decrease as flow rate increases

Rate of flow can itself affect concentrations of salivary constituents. This affects sodium and chloride concentrations because the shorter transit time through the striated ducts at higher flow rates reduces the resorption of these ions in this part of the ductal system. Hydrogen carbonate concentrations also increase at higher flow rates, primarily because of the greater production of carbon dioxide by the active glands, and the increased buffering power of the saliva pushes the pH up towards 8.0. Amylase concentrations tend to increase at higher flow rates (Fig. 2.12). Components which reach saliva by diffusion across the gland tissue, or are secreted in the ducts rather than in the acini, will decrease in concentration because the output remains steady whilst the saliva volume is increasing. Thus urea, which diffuses into saliva, and the immunoglobulins, which are secreted in the ducts, are both present at the higher concentrations in unstimulated saliva.

Duration of stimulation affects composition

Duration of stimulation is another variable affecting flow rate and composition. As stimulation is maintained, the flow rate falls slightly and the protein content is reduced, presumably because the stores of secretory material in the acinar cells are not replenished quickly enough. Hydrogen carbonate concentrations rise and chloride concentrations tend to fall. If saliva is being collected for analysis it is important that the collection should take place sufficiently long (at least 1 h and preferably 2 h) after previous stimulation, such as intake of food or drink, for such effects to have disappeared.

There are circadian rhythms of flow rate and concentration

Salivary flow rate, like many other physiological variables, differs at different times of day. In general the lowest flow rates of unstimulated or stimulated saliva are observed in the early hours of the morning (04:00–06:00 h) and the peak flow rates are seen in the afternoon (16:00–20:00 h). Although this does affect the sodium concentrations, they are influenced mainly by the circadian rhythm of aldosterone, which increases activity of the sodium-potassium-ATPase. This causes peaks and troughs of sodium concentration and therefore chloride concentration at opposite times to those of flow rate. The aldosterone rhythm induces a circadian pattern in potassium concentrations the reverse of that in sodium concentrations. Protein concentrations are also highest in late afternoon. Standardisation of times of collection eliminates this source of variation in saliva composition.

Although there are reports of rhythms in salivary flow rate or composition over periods of months or years, most observers have found the day-to-day variation in concentrations of salivary components in any one subject is such that it is difficult to find any consistent pattern. Even reports that saliva ionic composition varies in women during the menstrual cycle have not been confirmed by subsequent studies.

Saliva composition is little affected by changes in plasma composition, by diet or by changes in circulating hormones (except for aldosterone)

As saliva is the product of a process of secretion, rather than an ultrafiltration of plasma, it is not surprising that plasma composition has little effect on salivary composition. There is some correlation between plasma urea and glucose concentrations and those in saliva, and the ions which diffuse into saliva in the ductal system, such as fluoride and iodide, undergo similar concentration changes in the two fluids. Diet affects saliva only inasmuch as different foodstuffs stimulate salivary flow to different degrees and hence alter composition in a flow rate dependent manner.

Saliva flow rate and composition are unaffected by circulating hormones, except for aldosterone, as described above. The steroid hormones, being lipid-soluble, can diffuse across the secretory epithelium and are found in saliva in concentrations mirroring the concentration of free (unbound) hormone in plasma.

Infants have higher calcium, magnesium and chloride and lower phosphate concentrations in saliva, old people have lower submandibular saliva flow rates and parotid saliva sodium, calcium and chloride concentrations

In infants, unstimulated flow rates appear to be higher than in adults. The concentrations of calcium, magnesium and chloride are significantly higher than in adult saliva, whilst those of sodium and potassium are higher but not significantly so. Concentrations fall to adult levels by the end of the first year of life. Phosphate concentrations are at first low, but rise to adult levels over the first year. At the other end of the age spectrum the data are confusing, partly because few studies have examined non-medicated subjects. Although the salivary glands show histological evidence that suggests decreased function, the parotid glands appear to have a substantial secretory reserve and their saliva flow rates are not significantly affected by age. However, the submandibular and the minor glands do show decreased flow rates. The flow rate of oral fluid is within the wide range of values reported for younger adults. Two studies have reported that sodium, calcium and chloride concentrations are lower in stimulated parotid saliva collected from non-medicated subjects aged over 70 years.

Pharmacological variations in salivary flow rate and composition

Drugs affecting autonomic function and the diuretics reduce salivary flow rates

Drugs which affect the autonomic nervous system would be predicted to cause changes in salivary flow rate and composition. This is indeed the case. Of the drugs which are more commonly prescribed the diuretics are a key group. As these achieve their effects by modifying the transport of ions in the kidney, they also produce similar effects in the salivary glands. Thus inhibitors of the sodium–potassium–chloride transporter in the loop of Henle also inhibit this transporter in the salivary glands and markedly reduce salivary secretion.

The use of saliva as a diagnostic fluid

There has been a continuing hope over many years that saliva could provide an alternative to blood for tests which might help in the diagnosis of disease. This could occur only if a blood component was transferable across the salivary gland epithelium in proportion to its concentration in blood. This is true for urea, glucose and the unbound steroid hormones. Only for the last of these has saliva proved a useful medium for monitoring concentrations. Glucose is used by the gland cells and appears in saliva at around one-hundreth of its plasma concentrations – too low for easy measurement.

Changes in salivary composition in salivary gland disease

Salivary flow rate and/or composition is affected in sialadenitis, Sjögren's syndrome and radiation damage to the glands

Sodium and chloride concentrations in the affected gland secretions are raised in sialadenitis, suggesting that inflammation particularly affects the ductal system. This possibility is reinforced by the observation that phosphate concentrations are usually lowered.

Sjögren's syndrome is a connective tissue disease which usually involves reduced secretion from the lachrymal and salivary glands. Reduced salivary secretion causes a dry mouth and so is termed xerostomia. Again the principal changes in ionic composition of saliva are increased concentrations of sodium and chloride and decreased concentrations of phosphate. In addition, there are changes in the relative concentrations of some minor salivary proteins. These may have some diagnostic value. Salivary gland neoplasms are uncommon and there are few data available on their effects on salivary composition.

Radiation used in the treatment of neoplasms in the head and neck region often results in radiation-induced damage to salivary glands. This is seen as a marked reduction in flow rate, leading to xerostomia. The small amount of saliva secreted has high concentrations of sodium, chloride, calcium and magnesium but low concentrations of hydrogen carbonate. The low volume of saliva and its poor buffering power are associated with rampant dental caries in these patients. The best treatment for them seems to be frequent use of mouthwashes with a high fluoride concentration.

The relationship of saliva flow rate and composition to oral disease

There is no correlation of salivary ionic composition with dental caries or periodontal disease

Despite repeated attempts for over 60 years to link salivary calcium and phosphate concentrations with susceptibility to dental caries, no correlations have been established. This may be because of the wide variation in concentrations between different subjects, but may also demonstrate that it is dental plaque fluid concentrations and not saliva concentrations which are ultimately important in dental caries.

Salivary IgA concentration is higher in subjects with more dental caries. Tests of susceptibility to dental caries have been developed. They depend either upon measuring salivary buffering capacity (see above under hydrogen carbonate concentrations) or on cultivating bacteria from oral fluid samples (lactobacillus or streptococcal species). Individual variation has again rendered these tests less useful than was hoped.

There is no evidence of any differences in salivary flow rate or composition being significantly related to or due to periodontal disease.

Salivary changes in systemic disease

Salivary flow rate and composition is affected by generalised immunological reactions, cystic fibrosis, Addison's disease, Cushing's syndrome and hyperparathyroidism

Generalised immunological reactions, such as those seen in transplant rejection, may affect the salivary glands, reducing the rate of secretion and raising sodium and chloride concentrations.

Cystic fibrosis is a disease affecting the lungs and pancreas which results from a defective chloride transport protein. It has little effect on the parotid glands but causes decreased secretion from the submandibular, sublingual and minor glands and causes a marked increase in calcium concentrations in the saliva from these glands.

The only endocrine disturbances with noticeable effects on the salivary glands, with the possible exception of hyperparathyroidism, are those of the adrenal cortex. Aldosterone increases the reabsorption of sodium in the striated ducts of salivary glands, reducing the salivary sodium concentrations, and may also increase potassium concentrations in the saliva. The sodium:potassium ratios in saliva can therefore indicate normal, excess or deficient aldosterone secretion.

Calcium and phosphate concentrations in saliva are said to be raised in patients with hyperparathyroidism.

Further reading

Saliva and Oral Health, 2nd edition. Edgar, W.M., O'Mullane, D.M. (editors). British Dental Association, London, 1996

Human Saliva: Clinical Chemistry and Microbiology. Tenovuo, J.O. (editor). CRC Press, Boca Raton, 1989

Aspects of Oral Molecular Biology. Ferguson, D.B. (editor). Karger, Basel, 1991

7 Gingival crevicular fluid

The gingival crevice

The gingival sulcus is the soft tissue groove around a tooth. At its base is the epithelial attachment which seals the soft tissue to the hard tissue

The gingival sulcus or crevice is the groove in the soft tissues around a tooth. It is bounded by the tooth surface, usually enamel, but later in life or after periodontal tissue destruction, it may be cementum and the oral sulcular epithelium, a less well-keratinised continuation of the oral epithelium of the gingiva. At the base of the groove the epithelium becomes only a few cells thick and then extends down parallel with the tooth surface for a short distance (Figs 5.3 and 5.4). This is the junctional epithelium; it is attached to the tooth surface by hemidesmosomes and a thin layer of granular organic material. It is also known as the epithelial attachment. The junctional epithelium has a flat basal layer; it is non-keratinising and desquamates only at the base of the sulcus. Embryologically it derives from the dental epithelium and on the erupting tooth is part of the remains of the ameloblast layer. The cells have wider intercellular spaces than those of the sulcular epithlium and their rate of turnover is higher.

Development of the sulcus

The sulcus develops in response to bacterial irritation

Four stages of sulcular development are described. In the absence of any plaque or gingival inflammation the sulcus is non-existent. In a normal human subject with good oral hygiene the sulcus is less than 0.5 mm in depth. If the depth of the sulcus exceeds this it is usually referred to as a gingival pocket. The connective tissue beneath the oral sulcular and the junctional epithelium is infiltrated with white blood cells, mainly lymphocytes, and a few neutrophil leucocytes migrate through the epithelium to reach the sulcus. The lymphocytic infiltration represents a mild inflammatory reaction and increases or decreases according to the health of the gingival tissue. If acute inflammation develops the epithelium may show minute ulceration. Continuation of this process leads to a deepening of the sulcus: the junctional epithelium migrates down the tooth surface and an irregular ulcerated epithelial layer develops as a lining to the sulcus. This is termed pocket epithelium in distinction from the normal sulcular epithelium in continuity with the oral epithelium and the junctional epithelium at the base of the sulcus. Finally, when the inflammation extends down to reach the periodontal ligament, the junctional epithelium breaks up and most of the sulcus is lined with pocket epithelium.

Gingival crevicular fluid

Any stimulation of the gingiva by mechanical or chemical means results in the production of a sulcular or crevicular fluid which can be collected on filter paper strips or in fine plastic capillaries inserted into the sulcus. Although the fluid was originally called gingival fluid, the term crevicular fluid came into use; the compromise term gingival crevicular fluid is now generally used and often abbreviated to GCF. This fluid in a healthy sulcus is similar in composition to interstitial fluid. It reaches the sulcus by intercellular routes across the epithelial wall. The junctional epithelium in particular is characterised by wide intercellular spaces. The sulcus probably contains more osmotically active material than the interstitium and hence the fluid can move down an osmotic gradient. The organic compostion of the fluid may be modified in its passage across the basement membrane of the epithelium.

Gingival crevicular fluid is a transudate of plasma through the sulcular epithelium

More intense stimulation results in increased permeability of the flat layer of blood capillaries which lies beneath the sulcular epithelium, and the composition of the crevicular fluid then becomes similar to that of plasma.

Flow rate

The rate of production of gingival fluid depends upon the degree of local gingival inflammation

The rate of flow of gingival crevicular fluid is related to the degree of gingival inflammation as assessed clinically. In human subjects with minimal apparent inflammation, flow rates have been measured at between 0.05 and 0.20 µl/min. The fluid content of the sulcus has been assessed at 0.43–1.56 µl in molar interproximal spaces, and 0.24–0.43 µl in anterior teeth. The total flow of fluid is between 0.5 and 2.4 ml/day. A meter is commercially available for clinical use (the Periotron) which measures the amount of fluid taken up by special filter paper strips which can be inserted into the sulcus to give a numerical assessment which is related to the degree of gingival inflammation.

Composition

Cells

Gingival crevicular fluid contains desquamated epithelial cells derived from both the sulcular epithelium and the junctional epithelium. Junctional epithelium, perhaps because its free surface is small compared with its total area, has a higher rate of desquamation than the sulcular epithelium. It is thought that inflammation increases the rate of turnover of the epithelium.

The gingival crevice is the main route by which leucocytes reach the oral cavity. Crevicular fluid contains intact functionally active polymorphonuclear leucocytes (neutrophils); the only other leucocytes present are lymphocytes and monocytes which together make up less than 5% of the crevicular fluid white cell count. The numbers follow the gingival index of inflammation but leucocyte migration and crevicular fluid formation are not linked. The main stimulus for leucocyte migration into the sulcus, as elsewhere in the body, is the presence of chemically attractive substances. Extracts of dental plaque, the protein casein and other substances increase the numbers of leucocytes in the sulcus.

All samples of crevicular fluid contain bacteria similar to those in the adjacent dental plaque but the numbers do not correlate with the amount of supragingival plaque present.

Inorganic ions

Concentrations of inorganic ions in gingival crevicular fluid are similar to those in blood plasma

Almost all the analyses which have been carried out on human gingival crevicular fluid have been on fluid from areas with some degree of gingival inflammation. This is because the volumes of fluid obtainable from areas with very low levels of inflammation are too small for analysis. The composition of the fluid, therefore, would be expected to be similar to that of plasma but might be modified by the local environment of the sulcus. When samples from areas with minimal inflammatory involvement have been assayed for a particular component the concentrations have been much more similar to those in interstitial fluid than in plasma. A further problem is that many analyses have been carried out on these small samples which have been collected on filter paper strips: there is evidence that fluid evaporation from these strips is rapid and hence concentrations may appear higher than in actuality.

Of the ions which have been measured in gingival crevicular fluid (Table 7.1), calcium, magnesium, phosphate and fluoride are within the normal ranges for plasma concentrations. This means that crevicular fluid calcium concentrations are higher than those in saliva, both for total and ionised calcium, and this may have some significance for the deposition of pellicle and plaque at the gingival margins since calcium enhances salivary protein

Table 7.1
Composition of gingival crevicular fluid (GCF)

Component	GCF	Oral fluid	Plasma
Sodium	91.6 + 31.1	6–26	152
Potassium	17.4 + 11.7	13–40	4
Calcium	5.0 + 1.8	0.5–2.8	2.5
Magnesium	0.4 + 0.2	0.3–0.6	1.6
Phosphate	1.3 + 1.0	0.4–5.0	2.1
Protein (g/l)	70	1.2–1.7	70
Albumin (g/l)	35	0.025	35
Gamma globulins (g/l)	7.4	0.050	6–12

Concentrations in mmol/l unless otherwise stated.

precipitation and the aggregation of salivary bacteria. Although in the absence of inflammation calcium concentrations might be expected to be lower than those in plasma, most of the calcium in interstitial fluid is in an ionised form and therefore the concentration of active calcium in the gingival fluid would still be higher than that in saliva.

The concentrations of both sodium and potassium in gingival crevicular fluid are higher than those in plasma. Sodium concentrations in fluid from minimally inflamed gingivae are close to plasma levels but other observations give values 10–40% higher than in plasma. The most likely explanation of the very high values in early reports is the possibility of fluid evaporation from the samples before analysis. It is interesting to note that the sodium concentrations in supragingival plaque fluid are at a much lower level and in the range for saliva. Potassium concentrations are at least twice those in plasma and some reports put them even higher. As gingival crevicular fluid is in contact with cells and some of the leucocytes may also be breaking up, the release of intracellular potassium could be the cause of higher potassium concentrations. This possibility is supported by the observation that potassium concentrations are higher in fluid from deeper pockets. Even then, concentrations are lower than in saliva and very much lower than in plaque fluid.

Organic components

Concentrations of organic components are similar to those in plasma

In general the concentrations of organic components in gingival crevicular fluid are similar to those of interstitial fluid at low levels of gingival inflammation and to those of plasma in more inflamed gingivae. Thus a value of 5 g/l has been given for the total protein content of crevicular fluid from minimally inflamed gingiva and 68 g/l for that from inflamed gingiva.

The carbohydrate composition of gingival fluid is essentially similar to that of plasma. In diabetic patients the glucose content is high, as in plasma.

The major protein of gingival crevicular fluid is serum albumin and its concentration in most samples is similar to that in plasma. It is therefore in much higher concentration than in whole saliva and there is experimental evidence that most of the albumin in whole saliva derives from the gingival crevicular fluid. However, electrophoresis of single gland saliva also shows small amounts of serum albumin. Although many of the plasma globulins and fibrinogen have been detected in crevicular fluid samples, most workers have concentrated on measuring the immunoglobulins. IgA, IgG and IgM have been identified at levels similar to those in plasma and radio-labelled immunoglobulins injected into the bloodstream have been shown to pass into crevicular fluid. There are reports which suggest that the immunoglobulins are present in lower concentrations than in plasma when the fluid is collected from minimally inflamed gingivae, and this would be consonant with the higher albumin:globulin ratio of interstitial fluid. However, some IgG and IgA may be derived from the plasma cells of the gingiva itself. The immunoglobulin concentrations are higher than those in saliva and these proteins would be expected to contribute to the defence of the gingival area.

Complement components of both the classical and alternative pathways may be damaging to tissues as well as to bacteria because they can cause release of lysosomal enzymes from leucocytes and mediate cell lysis.

Protease inhibitors such as alpha-1 antitrypsin, alpha-2 macroglobulin and alpha-1 antichymotrypsin may also act as protective agents.

The small amount of lipid in gingival crevicular fluid is probably derived from plasma, although there may also be a contribution from the cells or bacteria.

Small organic molecules

Gingival crevicular fluid contains lactic acid, urea, hydroxyproline and PGE_2

The pH of the gingival sulcus is stated to be similar to that of resting supragingival plaque at 7.5 up to 8.0. The lactic acid content increases with the severity of inflammation. In contrast, urea, which is present at concentrations several times higher than those in plasma or saliva, decreases in concentration in more severe gingivitis. It is suggested that the high pH of the sulcular area may be due to metabolism of urea by micro-organisms to form ammonia.

Hydroxyproline levels in gingival crevicular fluid have been monitored as a possible means of assessing the breakdown of collagen, and therefore the severity of periodontal breakdown, but have so far proved inconclusive. In similar fashion, though with more success, the concentrations of prostaglandin E_2 (PGE_2) have been measured as an indication of the extent of gingival inflammation.

The gingival sulcus contains potentially pathogenic bacteria; the gingival crevicular fluid, therefore, might be expected to contain bacterial products as well as antibacterial factors from the host. In the first category are the lipopolysaccharides and endotoxins from both live and lysed bacteria and bacterial proteases. Hydrogen sulphide has been detected in crevicular fluid. Antibacterial systems include the immunoglobulins, the lysosomal enzymes from the leucocytes and a peroxidase system similar to that in saliva.

Enzymes of crevicular fluid

Gingival crevicular fluid contains a wide range of enzymes derived from bacteria, leucocytes and squames

Lysosomal enzyme concentrations correlate with pocket depth

The enzymes present in crevicular fluid (Table 7.2) could come from three possible sources: the plasma, bacterial cells or host cells – particularly the polymorphonuclear leucocytes, but also the epithelial squames. Of particular interest are the so-called lysosomal enzymes which can attack cells. Of these, acid phosphatase, beta glucuronidase, lysozyme, hyaluronidase and a number of proteases are found in crevicular fluid at around ten times the concentrations in plasma. All of these are produced by polymorphonuclear leucocytes, bacteria and epithelial squames. All except acid phosphatase occur at concentrations which show a positive correlation with pocket depth. There is evidence that this enzyme may derive particularly from the epithelial squames. The proteases of host origin are all endopeptidases which split protein chains: they include the carboxyendopeptidase cathepsin D, the serine proteases elastase, cathepsin G and plasminogen activator (possibly urokinase), and the metalloendopeptidase collagenase. There are bacteria within the gingival sulcus and in nearby dental plaque which can produce enzymes similar to all these. The adverse effects of these proteases within the sulcus will be moderated or even suppressed by the presence of the protease inhibitors referred to above. In addition to the acid phosphatase there is also alkaline phosphatase in crevicular fluid. It also is probably derived from the

Table 7.2
Enzymes of gingival crevicular fluid

Enzyme	Indicative of disease severity	Prognostic
Acid phosphatase	No	No
Alkaline phosphatase	Yes	No
Cathepsin B	Yes	Yes
Cathepsin D	Yes	?
Cathepsin G	No	No
Collagenase	Yes	No
Dipeptidylpeptidases II and IV	Yes	Yes
Elastase	Yes	Yes
Beta glucuronidase	Yes	Yes
Hyaluronidase	No	No
Lactate dehydrogenase	No	No
Lactoferrin	No	No
Lysozyme	No	No
Plasminogen activator	No	No

polymorphonuclear leucocytes since its concentration is around twice that in plasma. Alkaline phosphatatse is frequently associated with the process of calcification and there is a slight correlation of crevicular fluid alkaline phosphatase concentration with the amount of supragingival calculus. There are no data on the more interesting, and possibly more relevant, correlations with amounts of subgingival calculus. Concentrations of the metabolic enzyme lactate dehydrogenase (LDH), are 10–20 times as high as those in plasma, and the main isozyme present is LDH5, an enzyme characteristic of the anaerobic glycolysis often observed in inflamed tissues.

Functions of gingival crevicular fluid

Gingival crevicular fluid provides a protective flow of fluid towards the oral cavity, and its antibacterial contents assist in this. However, its enzymes are potentially harmful to tissues, and its calcium content may contribute to calculus formation

Gingival crevicular fluid may be protective to the tooth and gingival tissues or it may have adverse effects upon them. It has a protective role in washing potentially harmful cells and molecules out of the gingival sulcus. The immunoglobulins and any other antibacterial substances help to reduce bacterial invasion of the sulcus and may contribute to antibacterial effects in nearby dental plaque and even in saliva. Ionic calcium in the fluid has been suggested to assist in pellicle and plaque formation at the gingival margin. On the negative side, calcium may contribute to calculus formation and this is also promoted by the presence of alkaline phosphatase. The proteolytic enzymes of crevicular fluid are potentially damaging to the wall of the sulcus and the underlying tissues.

In considering these functions it should be remembered that the production of gingival crevicular fluid appears to be a response to inflammation rather than a fluid produced by completely healthy gingival tissue. In this context crevicular fluid may well have a use rather than a function: a number of potentially useful clinical tests have been considered. These range from the use of the Periotron to evaluate crevicular fluid flow to measurement of particular components which give information about the degree of inflammation. At the moment these tests simply confirm clincical assessment (although the Periotron reading is a good patient educator and motivator). There is a hope that tests can bc evolved which will be prognostic as well as diagnostic, and at least one test is now available commercially.

Further reading

Crevicular Fluid Updated. Cimasoni, G. Monographs in Oral Science, Vol. 12. Karger, Basel, 1983

Advances in Periodontal Diagnosis. Eley, B.M., Cox, S.W. British Dental Journal 184: 71–74, 109–113, 161–166, 220–223, 268–271, 323–328, 373–376; 1998

8 Deposits on the surface of teeth

The tooth crown is separated from saliva or air by a thin layer of protein which may be colonised by bacteria

It is probable that the enamel of the tooth surface is rarely exposed directly to saliva or to air except immediately after brushing or perhaps on the contact areas with other teeth during mastication. A newly erupted tooth is still covered by the dental cuticle arising from the remains of the enamel organ. This has an inner amorphous layer, thought to be the last secretion of the ameloblasts, and presumably made up of matrix-like proteins, and an outer cellular layer made up of the condensed outer layers of the enamel organ itself. This cuticle is generally lost rapidly in the oral environment although at the gingival margin it may persist longer.

Enamel pellicle

Pellicle is derived from salivary proteins

The cuticle is replaced by an amorphous layer of glycoproteins derived from saliva. This layer forms on cleaned enamel surfaces within minutes; whole tooth surfaces may be covered within some 20 min and the layer is 1–10 μm thick within 2 h. It is known as the enamel pellicle and, like the cuticle, can be floated off the enamel surface with dilute acids. It is formed by the interaction of negatively charged groups from salivary proteins interacting with the positively charged enamel surface. Such binding probably includes some specific binding to calcium ions on the apatite surface. Proteins in monolayers tend to denature, and this process helps to maintain them on the surface. Teeth alternately dipped in saliva and exposed to air develop a layer of salivary protein dried on the surface which resembles pellicle; it seems unlikely, however, that alternate wetting with saliva and drying would be a mechanism operating in the mouth under normal circumstances. The salivary proteins identified in pellicle include the proline-rich proteins, the histidine-rich proteins and MG1, the larger of the glycoproteins in submandibular saliva. About one-third of the protein in the first-formed layers of pellicle is proline-rich proteins, but these are then degraded by proteases, first to simpler proteins but then further so that in older pellicles proline-rich proteins are barely detectable. The proline-rich proteins not only form part of the pellicle but they also modify the further deposition of other salivary proteins: accumulation of MG1 in dental plaque is inhibited by them.

Pellicle contains specific proteins which may interact with each other and with calcium

In general, phosphoproteins are more tightly bound to apatite.

Accumulation of pellicle and plaque is assisted by the binding of divalent cations (usually calcium ions) to give bridging between proteins and between protein and bacterial cell wall components. The initial stage in the transition from pellicle to plaque may involve proteins which act as bacterial recognition factors – behaving like signal molecules and binding to specific receptor molecules on the bacterial surface. MG1 may be one such bacterial recognition factor; secretory IgA (sIgA) and lysozyme are also bound by bacterial cell walls.

The deposition of particular proteins may be facilitated or inhibited by others: thus alpha amylase and salivary cystatin SA1 bind cooperatively, as do MG1 and sIgA. MG1 deposition is inhibited by glycolipids as well as by the proline-rich proteins. Loss of proline from these latter will abolish their inhibitory influence. The smaller of the so-called mucoproteins of saliva that have been isolated and studied, MG2, has not been found in pellicle: the low sialic acid content suggests that it can be there in very low concentrations if at all. In experiments with apatite binding of proteins, MG2 binding is inhibited by the presence of cysteine-containing proteins.

Development of dental plaque

Dental plaque can be seen forming on a clean tooth surface in about 20 min

Observation of pellicle formation on cleaned enamel surfaces shows that bacterial colonisation begins rapidly near the gingival margin – as early as 20 min after cleaning – and other bacteria spread out either from isolated colonies left in pits and fissures or from foci of salivary bacteria which have attached to the pellicle (Figs 8.1–8.3). By 24 h a uniform covering of bacteria has formed

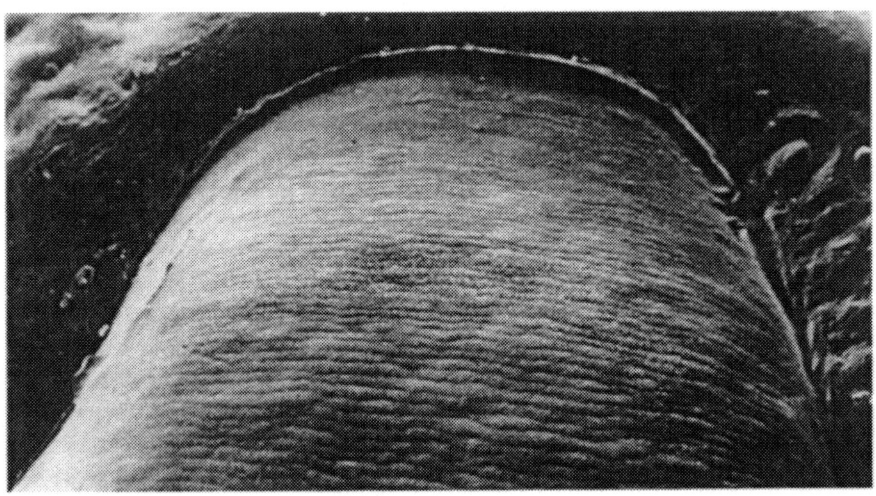

A low power scanning electron micrograph showing the naturally occurring ridges on the smooth surface of an incisor.

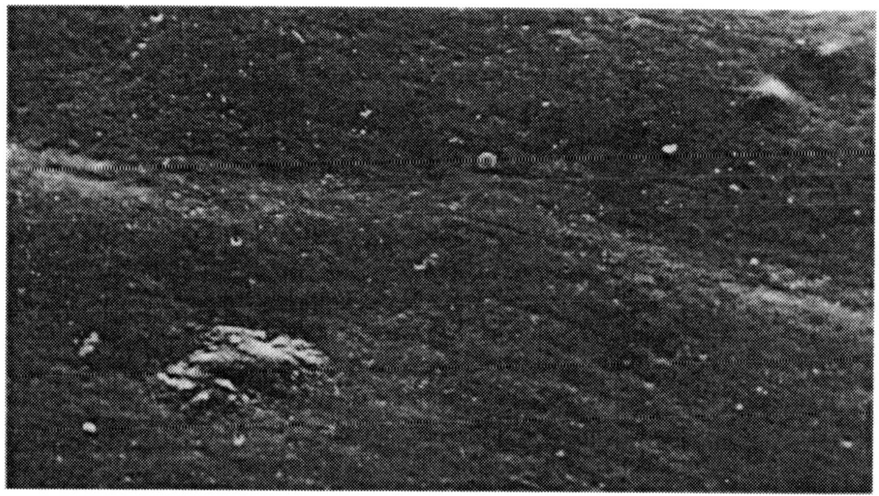

Fig. 8.2
The tooth surface presents a smooth appearance because of the deposition of a layer of pellicle and this is now being colonised by isolated colonies of bacteria.

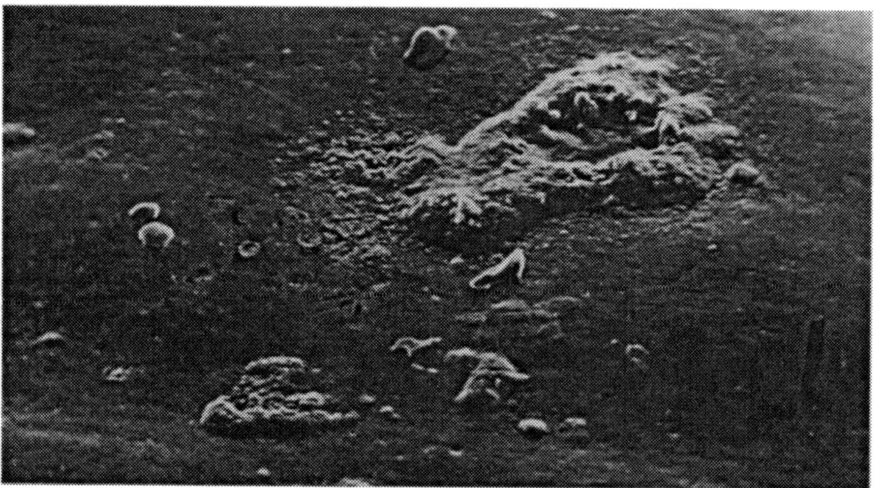

Fig. 8.3
The bacterial colonies fuse together and in this higher power scanning electron micrograph the individual organisms can be seen to be cocci.

and the pellicle plus plaque layer is around 10 µm thick. The range of variation is great and some investigators have reported thicknesses of up to 80 µm in some mouths. If the plaque is undisturbed by brushing it continues to accumulate, reaching 8–35 µm by 48 h and 6–45 µm by 72 h. This initial bacterial colonisation is by Gram-positive cocci and short rod forms with a high proportion of streptococci (Fig. 8.4). Typically, a 24-h plaque would be made up of two layers of streptococci. The bacterial composition changes as the plaque ages, firstly because in deeper regions only anaerobic organisms can survive and cell death of other organisms ensues, and secondly because bacteria develop interdependent colonies with symbiotic relationships. Thus the lactate produced by some veillonellae provides an energy substrate for some streptococci, and the two groups of organisms thrive in association with each other. The 'corncob' appearance described in mature plaque is probably an example of such an association (Fig. 8.5).

The chemical composition of dental plaque

Plaque contains some 80% water, proteins, carbohydrate and inorganic ions. Most of the components are within bacterial cells

The overall chemical composition of dental plaque has been thoroughly investigated. Table 8.1 and Fig. 8.6 give typical values for so-called 'starved' plaque, indicating how bacterial storage of carbohydrate in polymeric form will change the relative composition. The figure of 80–85% water is very similar to that obtained for centrifuged bacterial suspensions. Analyses of this kind ignore any non-homogeneity of dental plaque with its bacteria

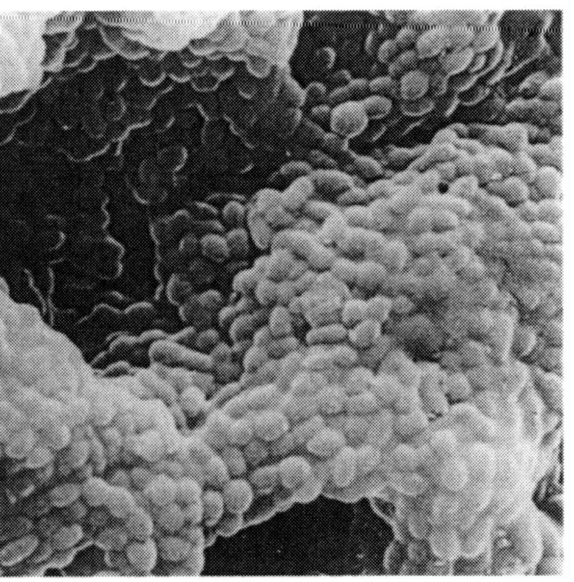

Fig. 8.4
The coccal layers build up to form a thick plaque.

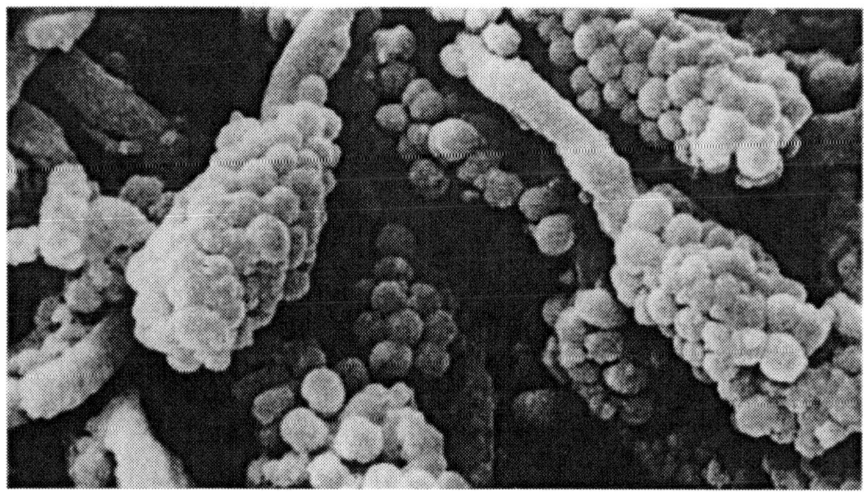

Fig. 8.5
As the plaque ages, rod-like forms appear and complex symbiotic relationships develop. Thus the veillonellae are able to utilise the lactic acid produced by the streptococci and grow together with them. The corncob appearance shown here demonstrates the symbiotic relationship.

Table 8.1
Plaque composition

	Typical values	Range
Inorganic (10% dry weight, approximately 2% wet weight)		
Calcium	8 μg/mg (0.2 μmol/mg)	5–15 μg/mg (0.12–0.38 μmol/mg)
Phosphate	16 μg/mg (0.5 μmol/mg)	
Inorganic P		4–9 μg/mg (0.12–0.24 μmol/mg)
Fluoride		20–100 ppm (1–5 μmol/g)

suspended in a matrix (see Table 8.3 for an example of the gross variation important in dental calculus formation). The matrix is made up of protein, carbohydrate and water. The proteins are partly of salivary origin but probably also of bacterial synthesis. Salivary proteins accumulate in the plaque as a result of pH changes which cause denaturation, and the presence of neuraminidase which cleaves sialic acid from glycoproteins, rendering them less soluble. There is probably also some attachment to bacterial receptor molecules. Of the bacterial proteins the enzyme glucosyl transferase is an important extracellular molecule. Alkaline phosphatase is also at the cell surface.

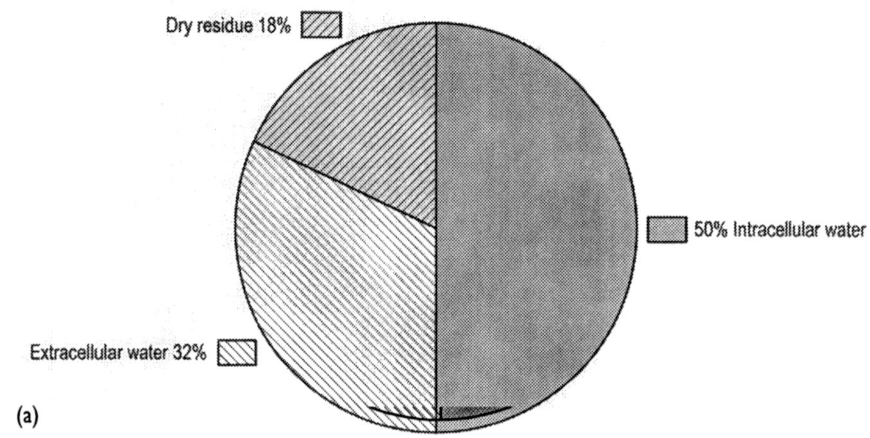

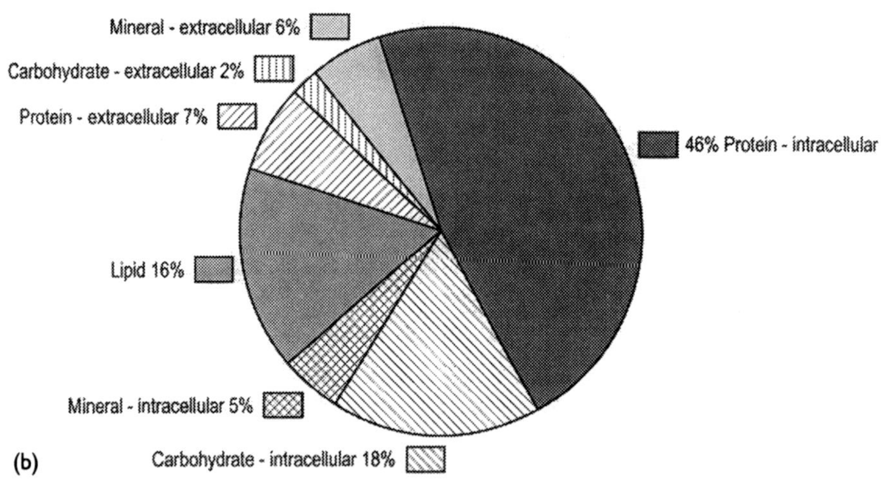

a The distribution of water and solids in 3-day dental plaque. **b** Composition of the residue obtained by drying dental plaque samples which have not been exposed to food for 8 h.

Plaque fluid

Plaque fluid is the extracellular part of plaque obtained by centrifugation. It is the actual chemical

Centrifugation of dental plaque in capillary tubes enables an aqueous layer to be separated. This is known as plaque fluid, and its composition has been investigated as representing the actual chemical phase in equilibrium with the tooth surface. This assumes that diffusion of components through the plaque is relatively free and that protein and carbohydrate between the cells or on the *environment of the oral surface of the tooth*

enamel surface do not form an appreciable barrier. Studies of diffusion tend to support this view: molecules as large as sucrose and lactic acid appear to diffuse easily. The composition of plaque fluid is given in Table 8.2. It will be noted that the potassium levels are high. This may be due to damage to cells as a result of centrifugation or may simply reflect the number of dead or leaky bacterial cells in the plaque. Calcium and phosphorus levels are high – in excess of the solubility product of hydroxyapatite. Calcium and phosphorus concentrations vary from site to site in the mouth, being highest in plaque collected from the lower anterior teeth (Table 8.3). Further, the concentrations of calcium and phosphate increase with the age of the plaque (Fig. 8.7). It is

Table 8.2
Plaque water (data from Tatevossian)

	Range	Mean	Oral fluid
pH	5.7–6.8		6.0
Potassium	30–85	70	21
Sodium	18–35	20	8
Inorganic P	11–54	16	5.5
Organic P		4	
Calcium	0.9–2.3	1.5	0.7
Total Ca	3–12	5	1.35
Magnesium	3.7–4.1	4	0.3
Fluoride (μmol/l)	2–29	2	1.5
Amino acids		17.7	
Carboxylic acids	90–100		
Carbohydrate		14	
Protein (g/l)		15	1.7
Ammonia		36	0.65
Hydrogen carbonate		5	3
Chloride	28–43	35	24

Concentrations are in mmol/l except where otherwise stated.
Albumin is present in greater concentration than in saliva but less than that in blood plasma.
IgA, and secretory IgA concentrations are approximately equal to those in submandibular saliva.
IgG concentrations are greater than those in saliva but less than those in blood plasma.

Table 8.3
Calcium and phosphate concentrations (mg/g) in dental plaque from different sites in the mouth

	Calcium	Phosphate
Lingual of lower incisors	18	21
Labial of upper incisors	6	14
Buccal of lower molars	7	15

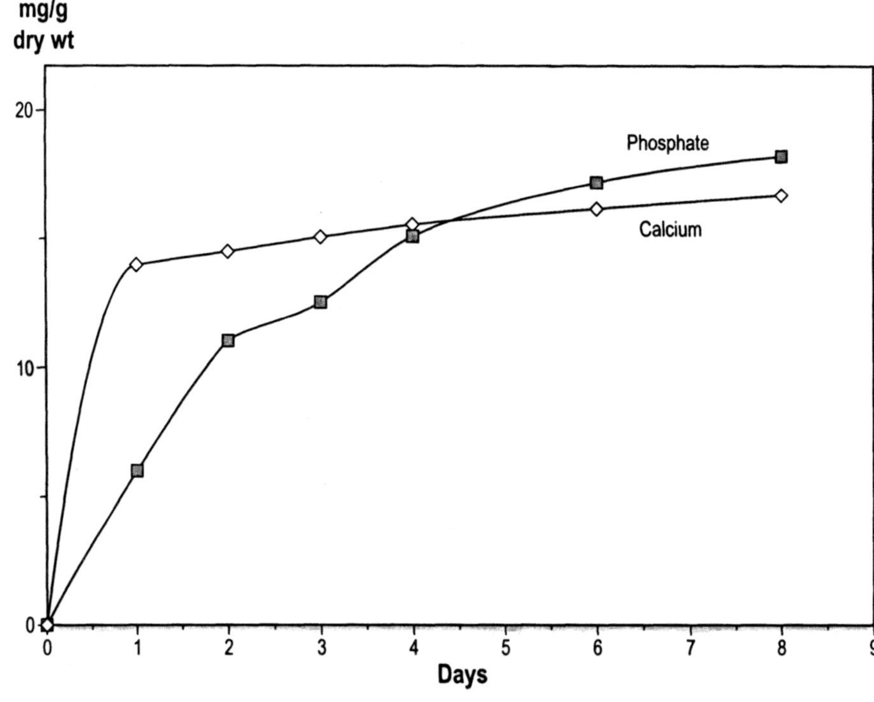

Typical changes in the calcium and phosphate concentrations in dental plaque allowed to remain on the teeth for several days.

not known whether this is true of plaque fluid as well as whole plaque. The carbohydrate content varies according to the time elapsed since the last meal.

Metabolism of dental plaque

Acid production in dental plaque

The metabolic activity of dental plaque relevant to dental health includes acid and alkali production, the synthesis of polysaccharides as well as the production of bacterial toxins and proteolytic enzymes

It is now generally accepted that oral plaque bacteria produce acid from carbohydrate substrates – usually mono- or disaccharides – in the diet, as well as from carbohydrate stored as glycogen within bacteria or glucans (dextrans) stored extracellularly (Fig. 8.8). Of the dietary sugars sucrose appears to be the most harmful because of its relative abundance in the diet and its role as a substrate for dextran production. The anaerobic metabolism results in the production of lactic acid, although other acids are also produced. In plaque fluid the two acids found in highest concentration are acetic and propionic acids. Butyric and formic acids have also been reported in concentrations in excess of lactic acid. At rest plaque contains up to 12 mmol/l lactic acid and this increases up to around 35 mmol/l after sucrose exposure. Acetic acid concentration varies little (normally around 45 mmol/l); propionic acid concentration is usually low.

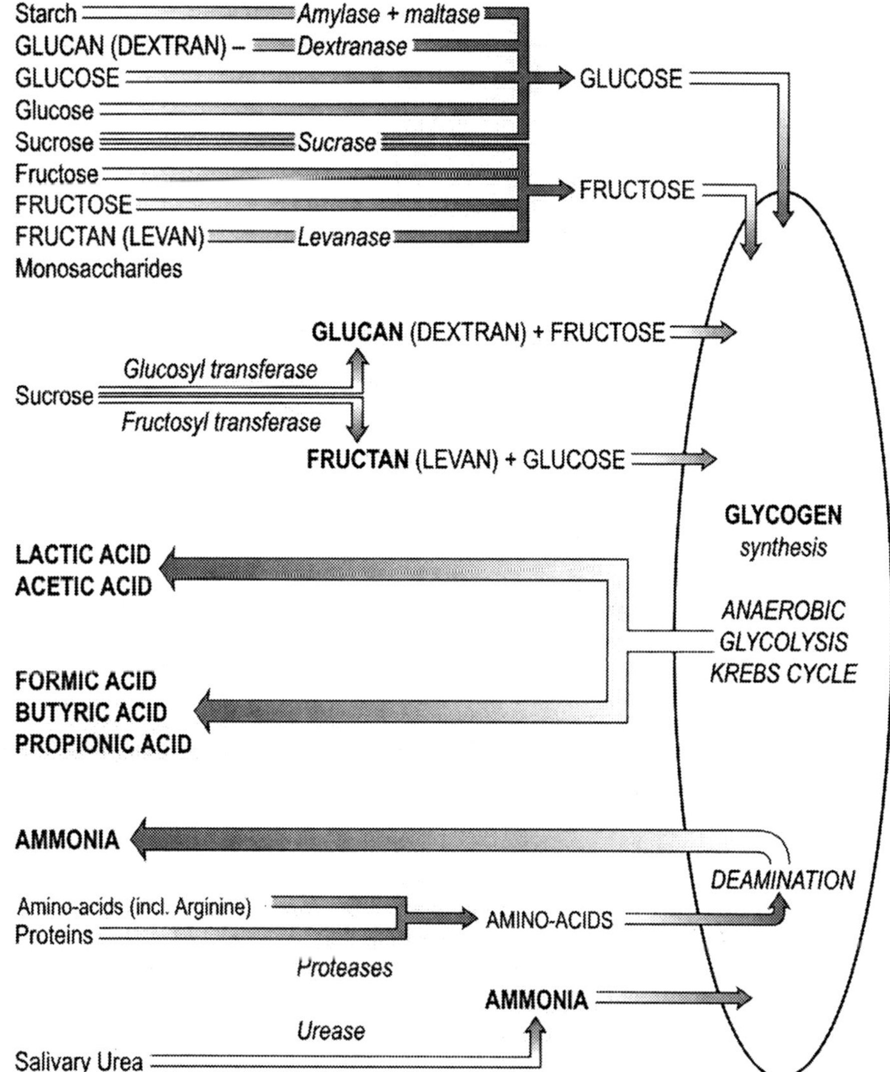

Fig. 8.8
Metabolic activities in dental plaque. Lower case letters are used to denote dietary constituents, bold upper case letters to denote final products within the plaque, and italic letters to denote enzyme activity. Intracellular events are shown in the ellipse on the right; all other events can occur extracellularly. The term glycosyl transferase is used to include both glucosyl and fructosyl transferases.

The pH attained in dental plaque after sugar fermentation may be as low as 4.0. Intake of sugar leads to a rapid fall in pH followed by a slower rise back to the original level over 20–30 min. The typical curve was first described by Stephan and is therefore known as the Stephan curve (Fig. 8.9). There have been repeated attempts to model this curve on the basis of the diffusion of sugar into the dental plaque and diffusion of the hydrogen ions outwards, and computer

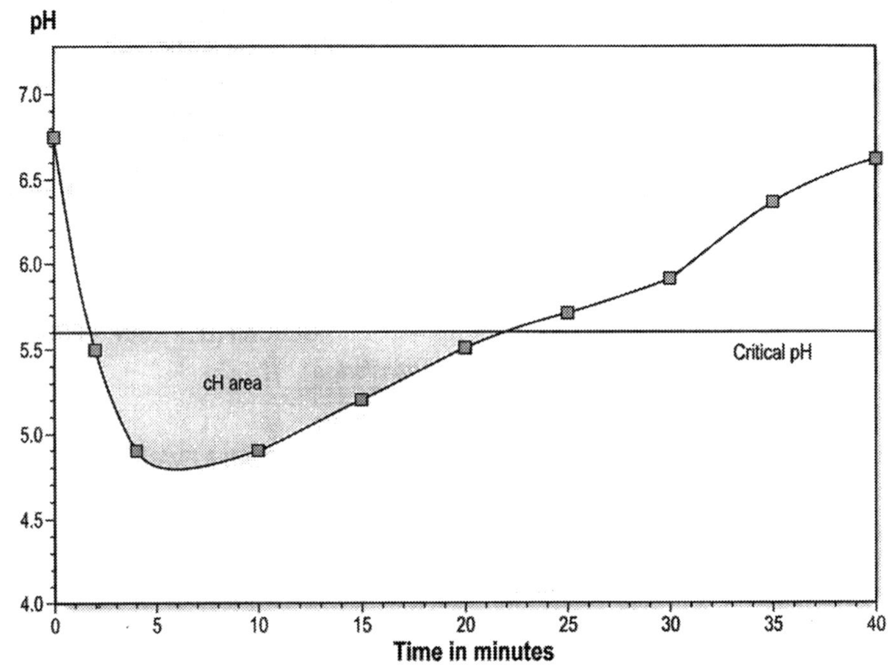

The curve of pH change in dental plaque following exposure to a sugar solution at time 0, usually known as a Stephan curve.

models are now beginning to resemble the observed curves. The lowest pH depends upon these factors and also upon plaque buffering. The buffering capacity is greater than that in saliva and probably depends largely upon phosphate buffering, although acetate/acetic acid itself could be an important buffer. The importance of the hydrogen carbonate buffering from saliva is, however, shown dramatically when saliva is excluded from the plaque (Fig. 8.10).

The pH of dental plaque determines whether enamel passes into solution. A critical pH for this process was calculated in a rat model of caries many years ago, which was based on the calcium and phosphorus concentrations in rat saliva. The figure of 5.6 has been quoted many times in relation to human dental caries despite the recognition that the calcium and phosphorus concentrations in human saliva differ from those in rat saliva. Fig. 8.11 shows the solubility lines for hydroxyapatite with the normal ranges of relevant salivary ions. The lower line of salivary ion products crosses the solubility line between pH 5.5 and 5.6. The most recent calculations of a critical pH in human dental plaque are based on measured calcium and phosphate concentrations in plaque fluid. Unfortunately the simple assumption that the mineral likely to dissolve is entirely hydroxyapatite is complicated by variation in the composition of the enamel surface, the presence of other calcified components and the wide variation in calcium and phosphorus concentrations in plaque fluid. A range of values from 6.4 down to 5.0 has therefore been given. If enamel were pure hydroxyapatite, the figure would be around 4.6. Some of the more recent computer models predict values below 5.0 at their lowest points.

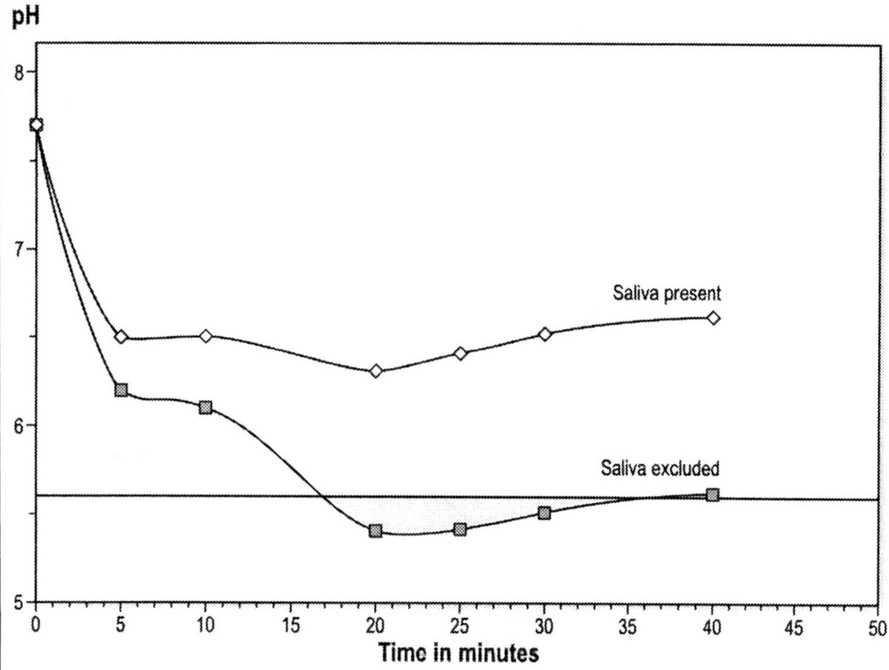

Fig. 8.10
Stephan curves in the presence and absence of saliva, demonstrating the buffering effect of salivary hydrogen carbonate.

Production of alkali in dental plaque

Dental plaque exposed to urea solution produces ammonia, and its pH therefore rises. Plaque proteases are able to degrade protein to yield amino acids which can serve as substrates for plaque metabolism to yield ammonia. Arginine in particular appears to be an important source of ammonia, and a tetrapeptide containing an arginine residue, known as sialin, which is normally found in saliva, probably functions as a plaque pH raising agent.

Whilst some metabolism of this kind could occur in parallel with acid production and perhaps reduce its impact on the plaque pH, the main period of alkali production is during periods of carbohydrate starvation – overnight, for example. Plaque pH values before breakfast were found in many subjects to be high. However, utilisation of carbohydrate stored as dextran could negate the effect of alkali production.

The pH of dental plaque will depend upon the mixture of foods to which it is exposed and the effect of pH upon dental enamel may be modified by other components

Plaque pH changes during food consumption

Studies of plaque pH during and after the consumption of various foodstuffs give complex pH curves and demonstrate the effects of acid- and alkali-generating substrates. Diffusion within plaque and into saliva complicate the picture – many acidic foodstuffs may actually raise plaque pH by

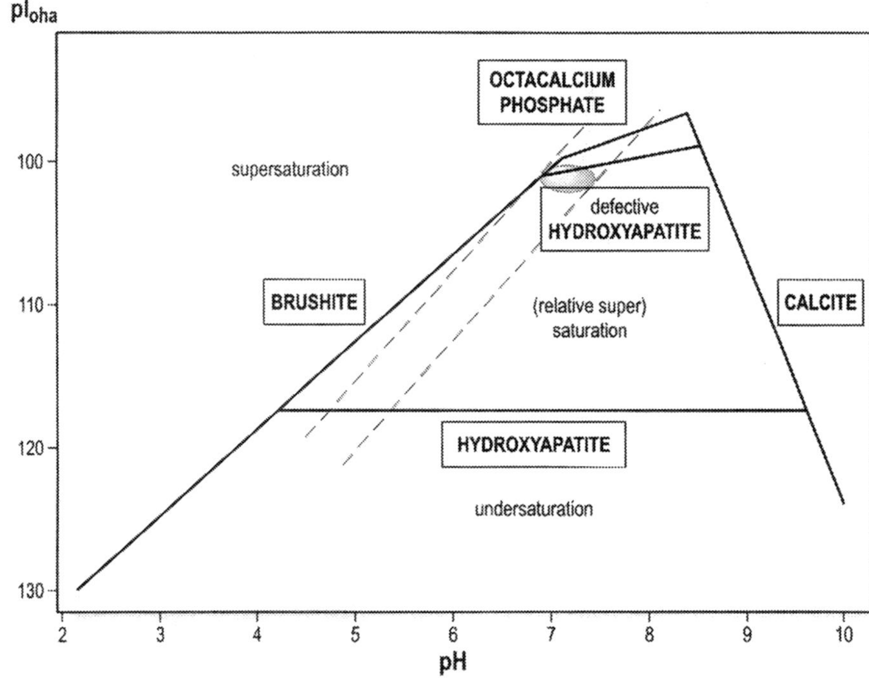

The hydroxyapatite phase diagram with a coloured ellipse showing the normal range of ion concentrations in saliva. The coloured dotted lines show how the ellipse would move at different pH values. In dental caries the ellipse moves down into the zone of hydroxyapatite dissolution, whilst increasing concentrations of calcium, phosphate and hydroxide move the pI upwards in the diagram, favouring precipitation, particularly as the pH becomes more alkaline.

stimulating saliva flow and increasing outward diffusion of acid. Cheese may have an effect in this way whilst simultaneously increasing intraoral calcium levels.

Polysaccharide synthesis in dental plaque

A characteristic feature of bacterial plaque metabolism is the synthesis of carbohydrate polymers from the simpler sugars. Like most cells, plaque bacteria store glucose in the form of glycogen and this intracellular store provides substrate for later metabolic activity. However, the bacteria of dental plaque, particularly *Streptococcus mutans*, also synthesise two other carbohydrate polymers when given access to sucrose. The glucosyl transferase enzymes break down sucrose to its constituent monosaccharides of fructose and glucose and then use the energy derived to build up fructose and glucose polymers. The glucose polymer is known as dextran or glucan: the glucose linkages are all alpha-1,6 bonds. Other glucans with more complex linkages may also be formed. The fructose polymer, levan or fructan, is similar: the linkages are probably of the beta-1,2 type. Both glucans and fructans are deposited extracellularly and therefore provide a voluminous sticky environment for the plaque organisms: the ability of the oral micro-organisms to form plaque on the tooth surface is directly related to their ability to synthesise these polysaccharides. Most methods of plaque control that have been explored have been based either on the blockage of bacterial glucosyl transferase activity and the resultant reduction in bacterial colonisation of the tooth surface and inability of the bacteria to produce thick plaques which hold acid metabolites close to the tooth surface, or on ways of solubilising the gel-like polysaccharides so that the plaque can be easily washed off the tooth surface.

Other dentally important features of plaque metabolism

Two other aspects of plaque metabolism are of obvious importance in relation to the health of the oral soft tissues around the teeth rather than in relation to the teeth themselves. Plaque bacteria, like other bacteria, produce exotoxins and have antigenically active cell wall components which can induce adverse tissue reactions. They also produce enzymes which can break down tissue components: proteolytic enzymes such as collagenase and elastase can obviously break down the host tissues. Enzymes of dental plaque may be of importance in calculus formation both by breaking down inorganic phosphates and by releasing calcium bound to protein.

Calculus

Dental calculus forms as calcium and phosphate concentrations in plaque rise

As plaque matures on the tooth surface its calcium and phosphate concentrations rise (Fig. 8.7). At about 3 days, calcification may begin to occur (Fig. 8.11 shows the conditions for calcification). At this stage there is no evidence of apatite formation by X-ray spectrography, but from this time onwards a hand instrument gives a sensation of minute traces of hard particulate matter being present – a slight 'crackly' sensation. This is particularly noticeable in plaque collected from tooth surfaces close to the ducts of major salivary glands – mainly the lingual surfaces of the lower incisors, but also to a lesser extent the buccal surfaces of the upper first molars (Fig. 8.12) and the labial aspects of the lower incisor interdental spaces. It is probable that the first formed material is the so-called amorphous calcium phosphate and this is later spontaneously transformed into hydroxyapatite. Crystallisation is homogeneous: increasing local concentrations of calcium and phosphate exceed the solubility product. This would account for apparently random spicules of calcium phosphate seen in electron micrographs of forming dental calculus. If this explanation is correct it would imply that there are areas of dental plaque in which acid production is unlikely to produce decalcification of the enamel surface because the ion concentrations are in excess of the solubility product. However, it is not uncommon to find tooth

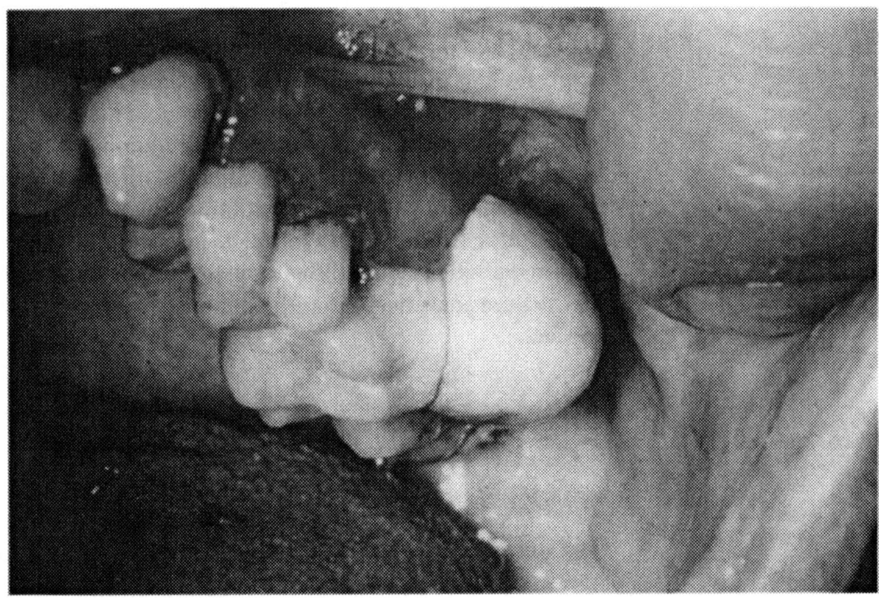

Fig. 8.12
An example of heavy calculus formation on the buccal side of an upper molar.

surfaces on which there is evidence of caries attack close to areas of calculus formation. This has led to the consideration of the possibility of calcification at lower concentrations of the relevant ions and possible mechanisms of very localised increases in ion concentration. There is no evidence of accumulation of calcium salts in structures like matrix vesicles by plaque bacteria. In some electron microscope pictures some bacteria can be seen with internal crystallisation which leads on to the total calcification of the bacterium in an apparently non-calcified matrix; when the bacterial wall is lost the crystalline mass can grow by apposition. However, the beginnings of crystallisation are more usually seen in the plaque matrix. Possible seeding substances have been suggested to be present. Collagen is clearly not a plaque constituent but there are glycoproteins and lipids present, both of which have been suggested as possible groups of nucleating substances in bone calcification. Many of the salivary proteins associated with dental plaque can bind calcium and may therefore be possible seeds for crystal formation. On the other hand, many research workers have identified proteolytic enzymes of bacterial origin in dental plaque and suggest that these may split the calcium-binding proteins of saliva to increase the local concentrations of calcium. The importance of salivary calcium-binding proteins is therefore unclear: they may maintain calcium in solution but they may also serve as substrates for bacterial enzymes and release their calcium in dental plaque or they may even accumulate calcium in dental plaque. One salivary component that has been associated with reduced levels of calculus formation is pyrophosphate. Calculus-inhibiting toothpastes have therefore been developed containing pyrophosphate. As in bone this inhibits calcification but it may be split by phosphatases. The predominant phosphatases of dental plaque are alkaline phosphatases rather than the acid phosphatases of saliva; alkaline phosphatases in tissues are often associated with mineralisation. One interesting observation on plaque from subjects who readily form calculus is that fibronectin levels are higher than in non-calculus formers. This raises the possibility that fibronectin may help in the attachment of calculus to the tooth surface – an attachment which can be exceedingly difficult to break.

Once crystallisation has been initiated, crystal growth can occur. Theoretically it should be possible for the enamel surface to act as a seeding surface, but sections of calculus always show a clear division between calculus and enamel – possibly because of the pellicle or the innermost layer of the plaque forming some kind of barrier. An alternative explanation is that calculus may indeed by intimately linked to the enamel in some places, but its greater organic content and lack of defined structure makes the distinction between the tissue and its covering clear.

Bacteria may assist in calcification by providing nucleating substances

Thus far the formation of calculus has been considered as a purely physicochemical event with calcium salts being bound and precipitated in an extracellular environment. Bacteria can be involved in this process by raising the local pH by urease activity, by increasing local ion concentrations, by splitting calcium-binding proteins and by removing local inhibitors of calcification such as pyrophosphate. However, many oral bacteria in media with high calcium and phosphate concentrations are capable of taking up these ions and themselves calcifying. Thus *Corynebacter matruchottii*, *Actinomyces israeli* and *Streptococcus salivarius* have all been observed to calcify intracellularly, whilst the veillonellae calcify extracellularly. *C. matruchottii* is a filamentous organism invariably present in calculus. Histological sections of forming calculus usually show needle- or plate-like crystals forming in the plaque matrix, but calcified bacteria are also seen in isolation or ahead of a mineralising front. *C. matruchottii* has been extensively studied as the most likely bacterium to be involved in calculus formation. In media with high calcium and phosphate concentrations it takes about 3 days for intracellular calcification to become visible. Proteolipids and high energy metabolites are necessary. The first formed crystals resemble those of brushite but these metamorphose into a poorly crystalline apatite. There is a specific bacterial proteolipid with a hydrophobic protein core of about 10 000 kDa and acidic phospholipid periphery which can function as a nucleating site. In association with another proteolipid it may form an ion channel in the bacterial cell membrane. The proteolipids are also capable of structuring cell membrane phospholipids to form calcium-binding complexes similar to those observed in chondrocytes and in matrix vesicles. Indeed *C. matruchottii* can itself secrete matrix vesicles. The other protein component of *C. matruchottii* which appears to have a role in mineralisation is alkaline phosphatase. Two interconvertable alkaline phosphatases are present in the cell membranes, one with an optimal pH between 7 and 7.5, the other with an optimal pH of 10. The presence of this enzyme is associated with phosphate transport.

All calculus is largely made up of apatite, although subgingival and supragingival calculus

The composition of fully formed calculus has been determined (Table 8.4). There are differences clinically between calculus formed above the gingival margin and that formed in the gingival crevice. Supragingival calculus is white or yellow; subgingival calculus is dark brown or greenish in colour and

Table 8.4
Composition of dental calculus

	Organic	CO_3	Ca	P	Na
Supragingival (80–89% mineral)					
Highly calcified	11%	2%	28%	16%	2.09%
Poorly calcified	20%	3.7%	26.9%	14.9%	2.58%
Subgingival (71–83% mineral)					
Highly calcified	17%	1.3%	31%	16%	1.77%
Poorly calcified	29%	3.6%	25%	14.6%	1.26%

Matrix 12–20% carbohydrate (6% hexose, 4% fucose, 2–3% hexosamine and glycosaminoglycans), 3% lipid (probably bacterial)

may vary in mineral composition. The gingivitis and periodontitis resulting from calculus accumulation may be due to mechanical irritation, but also to the products of bacterial plaque on the surface of the calculus

is much more firmly adherent to the tooth surface. These differences may arise from differences in formation – subgingival calculus being formed in a different, more anaerobic, bacterial environment, or being seeded by gingival fluid or plasma components rather than components of salivary origin – or differences in location after formation – the different nature of cementum or dentine surfaces and the frequency of bleeding in the gingival crevice. Thus the colour of subgingival calculus is most likely to be due to the presence of haemoglobin breakdown products such as bilirubin. The greater hardness of subgingival calculus as reported by clinicians is shown by the lower organic and higher inorganic content. The two types of calculus, however, are broadly similar in their inorganic composition and the crystalline forms detected in them (Table 8.5). It is interesting that calculus contains a relatively high proportion of whitlockite, a salt usually formed in the presence of magnesium ions. The magnesium content of saliva is higher than that of plasma. The hydroxyapatite of calculus readily exchanges with ions in its environment: its fluoride content is high and many trace elements have been identified in it. There is evidence that calculus contains some silica compounds.

The presence of calculus is frequently associated with inflammation and bleeding – gingivitis. Although this was thought to be due to the mechanical action of the calculus and the constant irritation of a hard rough surface against the thinly keratinised epithelium lining the gingival crevice, it is now believed that the bacterial endotoxins from the plaque on the calculus surface are the main source of the inflammatory response. The bacteria produce a variety of enzymes, many of which are proteolytic and contribute to the gingival fluid in the crevice.

Table 8.5
Distribution of different calcium phosphate crystal forms

	Supragingival	Subgingival
Apatite	58%	53%
Brushite	9%	6%
Octacalcium phosphate	21%	12%
Whitlockite	21%	30%

Further reading

Oral Microbiology, 3rd edition. Marsh, P., Martin, M. Chapman & Hall, London, 1992

Symposium on the Chemical Control of Plaque and Gingivitis. Journal of Dental Research 71: 1423–1449; 1992

Symposium on Plaque Fluid: Biochemistry and Properties of the Plaque/Enamel Interface. Journal of Dental Research 69: 1307–1342; 1990

9 Nutrition and diet in relation to oral health

Nutrition is the nutrient intake

Nutrition is the supply of essential foodstuffs and water to the body. It can be expressed in terms of the intake of proteins, fats and carbohydrates, vitamins, essential minerals and trace elements. Recommended values exist for minimum daily requirements and these are published as tables (Table 9.1). The data from which these tables are generated are based on Western diets and may not be universally valid; and even in Western countries the recommendations should always be checked to see if they are appropriate to the age and sex of the individual. The term diet is perhaps best reserved for the form in which the nutrients are supplied – that is say, the actual foodstuffs eaten. Table 9.2 gives analyses of a number of commonly consumed dietary items in terms of their nutritional value.

Diet is what we eat

Nutrition affects all tissues including those of the mouth

The nutrition of an individual will affect all tissues of the body, although some components may be particularly important for specific tissues – vitamin D and calcium for bone, for example. In the oral cavity nutrient intake will be important during development and growth, and then in the continued maintenance of tissues. The tissues which are unique to the mouth are the dental tissues, but these are embedded in fibrous connective tissue and bone, and the mouth itself is lined with epithelium. At all stages after weaning, the mouth is subject to contact with dietary constituents during feeding and the local action of these upon the oral and dental tissues is a special feature of this area. Thus the form in which nutrients are provided may have important consequences in the mouth but be much less important in relation to the rest of the body. This chapter will deal first with the broad topic of nutrition, picking out oral implications, and then go on to some of the aspects of diet which relate to oral health and disease.

The oral tissues come into contact with all dietary constituents

Nutrition and oral health

Protein

Protein is essential as the source of amino acids from which the body's own proteins will be built up or replaced. The recommended daily allowance of 30 g is based partly on the amount of urea excreted from the body and is designed to maintain nitrogen balance. Clearly larger amounts may be necessary during growth when additional new protein is being formed. The

Table 9.1
Dietary reference values

	Child, 5 years		Adult, 25 years		Adult, 75 years		Pregnancy
	M	F	M	F	M	F	
Energy (MJ)	7.16 (1715)	6.46 (1545)	10.6 (2550)	8.1 (1940)	8.77 (2100)	7.61 (1810)	8.9 (2140)
Saturated fatty acids	10%	10%	10%	10%	10%	10%	
Total fatty acids	30%	30%	30%	30%	30%	30%	
Carbohydrate	47%	47%	47%	47%	47%	47%	
Protein (g)	19.7	19.7	55.5	45	53.3	46.5	51
Vitamins							
Thiamin (mg)	0.7	0.7	1.0	0.8	0.9	0.8	0.9
Riboflavin (mg)	0.8	0.8	1.3	1.1	1.3	1.1	1.4
Niacin (mg)	11	11	17	13	16	12	
B_6 (mg)	0.9	0.9	1.4	1.2	1.4	1.2	
B_{12} (μg)	0.8	0.8	1.5	1.5	1.5	1.5	
C (mg)	30	30	40	40	40	40	50
A (μg)	500	500	700	600	700	600	700
D (μg)	Only needed in diet if living entirely indoors						10
Minerals							
Calcium (mmol)	11.3	11.3	17.5	17.5	17.5	17.5	
(mg)	450	450	700	700	700	700	
Iron (μmol)	110	110	160	260	160	160	
(mg)	6.1	6.1	8.7	14.8	8.7	8.7	

Source: Dietary Reference Values for Food, Energy and Nutrients for the United Kingdom. HMSO, 1991.

Table 9.2
Nutritional values of commonly consumed dietary items

Food	Energy	Protein	Carbohydrate	Fat	Vit. A	Thiamine	Riboflavin	Niacin	Vit. B_{12}	Vit. C	Vit. D	Vit. K	Ca	Fe	P
Milk	63	3.4	4.9	3.4 (2.1)*	0.007	0.04	0.10	0.2	0.0003	1.0	0.001	0	123	0.4	112
Cream	198	2.6	4.1	19.1 (11.9)	0.44	0.04	0.17	0.1	0.0003	1.0	0.001	0	91	0.1	76
Cheese	395	24	1.5	31.9 (20.63)	0.65	0.07	0.40	0.4	0.0003	0	0.001	0.3	694	0.6	346
Butter	741	0.8	0	82 (50.8)	0.75	0	0	0	0	0	0.004	0	12	0.01	5
Eggs	155	12.6	1	10.6 (3.28)	0.4	0.06	0.42	0.4	0.005	0	0.0025	0.02	25	0.5	96
Beef	199	23	0	11.9 (5.0)	0	0.7	0.18	3.5	0.002	0	0	0.4	8	2.4	182
Ham	170	18.5	1.5	10 (2.1)	0	0.40	0.14	3.0	0.0004	15	0	0.1	4	0.5	140
Cod	74	16	0	1.0 (0.07)	0.006	0.1	0.1	2.0	0.002	2	0	0.01	5	0.2	148
Mashed potato	65	2	14	0.1 (0.05)	0	0.01	0.03	1.3	0	9.4	0	0.08	7	0.8	26
Carrot	40	1.1	8.5	0.2 (0.02)	2.95	0.07	0.04	0.67	0	7.0	0	0.01	34	0.7	32
Cauliflower	30	2.4	4.5	0.2 (0.02)	0.009	0.09	0.03	0.34	0	60	0	0.4	33	1.0	22
Apple tart	308	2.6	45	13.1 (6.9)	0	0.13	0.09	1.2	0	1	0	0.02	9	1.1	28
Apple	58	0.2	13.5	0.4 (0.08)	0.007	0.03	0.01	0.11	0	8	0	0.01	5	0.2	10
Orange	50	1.0	11.0	0.2 (0.05)	0.027	0.1	0.05	0.3	0	58	0	0.1	40	0.1	20
Bread	240	8.0	50.0	0.8 (0.5)	0	0.3	0.15	3.0	0	0	0	0.1	50	2.2	200
Fruitcake	413	6.4	54.8	18.7 (7.5)	0	0.2	0.2	2.0	0	0.5	0	0	40	2.0	110
Shortbread biscuit	457	5.5	75.0	15.0 (8.7)	0.024	0.2	0.2	1.6	0	0	0	0	80	1.5	260
Cornflakes	370	7.0	83	0.7 (0.3)	[illegible]	1.2	1.3	15.0	0.0008	0	0.0028	0	0.5	7.9	50

Energy values are expressed in kcal/100 g, values for protein, carbohydrate and fat in g/100 g, all other values are used in mg/100 g.
*Values in parentheses are for saturated fat.

Low protein intake during tooth development may lead to later caries experience

same may be true in recovery from illness or starvation when the body may have been losing nitrogen as protein was mobilised as an energy source. Protein is an essential part of all oral tissues, particularly in the form of collagen. The effects of protein starvation in early or foetal life may affect the later health of oral tissues. Rats on a diet inadequate in protein are more susceptible to dental caries in later life. Human beings have also been shown to be more susceptible to dental caries under similar circumstances. Proteins are also essential for the synthesis of immunoglobulins and other defence proteins: in chronic protein starvation there is reduced resistance to infection. The oral cavity has a large commensal bacterial population and minor injuries to the mucosa can lead to persistent and severe ulceration when defence mechanisms are weak.

Two types of protein deficiency are prevalent in developing countries. Kwashiorkor is a condition of protein deficiency per se, whilst marasmus is a consequence of protein-energy malnutrition. In the latter condition there is reduced secretion of IgA in saliva and this may contribute towards caries susceptibility. Acute starvation has been shown to reduce salivary flow rate and alter salivary composition – again favouring caries development.

Fat

Fat = energy+EFAs+fat-soluble vitamins

The supply of lipids is important for several reasons. Firstly, fat is a compact form of energy and can provide large amounts of energy in small bulk. Secondly, there are some essential fatty acids (EFAs) which are necessary for synthesis of lipid molecules in the body. Thirdly, there are a number of fat-soluble vitamins which will not be obtained naturally unless there are fats in the diet. Diets which are inadequate in fats, therefore, may result in vitamin deficiencies as well as having direct effects. Animals raised on low fat diets show poor calcification of dentine. This implies that some lipids are essential for calcification, as has been suggested in studies of calcification, although no specific component and no mechanism in which lipids could be involved have been identified.

Lipids may be essential for calcification

Carbohydrate

Carbohydrate = energy

Carbohydrates function solely as energy sources. Deficiency of carbohydrate alone is unlikely but would manifest simply as energy deficit; as both lipids and protein can be metabolised to provide energy, this would probably be unimportant.

Vitamins

There is considerable observational and experimental evidence on the effects of vitamin deficiency and vitamin excess on oral structures. In almost every example these effects are local manifestations of effects on the body as a whole. Vitamins are classified as water-soluble or lipid-soluble. Deficiencies of either type may be detrimental but excess is harmful only for the lipid-soluble vitamins. This is because an excess of a water-soluble vitamin is readily excreted via the kidneys whilst and excess of a lipid-soluble vitamin accumulates in the body. Vitamin B_6 appears to be an exception to this general rule since it can produce harmful effects when taken in excess.

The main water-soluble vitamins are those of the B group and vitamin C.

Vitamin B group

Deficiencies of the B vitamins may cause oral soft tissue symptoms

The B group are a diverse group of micronutrients which function as metabolic intermediaries or as regulators of red blood cell development. Vitamin B_2, riboflavine, is the precursor of the oxidation-reduction co-enzymes flavin mononucleotide and flavin adenine dinucleotide (FMN and FAD). It is rarely deficient in the diet by itself but deficiencies are usually associated with those of nicotinamide and often of other B vitamins. Nicotinamide is also a main component of co-enzymes such as the co-enzymes of dehydrogenation, nicotinamide adenine dinucleotide and nicotinamide dinucleotide phosphate (NAD and NADP). Oral symptoms of these deficiencies are pallor of the lips and loss of epithelium to give the red shiny appearance described as cheilosis, particularly marked at the angles of the mouth, where actual fissuring may occur (angular cheilitis), and a loss of epithelium on the tongue to give a red shiny glossitis.

Vitamin B_{12}, cyanocobalamin, and folic acid deficiencies both result in megaloblastic anaemia; the main oral symptom is a pale appearance of the mucosa, but there may also be local inflammation.

Vitamin C

Vitamin C is essential for collagen formation

Vitamin C deficiency, manifesting as scurvy, produces oral symptoms sufficiently marked to have been the diagnostic factor in many cases. Vitamin C, ascorbic acid, is a powerful anti-oxidant which can maintain iron as iron(II) in situations where iron(II) is a necessary co-factor for the hydroxylation of proline and lysine. It is therefore essential for the formation of the triple helix of tropocollagen from the procollagen peptides. Although deficiency of ascorbic acid produces marked effects in humans, the effects are even more dramatic in the guinea pig and there is much experimental data gained from this animal. Acute ascorbic acid deficiency in adult humans manifests first as swelling and redness of the interdental papillae, which progresses to purplish inflammation and loss of epithelium. There is spontaneous bleeding from small capillaries (petechiae). The red, swollen, bleeding gums are often the first sign of scurvy, but later there is petechial bleeding in the skin and other soft tissues. As collagen is a major component of the walls of small blood vessels their structure is weakened and they damage easily. Blood is lost into tissues to appear as bruises or frank bleeding occurs. The capillary fragility of scurvy seems to be due to deficiencies in basal membrane formation as well as to the poor quality of the supporting collagen. Collagen is a vital part of all connective tissues and a component of the matrix of bone, dentine, and cementum. In the scorbutic guinea pig (Fig. 9.1) there is poor bone formation with a deficiency of normal matrix and any bony defects are made good only by a loose, poorly organised fibrous network. The continuously growing incisors have deficiencies of dentine formation where the collagenous matrix

Vitamin C deficiency (scurvy) manifests as gingivitis and as bruising in response to minor trauma

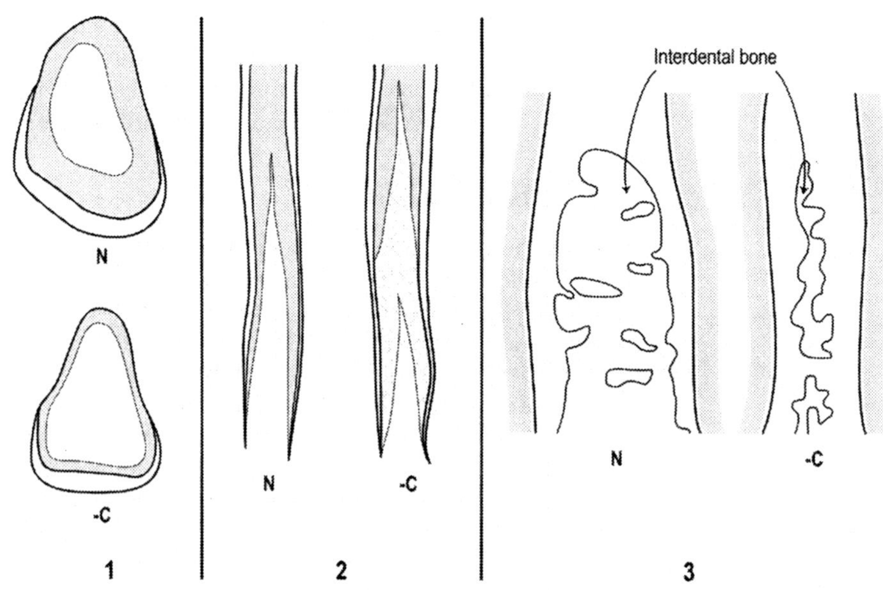

Effects of vitamin C deficiency observed in the guinea pig. The dentine is coloured in each diagram and the diagrams are marked N for normal and C for vitamin C-deficient. Diagram 1 is a section through a guinea pig incisor showing the poor development of the dentine in the deficient animal. The developing molars of a guinea pig in diagram 2 show the poor development of dentine and the substitution of a poorly calcified irregular secondary dentine in the rest of the pulp in the C-deficient animal. Diagram 3 shows poorly developed bone and periodontal ligaments between the molars of the C-deficient guinea pig.

Poor collagen formation affects fibrous tissues and bone remodelling

Anti-oxidants such as vitamins C and E may protect against harmful effects of superoxides

is absent or poorly formed. If the vitamin deficiency is present at the time of formation of the permanent molars these too will have dentine inadequate in quantity and quality. The human is less susceptible to vitamin C deficiency but all functions which require collagen will be impaired. Thus wound healing is poor and the fibrous tissue produced in the wound readily breaks down to re-open the wound. Tissues with a high rate of collagen turnover are weakened: the periodontal ligament is affected and teeth become loose in their sockets. Bone remodelling is impaired by the poor collagen matrix and bone fractures heal poorly. Fibroblasts migrate into areas of bone deficiencies and they fill with weak, poorly organised fibrous tissue. Most Western diets contain sufficient fresh fruit and vegetables to maintain an adequate supply of vitamin C but the vitamin is readily oxidised in cooking and storage. Acute cases of avitaminosis have been reported among older people living alone and subsisting on diets lacking in fruit and vegetables, and there are some suggestions that so-called subclinical deficiency may be not uncommon and manifest as gingivitis. Recent interest in the role of free radicals (superoxides) in the process of ageing and in carcinogenesis has led to suggestions that the intake of the anti-oxidant vitamins C and E may usefully be increased in the diet.

Vitamin A

The fat-soluble vitamins A, D and K have important roles in relation to the health of the oral tissues.

Vitamin A deficiency affects keratin formation and reduces saliva secretion

Vitamin A, retinol, in addition to its role in vision, is essential for the maturation and differentiation of epithelial tissues. Lack of vitamin A leads to hyperkeratosis of normally keratinised tissues and keratinisation of normally non-keratinised tissues. In the mouth there may be hyperkeratosis of the mucosa and the salivary glands are subject to hyperplasia of both acini and ducts. Keratin plugs may obstruct the ducts. Reduced salivary flow is usually a consequence and this may result in increased caries susceptibility. Animal experiments show that a lack of vitamin A may cause degeneration of ameloblasts (cells of epithelial origin) and consequent enamel hypoplasia. Vitamin A deficiency also adversely affects odontoblasts – causing atrophy and therefore poor dentine formation – and osteoclasts – resulting in a failure of normal bone remodelling and therefore no check on osteoblast bone deposition (Fig. 9.2). There is little evidence of any of these effects in the human, probably because deficiencies are rare and usually partial.
Cases of excessive vitamin A intake have been reported in relation to unusual diets. There have been instances of people living on high intakes of polar bear fat or carrot juice: the principal ill-effects are again on epithelial tissues.

Retinoic acid is a growth factor

Retinoic acid, a derivative of vitamin A, has now been identified as a powerful growth factor. It has been known for many years that vitamin A can be important in the development of cleft palate in rats although the significance of this to human cleft palate incidence is unknown. Retinoic acid has been shown experimentally to cause regression of some skin cancers.

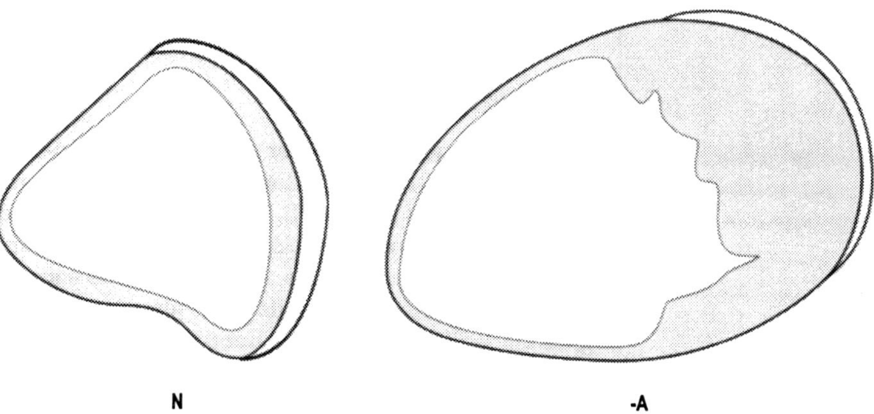

Effects of vitamin A deficiency in the rat. In this example the incisor shown in cross-section has not achieved its normal shape and the dentine is irregular and excessive in amount. In more severe cases the enamel covering would be incomplete and dentine would be exposed to the environment. N, normal; -A, vitamin A-deficient.

Vitamin D

Lack of vitamin D results in poor calcification of osteoid tissue and predentine

The importance of vitamin D is dealt with at more length in Ch. 1; here it is sufficient simply to outline oral effects of deficiency and excess. The vitamin is essential for the normal absorption of calcium from the small intestine and the formation and removal of bone. Lack of the vitamin results in low levels of plasma calcium so that calcium is not available for bone deposition. Matrix is laid down but cannot be calcified, resulting in large amounts of osteoid. Skeletal development and maintenance are also hindered by the stimulation of the parathyroid glands by the low plasma calcium and the consequent secretion of parathyroid hormone which promotes bone resorption by the osteoclasts. These two effects are manifested clinically in children as rickets (osteomalacia – literally soft bones) and in adults as osteitis fibrosis cystica (development in bones of spaces in-filled with fibrous tissue). Both these conditions may affect bones of the jaws although rickets is most commonly seen in the long bones. In dogs experimental deprivation of vitamin D causes changes in dental tissues as well as in bone. In these animals enamel is thin and hypoplastic, and dentine calcification is impaired. As in bone, matrix is laid down normally but fails to calcify. There is, therefore, a wide zone of predentine, and the border of predentine with calcified dentine is much more irregular than usual. The dentine is thin and contains more interglobular dentine. Although similar appearances are seen in relation to enamel hypoplasia in humans there is no evidence to link this with vitamin D deficiency. Suggestions that vitamin D might have a protective role against dental caries have not been substantiated. Equally there is little evidence that enamel hypoplasia necessarily implies a higher susceptibility to caries.

There is no evidence of enamel defects or increased dental caries in humans deficient in vitamin D

Excess of vitamin D, usually due to intake of too many vitamin supplements or foods supplemented with the vitamin, leads to hypercalcaemia and ectopic calcification. Renal calculi are one manifestation of this. There are no data on salivary calcium levels in this condition or on the incidence of salivary and dental calculi.

Excess of vitamin D results in ectopic calcification

Vitamin K

Vitamin K has been used to enhance blood clotting after extractions

Vitamin K is menaphthone or menadione, a lipid-soluble vitamin essential for the synthesis of the blood clotting factors which contain gamma-glutamic acid, prothrombin and factors VII, X and XI. Deficiencies result in the failure of blood to clot, or increased clotting times. Vitamin K is sometimes prescribed for patients after extractions, although it takes some time to induce synthesis of the clotting factors. The vitamin is also necessary for synthesis of the glutamic acid protein of bone but there are no reports of deficiencies affecting bone formation or turnover.

Minerals

Calcium and phosphate

There is no evidence that low calcium or phosphate

It has often been supposed that a low intake of calcium, or phosphorus, or both might lead to poor calcification of teeth and possibly, therefore, to an

intakes during tooth formation lead to higher caries rates

increased risk of dental caries. There is no evidence in human beings of this being the case. Animal experiments using rats on diets with differing amounts of calcium and phophorus and different calcium: phosphate ratios suggested that the calcification of the teeth could be affected if calcium was very low in the diet. The effect was limited to dentine formation, and was seen as an increased thickness of the predentine layer and an increase in interglobular dentine. Reductions in the phosphate content of the diet had little effect on the amount of apatite formed but did affect its composition, resulting in a high carbonate apatite. Such apatite is more soluble in acid than low carbonate apatites. Variations in the calcium:phosphate ratio of human diets between 2:1 and 1:3 do not appear to affect significantly the proportion of carbonate in human apatite. Whilst deficiencies in calcium and phosphate intake do not affect tooth calcification they do reduce that of bone, and they result in mobilisation of calcium from already formed bone. There is evidence of loss of calcium from the mandibles of older women as part of a general osteoporotic change and current practice is to recommend calcium supplementation in their diet. In pregnancy, when the dietary need of the mother for calcium and phosphate are increased by the demands imposed by the growing foetus, there is mobilisation of bone calcium if the dietary supply is insufficient. Mobilisation of calcium from the teeth does not occur; the dental tissues appear to be protected from the action of parathyroid hormones. There is evidence of increased dental caries in pregnant mothers, but this is not indicative of any systemic loss of calcium from enamel as dental caries is an occurrence at enamel surfaces and enamel, separated by dentine from the blood supply to the tooth, is not in exchange with systemic extracellular fluids.

Calcium is not lost from the teeth during pregnancy

Magnesium

In animal experiments magnesium is an essential mineral for calcification of dentine. Human diets are rarely so deficient in magnesium that any effect might be expected. Substitution of magnesium in enamel is associated with increased susceptibility to dental caries, but the mechanisms by which magnesium levels in apatite are increased and the way in which this affects enamel solubility are unknown.

Iron

Iron deficiency anaemia is manifested in oral tissues

Iron deficiency is fairly commonly observed, particularly in young women and during pregnancy. The deficiency is relative in that menstruation and foetus formation result in an effective loss of iron from the body and therefore a greater intake is required to maintain iron balance. The anaemia resulting from iron deficiency may be recognised by the pale colour of the gingivae and other oral soft tissues. Because the epithelium is thinner and less keratinised than that of skin, its colour is even more dependent upon the amount and haemoglobin content of the blood flowing through it. Oral mucosa therefore demonstrates anaemic loss of colour more dramatically. The poorer supply of oxygen to the oral soft tissues leaves them more susceptible to injury and infection; the loss of papillae on the tongue surface is probably a manifestation of this.

Trace elements

Fluoride, molybdenum, boron and strontium in water are associated with lower caries incidence, selenium and vanadium with higher

After the recognition that water-borne fluoride was responsible for the lower incidence of dental caries in subjects from areas with water supplies containing at least 50 µmol/l (1 ppm) of the element, extensive surveys were carried out of the relationship between other trace elements in water supplies and the incidence of dental caries. Much data was obtained from US servicemen called up for national service. The results show that molybdenum, boron and strontium are associated with low caries levels while selenium and vanadium are associated with high caries levels. The mechanisms of such effects are unclear and such data as exist on the amount of these ions in surface enamel do not indicate meaningful variations. Molybdenum has been studied more extensively than the others: it has an additive effect to that of fluoride.

Diet and dental caries

Dietary acid causes erosion of enamel

Foodstuffs and drinks can be harmful to enamel in two ways: acid foods or liquids may dissolve the apatite surface whilst other foods or drinks may contribute to dental caries. The dissolution of surface enamel by acids is termed erosion: dramatic examples of it may be seen in patients who drink lemon juice regularly or eat large quantities of citrus fruit and lose the whole of the labial enamel surface of their incisors. Such erosion of enamel is purely a physicochemical process.

Dental caries results from bacterial acid production from simple sugars

Sucrose is cariogenic

Dental caries is a bacterial disease in which the bacterial attack is external to the body surface – an attack initially on the surface of enamel (or cementum or dentine in root caries) by bacteria within the mouth but not inside the body cavity proper. As such it is influenced by nutritional state only in that poor nutrition during tooth development may result in enamel which is less resistant to carious attack. However, diet – the manner of presentation of the nutritional components – is of great importance. Indeed it is not only what is eaten, but how and how often. Thus carbohydrate as such may be unrelated to dental caries incidence whilst high intakes of one specific carbohydrate, sucrose, are usually associated with a high caries incidence. Foods which are retained in the mouth may be more harmful than those cleared quickly. The order in which foods are eaten during a meal may be important. Some foods which might be thought to be harmful in fact stimulate a copious flow of saliva which washes them away or neutralises their effects.

Studies of the relationship between diet and dental caries have been carried out by epidemiological surveys, by altering diets to see how this affected caries rates, and by exposing animals to different dietary regimes. Tests of individual foodstuffs have been carried out by measuring pH changes in dental plaque exposed to the foodstuff in the mouth or in the laboratory, by assessing the solubility of enamel powder or calcium phosphate in saliva foodstuff mixtures, and by measuring the loss of mineral from enamel blocks embedded in dentures or tooth restorations.

Epidemiological studies

Cross-sectional studies

Most epidemiological studies are cross-sectional: they compare two or more groups of people and assume that the difference in diet is the only variable. Obviously, the more closely the groups can be matched, the more valid will be the conclusion as to dietary effects. There is now a considerable body of data available as to caries incidence in different countries at particular ages – 5-year-olds or 12-year-olds, for example. The earliest observations of this kind were of people from Western countries and those from less developed African countries. Studies of Eskimo populations before they had extensive contact with other cultures, and of isolated groups such as the South African Bushmen, furnished evidence that dental caries could be regarded as a disease of Western civilisations, and the principal difference between the high and low caries experience lay in the greater consumption of refined sugars in the caries-prone populations. This conclusion was supported by studies of caries incidence in populations which had experienced a major change in diet from a low sugar diet to a high sugar diet: the Alaskan Eskimos, urbanised groups in Ethiopia and Nigeria, and the very significant experience of the inhabitants of Tristan da Cunha who were evacuated from the island when a volcanic eruption occurred. Similar evidence was adduced from studies of the caries incidence in Norway, Britain and other European countries for the period before World War II, the period of the war, and the post-war period from 1945 to 1950. Reduction in the supply of refined sugar during the war led to rationing of sugar-containing foods which was continued in countries such as Britain for several years afterwards. The effect of this rationing was to reverse the steady increase in dental caries in European countries which had been recorded from the beginning of the century. After 1950 the increase resumed. Analysis of wartime diets shows that the reduction in sucrose intake was the most noticeable change that might be associated with the reduction in dental caries, although the use of less refined flours led to increased amounts of phytate (inositol hexaphosphate) in the diet. Phytate has been identified as a protective factor as it reduces calcium phosphate solubility.

High sucrose intake is associated with high caries rates in populations

Low sucrose intake during World War II was accompanied by a reduction in caries rates

Phytate is a protective factor

Observations of subjects with a high dietary intake of sucrose, such as confectionery workers, indicated high levels of dental caries, although workers in sugar cane plantations had very variable levels. This latter observation has two possible explanations: very high sugar concentrations may be harmful to bacteria, and there is some debate as to whether sugar phosphates and other contaminants of unrefined sugar may act as protective factors. Some less refined sugars and molasses contain calcium salts which are added to precipitate contaminants from the sugar liquor during the precipitation of pure sucrose during cane extraction. Laboratory observations on such compounds show less dissolution of calcium phosphates in their presence.

A wholemeal flour and low sugar diet reduced caries incidence in children

The orphan children cared for in Hopewood House, New South Wales, receive a wholemeal flour and low sugar diet specified by the founder of the institution: their caries levels are very much lower than those of children of comparable age in Sydney. In 1980, 46% of 80 children were caries-free.

Although the observations are really cross-sectional this can also be regarded as a longitudinal study.

Longitudinal studies

Studies of diets over long periods identify foods as cariogenic or protective

All the observations quoted thus far (with the exception of the Hopewood House study) have been from cross-sectional studies and open to the objections to such studies. There are two longitudinal studies in which a group of subjects have been studied over a period of time. As it takes more than a year for a caries lesion to become evident these studies have to extend over relatively long periods. Bibby and his co-workers carried out a 1-year study in which they correlated snack food intake and caries development in American adolescents. In the most thorough study available, the diet and progress of dental caries was followed in 405 children in South Northumberland in England over a period of 2 years. This latter study showed a correlation of dental caries increments with sugars, with the number of items exceeding 10% sugar by weight, and with the foods exceeding 10% sugar by weight. Frequency of intake was less significantly related to caries incidence.

Dietary modification

Diets can be modified to reduce dental caries incidence

Clinical experiments in which diet has been modified and changes in caries rates observed have been few in number. There were attempts to reduce caries by reducing refined sugar intake in the 1960s, but these were monitored by changes in lactobacillus counts rather than by measurement of caries, and the conclusions are therefore uncertain. The most famous study is the Vipeholm study in which patients in a Swedish mental hospital were given confectionery in different amounts and in different time schedules. The results of the study showed that the amount and frequency of intake of confectionery was important, that confectionery eaten with meals was less harmful than that between meals, and that chocolate appeared to be less cariogenic than other confectionery. This study has been criticised because of, amongst other things, the small number of patients involved, and their age. A totally different study was the very large study in Turku, Finland, where the sugar alcohol, xylitol, was substituted for sucrose in confectionery supplied to schoolchildren. This showed a dramatic drop in the caries increment over the 1-year period of the study.

Substitution of xylitol for sucrose as a sweetener reduces dental caries incidence

Animal studies

Animal experiments have been used to identify cariogenic bacteria and cariogenic foodstuffs

Experiments with germ-free animals and then with gnotobiotic animals showed that caries was a bacterial disease, that the main bacteria concerned were the mutans streptococci, and that dietary sucrose and glucose were the most important substrates for bacterial acid production leading to dental caries. Other sugars such as fructose appeared to be less important. Various test foods have been used to feed rats and monkeys.

Laboratory studies

In vivo studies

Bibby attempted to estimate the cariogenicity of foods by first measuring their sugar content and then measuring the time taken to clear the remains of the food from the mouth after it had been eaten (Table 9.3). He derived a cariogenicity index from the product of the two measurements. This approach suffered from the inability of the method to predict whether the sugar remaining in the mouth was available as a substrate and to take into account any protective factors in the food.

Stephan curves show acid (or alkali) production from test foodstuffs

Stephan, using a glass pH electrode, showed that dental plaque produced acid when exposed to sugar solutions. Subsequently other workers used electrodes to touch into plaque on the tooth surface as food was eaten, or used miniature electrodes mounted in dentures either with wires extending out of the mouth or sending radio signals to receivers outside the mouth. Others removed small amounts of plaque to measure the pH in cup electrodes. Various foods have been tested in these ways (Fig. 9.3 and Table 9.4). Particularly interesting have been the studies in which a sequence of food and drink mimicking that of a typical meal has been studied. In order to compare foodstuffs some measure of the pH curve is required since foods may cause the pH to be lowered to different pH values and for different times. Although at first the lowest pH reached was taken as the measure of cariogenicity, most research workers now use a calculated variable termed cH. This is the area of the Stephan curve below an arbitrary line which is usually set at pH 5.6 – the so-called critical pH for enamel dissolution (see p. 168). Any comparison of pH and any averaging of pH values presents theoretical problems as pH is a logarithmic function. It is debatable whether one can calculate a standard deviation for pH values except by transforming them into the linear function of hydrogen ion concentrations.

Oral demineralisation tests are not solely dependent upon acid production

Another approach which began as a study of demineralisation resulting from caries has now moved on to considering remineralisation as well. A piece of dental enamel, either human or bovine, is mounted on some fixed device in the mouth and arranged so that it accumulates dental plaque. After exposure

Table 9.3
Retention times for various foodstuffs (mg of food remaining in the mouth at various times after eating)

Food	5 min	15 min
Peanuts	4.9	3.3
Chocolate milk	7.4	3.8
Potato crisps	12.3	4.9
White bread	16.1	10.0
Raisins	16.8	5.7
Sponge cake	18.8	6.0
Milk chocolate	19.0	6.8
Plain cracker	33.6	10.4
Cookie (biscuit)	35.0	8.4

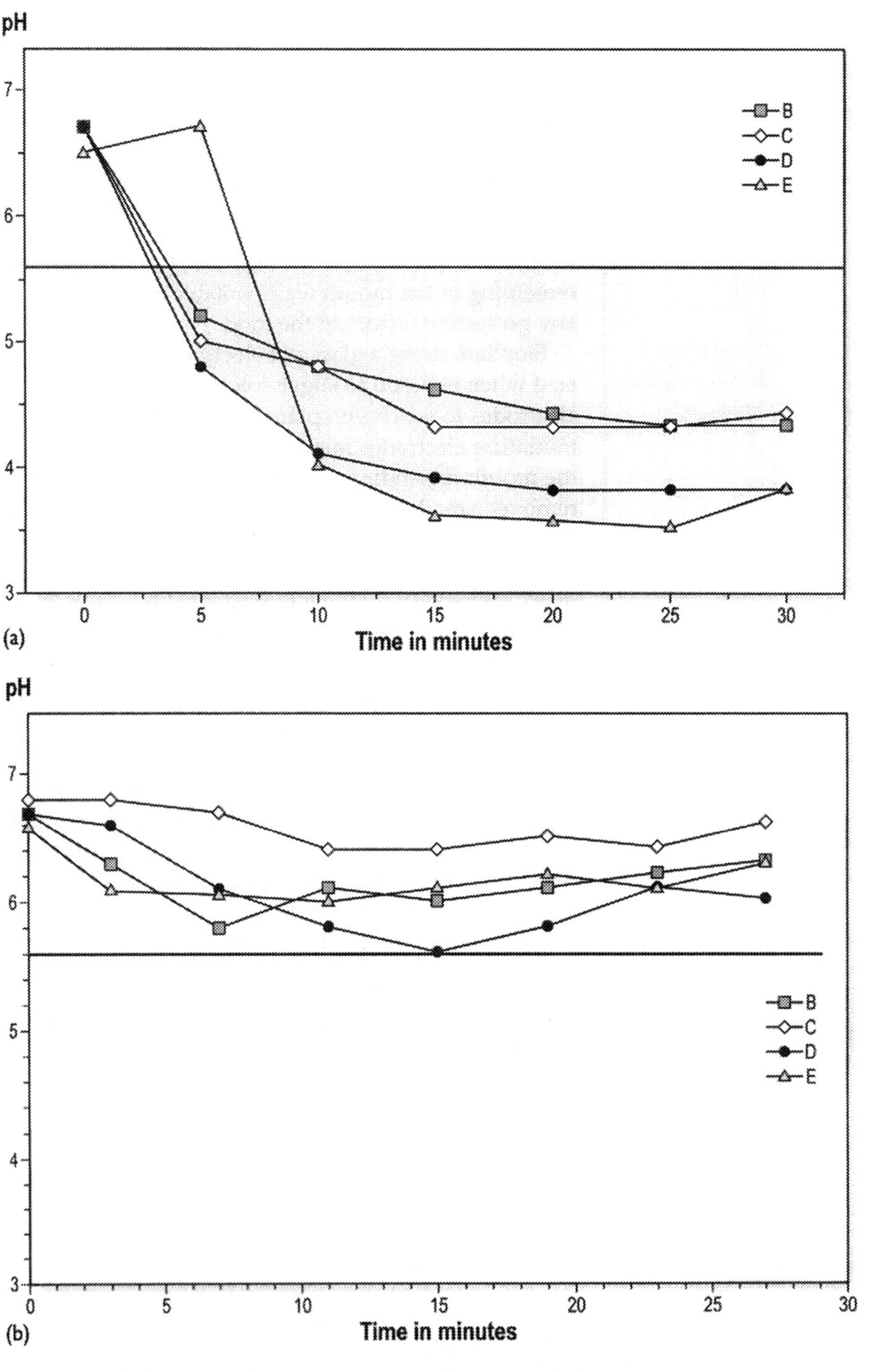

Stephan curves for some snack foods: **a** measured with an intraoral electrode, **b** with samples taken from mouth. In each case curve B is chocolate, curve C is bread, curve D is a biscuit (cookie) and curve E is an apple. In both diagrams curves C and E are rising at the end of the study time whilst curve D remains low.

Table 9.4
The minimum pH reached and the area of the pH curve below the line of critical pH (cH) at pH 5.6 after consumption of various foodstuffs

Food	Minimum pH	cH
Peanuts	6.5	0
Potato crisps (chips)	6.2	1.0
Bread and butter	6.3	0.8
Sponge cake	5.6	8.9
Chocolate	5.6	3.8
Plain biscuit	5.6	7.3
Chocolate-coated biscuit	5.6	6.0
Boiled sweet (candy)	5.3	12.1
Sugared coffee	5.4	10.8
Toffee	5.4	10.1
Ice cream	5	4.2
Apple	5.8	2.9
Orange juice	5.5	5.0

The values obtained are very dependent upon the particular method of measuring pH but show general agreement in rank orders.

to various foods the enamel can be removed and its hardness measured by indentation with a diamond point under a specified load. Hardness is used as an indication of the removal of calcium salts. This method has the advantage that it is measuring the actual effect upon enamel itself and therefore includes the influence of any protective factors in the foodstuff.

In vitro studies

In vitro tests may assay acid production or calcium phosphate dissolution

The cariogenicity of foods has also been studied by laboratory tests. These have the advantage of not requiring volunteers and being more highly controlled in relation to oral variables. In general they can be applied to two characteristics of the caries process: the pH change in saliva or plaque when the micro-organisms metabolise the foodstuff, or the dissolution of calcium phosphate salts in the acid produced.

Foodstuffs which might have a protective role can be tested by seeing if they inhibit the dissolution of calcium phosphate or enamel in acid buffers or in saliva–sugar mixtures.

pH change

Foodstuffs can be added to whole saliva (oral fluid) and the pH monit
over several hours. Alternatively, whole saliva can be centrifuged to
sediment – consisting of oral bacteria, epithelial squames and neut
and the sediment dispersed in water to which the foodstuff is ad
to approximate more closely to dental plaque in the mouth, sa
from the teeth can be collected and dispersed in a suitable flu
the same way. All these techniques are open to the same cri
studies in the mouth: they ignore the contribution of anti-

Solubility of calcium phosphate or enamel powders

The other method of studying cariogenic potential in the laboratory is to see if calcium phosphate powder, or enamel powder, or even enamel pieces, dissolves in mixtures of the foodstuff with saliva or any other above mixtures. This involves measuring the changes in phosphate concentration in the mixture as this can be done very accurately. The method is, however, best suited to assessing caries protective properties using acid buffers as attacking agents.

Results of dietary studies

Frequency of sugar intake may be an important factor in caries development

If sugars such as sucrose and glucose are metabolised by plaque to produce acid it might be predicted that repetition of the sugar exposure would maintain the plaque pH at a low level. Thus continuing or frequent intakes of sugars will accentuate their harmful effects. The observations in the longitudinal study in Northumberland, however, somewhat surprisingly, did not identify frequency of sugar intake as highly correlated with caries development. The slightly different variable of the number of sugar intakes per day was identified. The data available from the many studies of food cariogenicity implicate sucrose-containing foods as being most harmful to the teeth. Most snack foods and confectionery are high in sugar content. Savoury types of snacks, such as potato crisp type preparations and nut-based snacks are shown to be less harmful from the point of view of caries. It should be

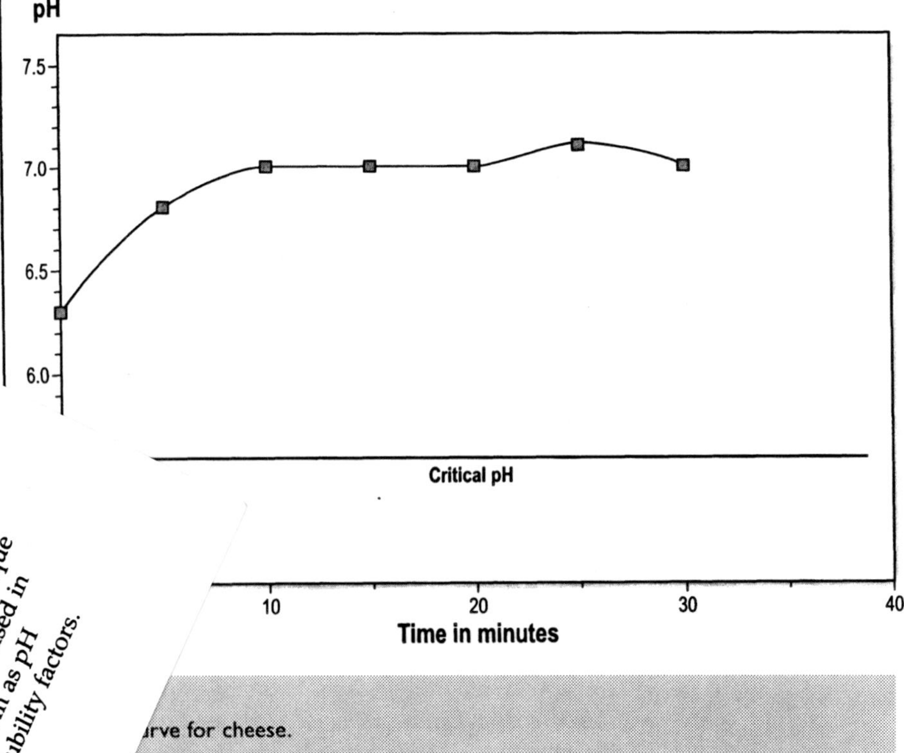

…rve for cheese.

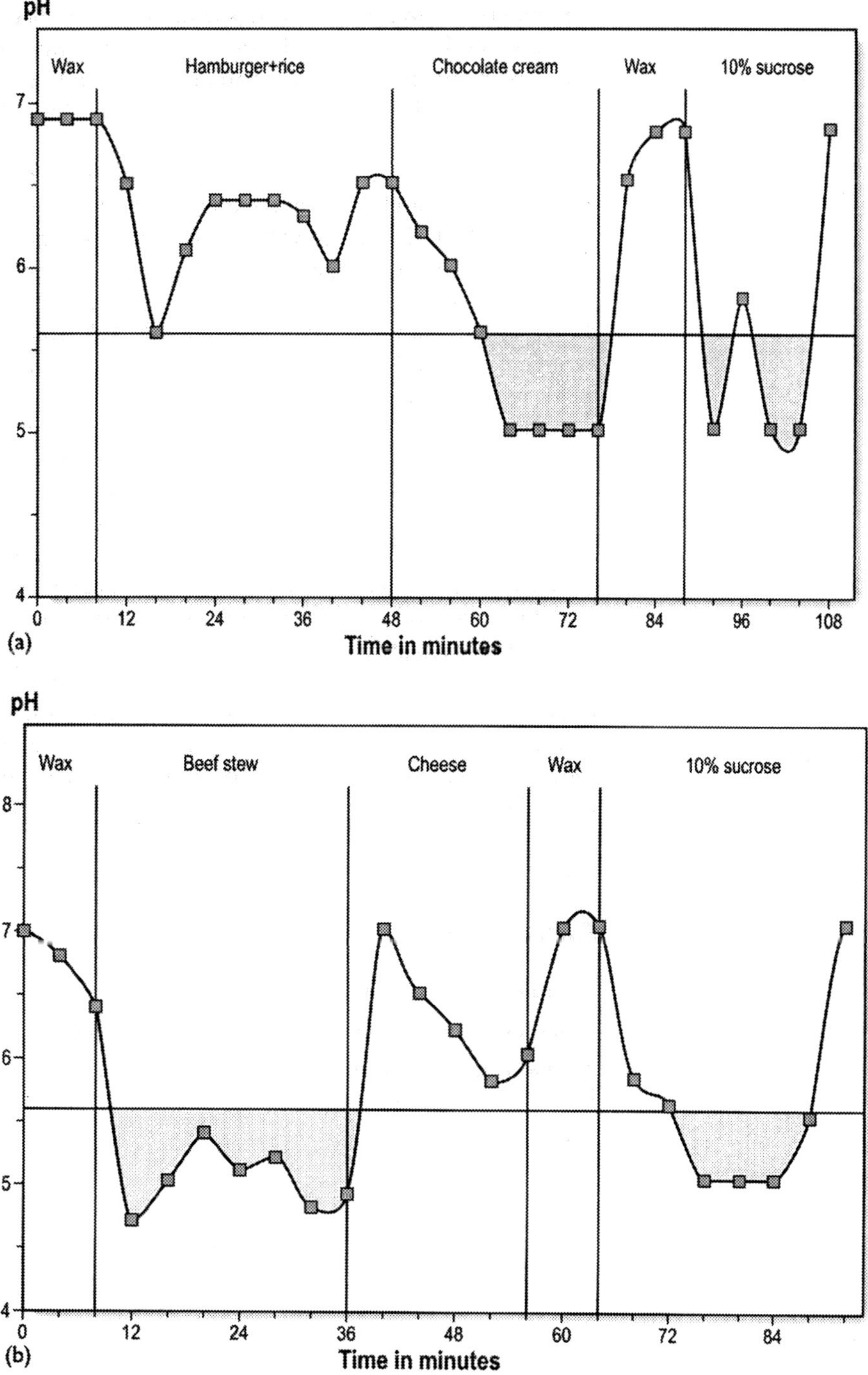

Fig. 9.5
Dental plaque pH changes recorded with an intraoral electrode during the sequential consumption of various foodstuffs. Paraffin wax was chewed between foods to return the plaque pH to a 'resting' range.

There are anti-solubility factors in nuts, brown flours and chocolate

remembered, however, that caries is not the only disease with correlations with diet, and the fat and salt content of crisps and some other savoury snacks may adversely affect lipid accumulation in blood vessels or raise blood pressure. Nuts show anti-solubility properties. The active factors seem to be localised in the surface layers of the nuts.

The evidence on starchy foods demonstrates them, on the whole, to be non-cariogenic, although in animal experiments starches can act as substrates for cariogenic bacteria. The phytate present in wholemeal flours contributes to protection of the teeth against carious attack since it reduces calcium phosphate solubility, possibly by forming a surface layer over the crystals. In the Vipeholm study there was evidence that chocolate confectionery was less cariogenic than other sweets or candies: it is possible that cocoa contains a factor reducing calcium phosphate solubility.

Cheeses, which might be expected to cause some demineralisation because of their acid nature, in fact are associated with lower caries levels for two reasons: the acid taste stimulates salivary flow and hence increases salivary buffering (Fig. 9.4), and the high calcium content lowers the solubility of apatite. This was the only food in the British Northumberland survey which showed a negative correlation with caries development.

Sequence of food presentation in a meal is important

All in vivo studies with enamel pieces in the mouth show that one cannot predict the cariogenicity of food simply from its sugar content: the physical presentation of the food and the combination of other components are also important. Experiments on meal-like sequences of food intake studied by plaque pH changes showed that the pattern of food intake was also important. Thus ending a meal with cheese or with non-sugar saliva stimulants could leave the plaque pH high or even alkaline. Excessively sweetened coffee could reverse this situation (Fig. 9.5).

Further reading

Standard texts on nutrition

Identification of Low Caries Risk Dietary Components. Imfeld, T.N. Karger, Basel, 1983

The Prevention of Oral Disease, 3rd edition. Murray, J.J. (editor). Oxford University Press, Oxford, 1996

10 Fluoride

Ionic fluoride either in water or as a constituent of toothpastes, mouthrinses and topically applied gels is the most effective anti-caries agent currently available. It is generally considered that the decrease in the incidence of dental caries in North America and Europe over the period 1980–1990 is directly related to the now almost universal use of fluoride toothpastes.

The discovery of the effects of fluoride

Fluoride in water supplies was observed to cause mottling of dental enamel early in the 1900s

The recognition of the association between water supplies which contained 1 ppm or more of fluoride (approximately 50 μmol/l or more) and a low incidence of dental caries dates back to 1931. Strictly, the association which Churchill reported at that time was one of high water fluoride levels with tooth mottling. This was the culmination of a search begun 30 years earlier when McKay had noticed a geographically defined incidence of tooth mottling in the Colorado Springs area and looked for its cause. Mottling manifests as defects in the enamel which appear at first as chalky white and then progress to brown. G.V. Black had examined children at Colorado Springs in 1909 and observed that, despite the imperfections in enamel formation, the teeth exhibited relatively little dental caries. Ainsworth in Maldon, England, in 1928 found that a water fluoride level of 4.5–5.5 ppm (225–275 μmol/l) was associated with a high incidence of mottling and a low incidence of dental caries. During the 1930s Dean was able to extend these observations with several surveys which led up to his survey of 21 American cities and the artificial fluoridation of the water supplies to Grand Rapids, Michigan. Other fluoridation studies followed in the USA, Canada, the Netherlands, New Zealand and Britain, all confirming that a reduction in dental caries incidence resulted from the fluoridation of pubic water supplies.

In the 1930s it was realised that fluoride at concentrations of around 1 ppm (0.05 mmol/l) reduced dental decay

The maximum benefit from fluoridated water in terms of caries reduction was achieved in the US studies with a little over 1 ppm (50 μmol/l), although the British observations favoured a higher concentration of 2 ppm (100 μmol/l). The level aimed at in artificial fluoridation has to reconcile the caries benefit with the least drawback in the form of mottling. The British observations of Forrest, combining mottling and caries data, suggested that a level of 1 ppm was suitable to reduce both these effects as far as possible (curves from US data show a similar relationship – Fig. 10.1).

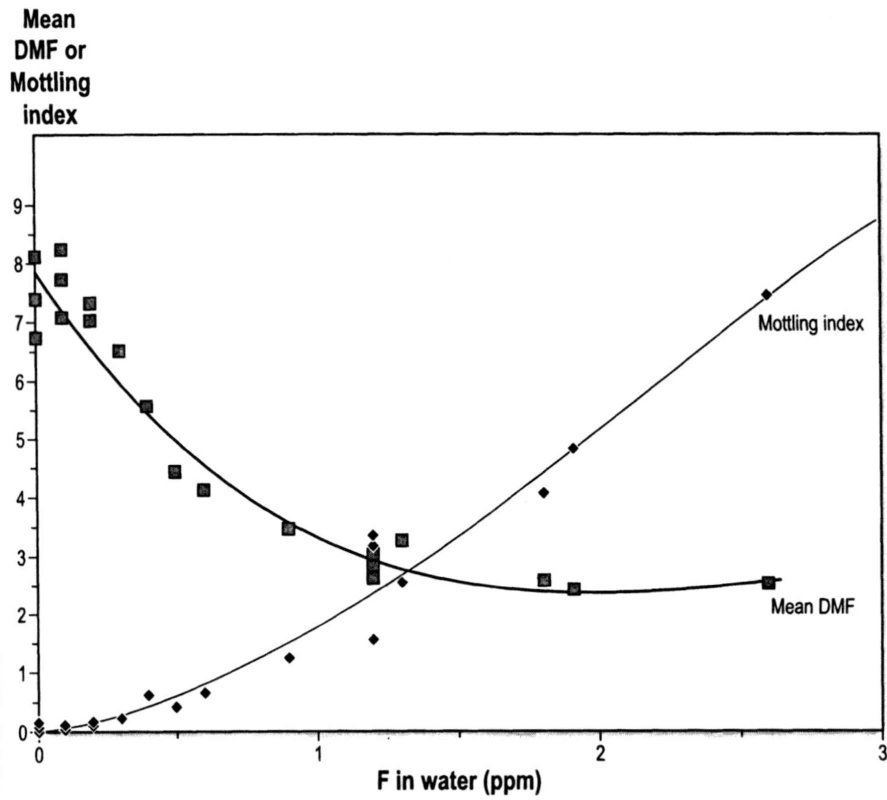

The relationships between concentrations of fluoride in the water supply, dental caries experience and incidence of mottled teeth. Data are from Dean's 21 cities study. The dental caries experience is the mean DMF (number of decayed, missing and filled teeth in each mouth) in 12–14-year-old children, whilst the mottling index is given as one-tenth of the percentage of children examined showing any grade of mottling. The two lines cross at about 1.3 ppm (0.07 mmol/l) of fluoride in the water supply, suggesting that this concentration gave least mottling and greatest protection from dental caries in these US cities. The recommended level of fluoridation (1 ppm or 0.05 mmol/l) reduces the incidence of mottling without seriously affecting the protection from dental caries.

The distribution of fluoride

Fluoride is widely distributed in human foodstuffs and drinking fluids, (Table 10.1), although in most geographical areas the concentrations are low – ppm or µmol/kg. The ultimate source of the fluoride is in fluoride-containing minerals, either in rocks or soil, and the fluoride is usually found in association with calcium or aluminium. As most fluoride salts are insoluble, the amounts leached out by water are small and the range of fluoride concentrations in ground water varies between 0.1 ppm (5 µmol/l) and 18 ppm (almost 1 mmol/l). It is usual to describe an area as a high fluoride area if

Table 10.1
Fluoride content of foods and drinks (in µmol/g or mmol/l)

Food	Fluoride
Water	0.05 in fluoridated supplies
Tea	0.05 average
Beer	0.01
Fruit juice	0.01
Coca-cola	Depends upon water supply
Milk	0.014
Cream	0.014
Cheese	0.014
Butter	0.014
Eggs	0.015
Beef	0.012
Ham	0.012
Mashed potato	0.020
Carrot	0.020
Cauliflower	0.015
Peas	0.028
Apple	0.003
Orange	0.003
Bread	0.022
Fruitcake	0.022
Shortbread biscuit	0.022
Cornflakes	0.022

The table lists the same foodstuffs as previous dietary tables; some of the data are extrapolated from analyses of similar foods.

the water supply contains 1 ppm or more of fluoride. In temperate climates the normal water intake is 1.0–1.5 litres/day and so the intake of fluoride from a 1 ppm fluoride water supply is between 1 and 1.5 mg/day. In hotter climates where a greater intake of water is normal, the intake of fluoride will therefore be higher unless the level in the water supply is reduced.

The amount of fluoride taken up by plants seems to be fairly constant and relatively unaffected by soil fluoride content. However, the treatment of plant foods before consumption will affect the final fluoride concentration: dried foods will have a higher concentration than before drying, and foods cooked in water tend to stabilise to concentrations similar to those in the cooking water. Animal tissues, with the exception of calcified tissues, also have uniformly low fluoride levels. Very high levels of fluoride intake may increase the concentration of fluoride in the kidney and, to a lesser extent, the liver. Neither meat nor fish, therefore, contribute much fluoride to the diet unless they contain bony tissue in an edible form. Fish in which bone is eaten – such as tinned mackerel, sardines, or salmon – may contain appreciable amounts of fluoride, as do some foods homogenised for infant feeding which include ground bone – e.g. some chicken dishes. Bone meal, advocated at one time as a caries preventing supplement, probably produced its effects mainly by virtue of its high fluoride content.

Fluoride intake

Total fluoride intake in the UK is around 2 mg/day in areas with 0.1 ppm in the water, and 3–4 mg/day where the water supplies contain 1 ppm

The total intake of fluoride from food (including the contribution from the cooking water) in UK adults is between 0.3 and 0.5 mg/day in a non-fluoride area. Figures obtained in from studies in USA and other countries range from 0.16 to 1.03 mg/day with a mean around 0.67 mg. In fluoride areas these figures rise to 0.8–3.4 mg/day, the average being approximately 1 mg/day higher than in the low fluoride area. All these figures are much below the intake from drinking water (1–2 litres of fluid intake gives 2 mg of fluoride in a fluoridated area) and in the UK the use of tea as the main drink results in higher intakes than in non-tea-drinking countries. Table 10.2 shows some calculated figures for fluoride intake.

The general availability of fluoride toothpastes in Western countries has added another source of fluoride intake. Although the deliberate eating of toothpaste is limited to a few children, both children and adults do swallow a proportion of the toothpastes they use. With the normal concentrations of 1000 ppm, the typical brushload of 0.5–1 g contains 0.5–1.0 mg of fluoride.

Other intakes of fluoride from therapeutic agents include those from tablets and rinses for prophylaxis of dental caries, and small amounts from fluoride-containing anaesthetic agents after longer periods of anaesthesia.

All the data so far are for amounts of fluoride ingested – not the amounts absorbed. As with any dietary component, balance studies can be carried out for fluoride. Such studies involve measurement of fluoride intake from all sources, fluoride output in faeces and urine, and possibly also the output in sweat and epithelial cell loss. These last are usually ignored and so figures for retention are usually higher than they should be, particularly in studies in hot climates. If the faecal output is assumed to represent the non-absorbed

Table 10.2
Estimated fluoride intakes (in mg) in the UK

Group	Low fluoride area		High fluoride area	
	Food	Total	Food	Total
Children	0.3	0.6	0.3	1.2
Women	0.4	1.3	0.4	2.2
Men	0.5	1.7	0.5	3.2
Tea drinkers (or heavy beer drinkers!)	0.4	3.0	0.4	4.0–5.0

The figures are indicative only, since the ranges reported are wide: figures from the USA range from half to twice these estimates. Despite this, the figures indicate the relatively small proportion of fluoride derived from food in comparison with that derived from water.

fluoride, a figure for amount absorbed is around 90% of that ingested. As fluoride is precipitated by excess calcium, increased calcium intake may reduce the absorption of fluoride. Indeed it has been estimated that the high calcium content of most toothpastes means that only 30–40% of the amount of fluoride ingested from this source is actually absorbed.

Metabolism of fluoride (Fig. 10.2)

Absorption of fluoride

Absorption of fluoride occurs in the stomach and small intestine. As HF is poorly dissociated the hydrogen ions of the gastric secretion and the fluoride ions form the lipid-soluble HF which can enter cells and be absorbed

Absorption occurs in the stomach and small intestine. Although there is no evidence of active absorption of any substances in the stomach, and few water-soluble substances are therefore able to cross the epithelium to reach the serosal side, lipid-soluble substances can be absorbed down concentration gradients. Fluoride ions themselves are not lipid-soluble but hydrogen fluoride (HF) is. In physicochemical terms hydrogen fluoride is a weak acid – i.e. it does not dissociate easily. In the presence of the excess of hydrogen ions in the stomach fluoride forms HF and this can then diffuse across the gastric mucosa. With high intakes of fluoride minute points of cell damage have been observed in the gastric mucosa of dogs and rats, and these have been attributed to the direct effect of hydrogen fluoride on the mucosal cells. There is no evidence of such effects in humans, probably because the human gastric mucosa is rarely exposed to sufficiently high concentrations of fluoride. In the small intestine fluoride uptake continues. Some earlier work suggested that there might be an active transport mechanism in the small intestine capable of

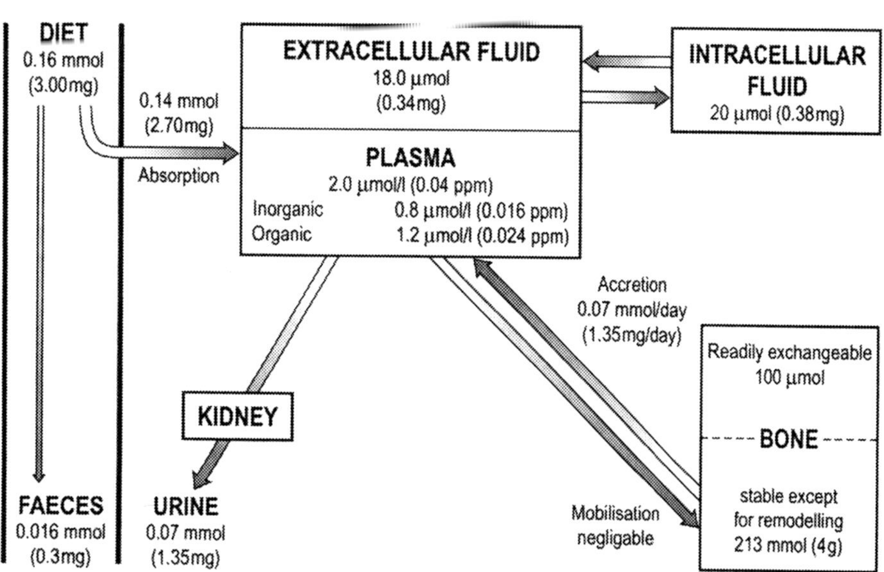

Fig. 10.2
The distribution and metabolism of fluoride in the body.

carrying fluoride ions, but it now seems more likely that the active secretion of hydrogen carbonate into the lumen of the small intestine may create a gradient of pH across the gut epithelium and favour HF formation on the serosal side of the cells. This would generate or increase a gradient for diffusion of fluoride ions across the mucosa. However, many of the channels for anion diffusion which are usually thought of as chloride channels are in practice fairly non-specific and would allow fluoride diffusion. This includes band 3 protein, the hydrogen carbonate–chloride exchanger. In the larger intestine it is possible that some secretion of fluoride into the lumen occurs; if this is so, the final amount of faecal fluoride will include secreted as well as unabsorbed fluoride.

Fluoride in blood plasma and other body fluids

Plasma fluoride is normally low at around 1 μmol/l or 0.02 ppm but rises to a peak over 30–60 min after fluoride intake

The absorbed fluoride passes into the portal circulation to reach the liver. Plasma contains fluoride in both ionised and non-ionised forms. These amount to 0.4–4.5 μmol/l and 1.2–2.4 μmol/l, respectively. Little is known about the non-ionised fraction, either chemically or biologically. The concentration of ionised fluoride varies according to the fluoride level in the water supply and is approximately 1 μmol/l at water concentrations of 0.05 mmol/l (1 ppm). After ingestion of a single dose of fluoride the plasma ionised fluoride concentration rises to a peak over 30–60 min and then declines again over some 3 h (Fig. 10.3). As fluoride is distributed throughout the extracellular compartment of body water the peak values in plasma are considerably less than if the ion were confined to the plasma water. After a 6 mg dose of fluoride, for example, the peak plasma level was 24 μg/l (1.3 μmol/l). The uptake into tissues varies, but in general the tissue plasma ratios vary between 0.4 and 0.9. Adipose tissue takes up much less than other tissues because of its low water content, whilst cerebrospinal fluid has a very low uptake because the blood–brain barrier is relatively impermeable to fluoride. The kidney shows a gradient of concentration from cortex to papilla similar to that for sodium and chloride ions. Calcified tissues accumulate fluoride as it is incorporated into the hydroxyapatite crystal to form fluorapatite.

As fluoride ions can pass across epithelial cell layers to a limited extent, they can be transferred into body secretions such as sweat, bile, saliva and milk. In human samples milk contains about 50% of the plasma level of fluoride; this is true also of cows' milk. An increase in plasma fluoride levels is followed by a later, less marked rise in milk fluoride concentrations. Bile contains roughly the same concentration as plasma. Saliva levels are between 70 and 95% of plasma levels (Fig. 10.3) and change rapidly to follow them. In gingival crevicular fluid the levels are slightly higher than in plasma. The secretion of fluoride into saliva and gingival crevicular fluid provides a second route by which ingested fluoride can affect the dental tissues. This fluoride can enter enamel from exposure to food and drink, from the blood during tooth development, and from saliva after eruption.

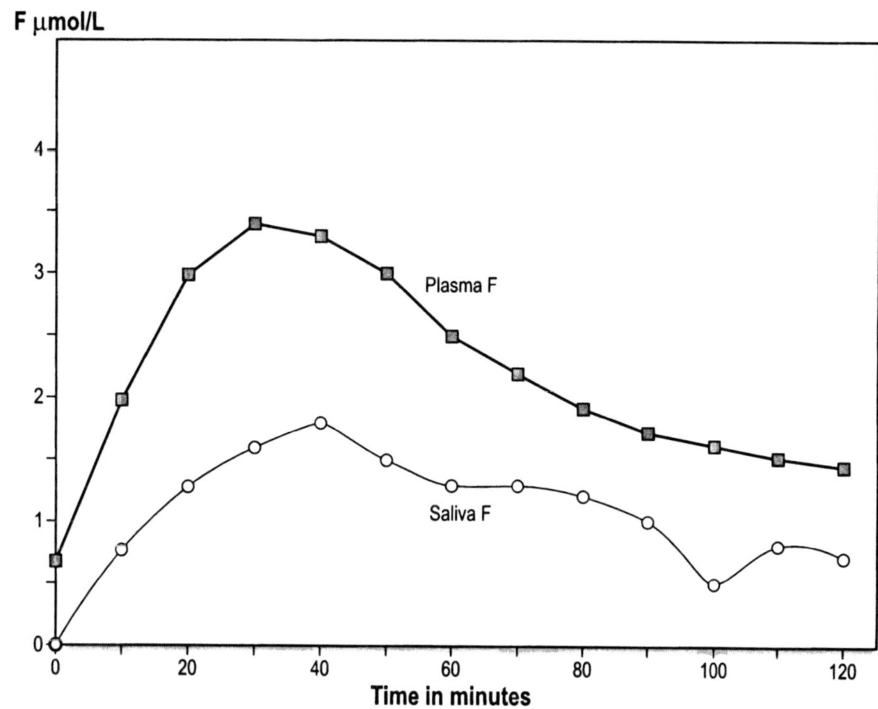

Fig. 10.3
Concentrations of fluoride in plasma and in saliva at time intervals after ingesting 1 mg of fluoride as sodium fluoride.

Fluoride uptake into calcified tissues

Most of the fluoride ingested is taken up into calcified tissues

From plasma and the extracellular fluids fluoride passes particularly to the calcified tissues. If these tissues are growing and calcification is occurring the fluoride is incorporated directly into the new apatite crystals. Where growth as such has ceased similar incorporation can occur in areas of bone turnover, but otherwise fluoride is taken up at the bone surface by ion exchange. Thus compact bone from individuals living in a low fluoride area (water supply 5 µmol/l, 0.1 ppm) increases in fluoride content from around 300 ppm at age 20 years up to 1500 ppm at age 70 years and over 2500 ppm at age 90 years (Table 10.3). The amount of fluoride taken up into a hard tissue depends upon the rate of apposition: in rapid apposition there is little time of exposure to the fluoride in the extracellular fluid whilst during slow deposition of calcium salts much more fluoride can be taken up. The bulk of dentine and cementum are formed at a steady rate during the initial development of the tooth and hence these tissues have a fairly uniform fluoride concentration throughout most of their thickness. However, both tissues increase slowly in thickness throughout life and therefore the surfaces in contact with the interstitial fluid of periodontal ligament or pulp accumulate much higher concentrations of fluoride (Fig. 10.4). Enamel also has a relatively constant concentration of fluoride throughout its thickness but shows great variation at its surface. In

Table 10.3
Fluoride concentration in hard tissues (ppm and, in parentheses, µmol/g)

Tissue	Low fluoride area		High fluoride area	
	Age 20 years	Age 60 years	Age 20 years	Age 60 years
Enamel	100 (5)	100 (5)	170 (8)	350 (17)
Dentine	100 (5)	400 (20)	400 (20)	1200 (60)
Cementum	400 (20)	2000 (100)		
Cortical bone	250 (12)	2000 (100)	500 (25)	4000 (200)

There is wide variation in reported data. All values are averages for the tissues and do not reflect the differences across the tissue. Data for enamel is especially variable because of the high concentrations on the surface and the loss of enamel by abrasion or attrition with age; earlier estimations suggested an increase with age but more recent data shows no relationship between age and fluoride concentration in this tissue. There do not appear to be any data on fluoride content of cementum from high fluoride areas but it is probably similar to that of cortical bone.

younger teeth the enamel surface has high concentrations of fluoride which have been acquired from food, water and saliva (Fig. 10.4a). In later years fluoride continues to accumulate on the enamel surface, but the surface is itself removed by attrition, erosion and abrasion. Hence the fluoride concentration in the outermost layers of enamel is very variable, depending upon the exact situation on the tooth surface and the degree to which the original surface has been lost. Fluoride concentrations in hard tissues are shown in Table 10.3 and Fig. 10.4. Bone concentrations increase throughout life but in areas where the intake of fluoride is high they tend to plateau at between 2000 and 3000 ppm. Some observations suggest that bone in older subjects continues to take up fluoride and does so even more rapidly than in lower age groups; the changes in bone density and alterations in the proportions of different types of bone may explain the apparent increases in bone fluoride in these subjects.

Fluoride in dental plaque

Fluoride is present in dental plaque at higher concentrations than in saliva

Dental plaque accumulates fluoride by taking it up from saliva and gingival crevicular fluid. The mechanism of accumulation is still not clear. It may be related to the high calcium and phosphate levels in dental plaque even before calculus formation begins. Thus some investigators believe that micro-crystals of calcium fluoride and/or fluorapatite may be present in dental plaque. There is evidence that some plaque bacteria take up fluoride, a process which would be favoured by the low pH values present in plaque after acid production from sugars. Attempts at extraction of fluoride from dental plaque have led to the identification of three fractions termed free, loosely bound and tightly bound. The free fraction is that present in the plaque water. Separation of the plaque fluid by centrifugation of plaque and estimation of fluoride in the supernatant gives values of ionic fluoride around 2 µmol/l. All the fluoride appears to be in an ionic form. The loosely bound fraction is defined as that which can be released by acidification to a pH of 4–5 and is thought to be

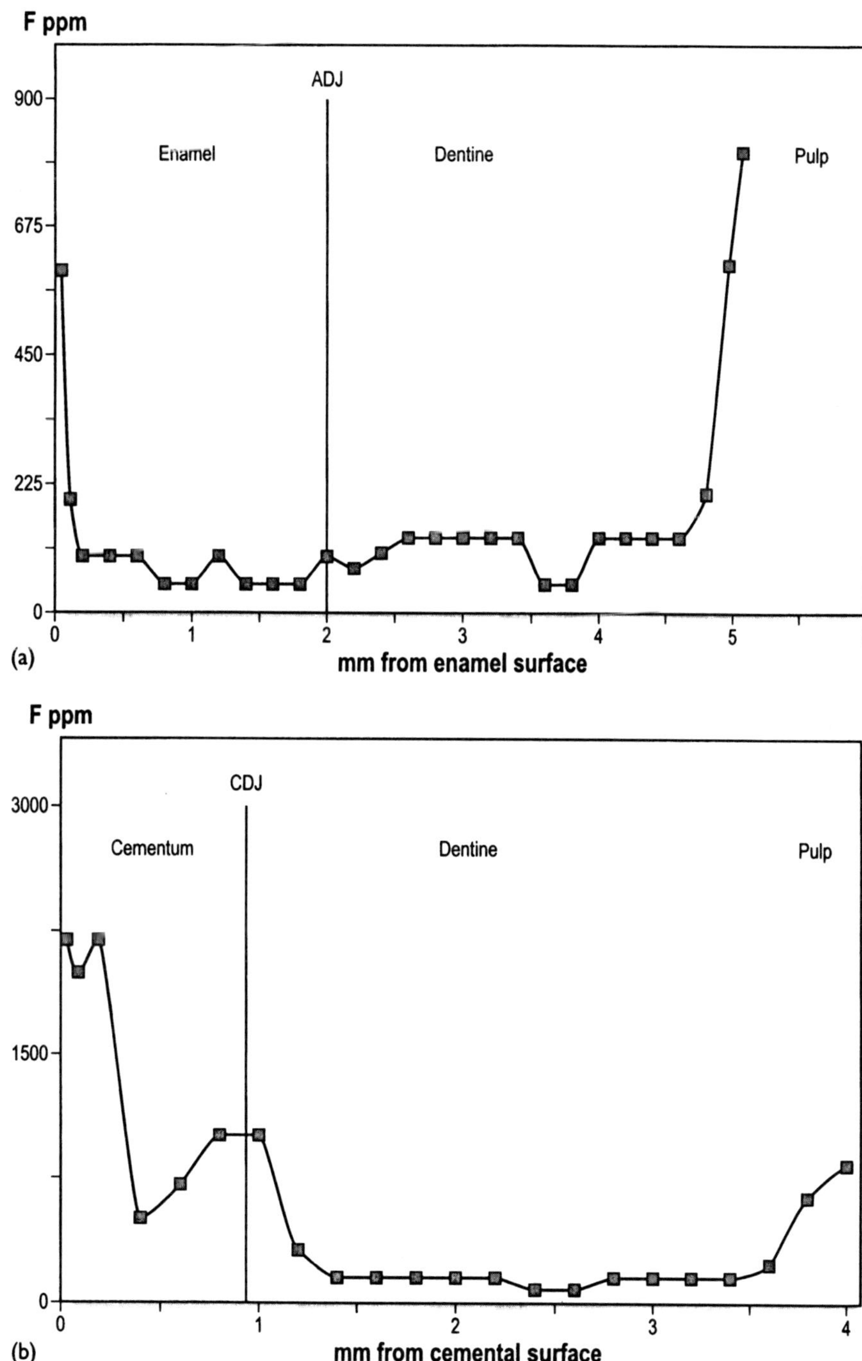

Fig. 10.4
Concentrations of fluoride in dental tissues: **a** from the enamel surface to the pulpal surface of dentine (ADJ marks the amelodentinal junction), and **b** from the periodontal ligament surface of cementum to the pulpal surface of dentine at a level approximately half way down the root (CDJ marks the cementodentinal junction).

present either as insoluble calcium salts or in some form of binding to bacteria. The firmly bound fraction is thought to be that taken up by bacteria and therefore only extractable after ashing. Estimates of this fraction vary between 0.5 and 50% of the total plaque fluoride. Many species of oral bacteria, including *Streptococcus mutans* and some other streptococci, have been found to take up fluoride from culture media to levels in excess of those in the media. This has been taken as evidence that the tightly bound fraction in plaque is probably within bacteria, but this conclusion has been questioned. The fluoride content of dental plaque was reported some years ago to vary from around 25 ppm in a low fluoride area to between 40 and 100 ppm in a high fluoride area. More recent data suggest that these estimates were high and values of 5–10 ppm have been obtained in plaque from low fluoride areas.

Excretion of fluoride

The main route for fluoride excretion is in the urine

Fluoride which is not taken up into the calcified tissues or lost in secretions is finally excreted by the kidneys. Within the kidney tubules the same general rules apply to fluoride reabsorption as to its transfer across epithelial cells elsewhere. A proportion of fluoride ions pass through chloride ion channels – including the sodium–potassium–chloride exchanger – but otherwise fluoride can cross the lipid cell membranes only as undissociated HF. The amount of fluoride reabsorbed, therefore, depends upon the acidity of the tubular fluid and a large proportion is absorbed in the distal parts of the tubules where the acidity is highest. The non-reabsorbed fluoride is excreted in the urine. This amounts to about 50% of an ingested dose. In experiments with young growing animals where the proportion of fluoride incorporated into bone was much greater than in adults, the fraction excreted in the urine was around 10% of the ingested dose.

Fluoride and dental caries

A total fluoride intake of 2–4 mg/day reduces dental caries experience by some 50%

Observations in populations living in areas with water supplies containing 0.05 mmol/l or 1 ppm fluoride and controlled experiments on large populations given fluoride in their water supplies have established that a total intake of fluoride of around 2–4 mg/day results in a decrease in dental caries experience of some 50%.

Despite the long history of observations of reduced caries experience, the mechanisms by which water-borne fluoride may affect dental caries are still not fully understood. At lease six possible mechanisms have been explored but their relative importance is still debated. Fluoride could act at three levels: in soft tissues to modify the developing teeth, in hard tissues to affect mineralisation, demineralisation and remineralisation, and on cariogenic bacteria to alter their metabolism or ecological relationships.

Fluoride and tooth morphology

Fluoride may alter tooth morphology

Teeth from fluoride areas tend to have wider and shallower fissures. Animal experiments have shown a similar effect of fluoride given during the period of tooth development. This would suggest that fluoride can in some way influence the development of the cells of the dental papilla responsible for delineating the final shape of the tooth crown. Although theoretically teeth with wider and shallower fissures should be less susceptible to dental caries in the fissures, there is no direct evidence of this. Indeed, it has consistently been reported that the main reduction in carious lesions has been on smooth surfaces rather than in pits and fissures.

Fluoride in dental tissues

Fluoride is incorporated into hydroxyapatite and makes it more resistant to acid dissolution. It also assists in the crystallisation of apatites

The effects of fluoride on the mineral component of dental enamel (or dentine or cementum) may be distinguished during mineralisation or at later stages. If sufficient fluoride is present in plasma during the mineralisation of teeth, fluorapatite rather than hydroxyapatite is formed (Fig. 10.5). Crystallisation of apatites occurs more rapidly in the presence of higher physiological concentrations of fluoride. By itself this should lead to larger crystal sizes and these are more resistant to acid dissolution because of their smaller surface to volume ratio. The more rapid crystallisation favours formation of apatite at the expense of octacalcium phosphate. The eventual transition of octacalcium phosphate to apatite tends to result in calcium-deficient apatites; fluoride

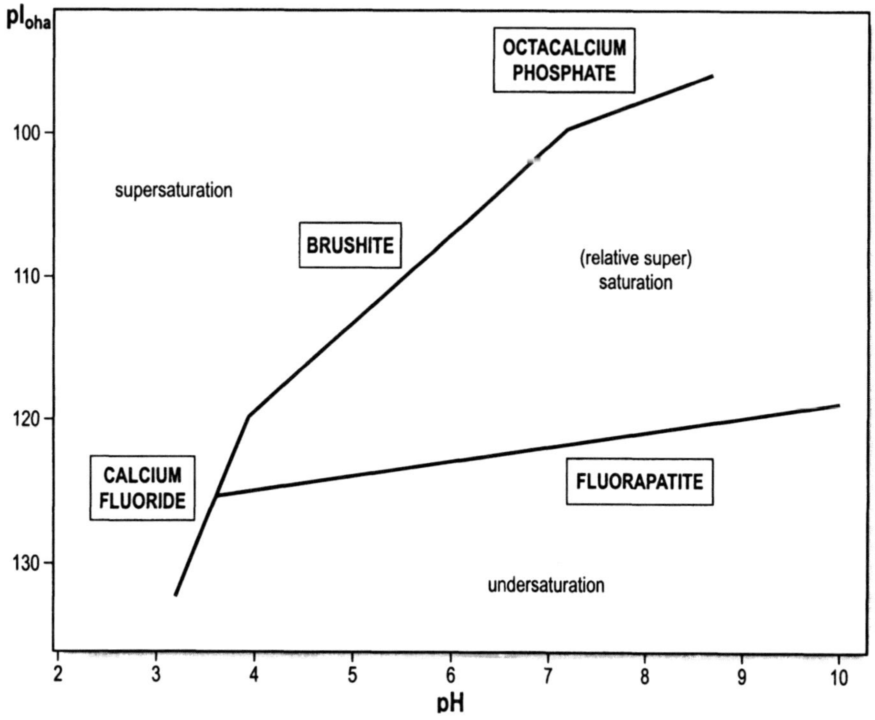

Fig. 10.5
Solubility curves for fluorapatite and other crystals when the aqueous phase contains calcium, phosphate, hydroxyl, carbonate and fluoride ions.

therefore favours formation of more perfect apatite crystals. Solubility is related to crystal size and to crystallinity; apatite from enamel is less acid-soluble than that from dentine which is turn less soluble than that from bone. The substitution of fluoride into the hydroxyapatite lattice changes its dimensions slightly (Ch. 2) and slows its rate of dissolution in acid. Apatites with a high fluorapatite content therefore dissolve more slowly than those with lower fluoride contents and are less soluble than those with high carbonate or magnesium contents.

After eruption the teeth are exposed to fluoride-containing liquids, foods and saliva, and so fluoride uptake continues on the enamel surface. This occurs by substitution for hydroxyl ions in the apatite lattice to form fluorapatite. High concentrations of fluoride from topical applications also lead to deposition of calcium fluoride on the enamel surface. This surface layer is not, however, integral to the enamel surface and is more soluble than hydroxyapatite and so is lost again over 24–36 h. There is, however, some exchange of fluoride ions from the calcium fluoride with the apatite until such time as the layer is lost.

Strictly, the immediate environment of each tooth is the layer of pellicle and/or dental plaque on its surface and it is through this layer that intraoral fluoride reaches the teeth. The plaque fluid is relatively high in fluoride concentration – about 3.5 μmol/l (0.7 ppm) – in comparison with saliva, and the plaque fluoride content is directly related to the fluoride intake. The enamel surface may be envisaged as being in equilibrium with the plaque fluid; pH changes in the fluid will govern the dissolution or remineralisation of the enamel. The presence of fluoride in the apatite crystals decreases their rate of dissolution, and the fluoride in the plaque fluid itself enhances the recrystallisation of the apatite when conditions become less acid. Further, the preferential dissolution of carbonate- or magnesium-rich apatite crystals and their replacement during remineralisation by fluorapatite crystals effectively increases the resistance of the enamel to acid attack. Current opinion is strongly in favour of the role of fluoride in remineralisation as being the major explanation of the posteruptive effect of fluoride in reducing dental caries.

Effects of fluoride in modifying plaque metabolism

Fluoride reduces the cariogenicity of plaque bacteria by reducing acid production

However, in addition to its protective effects on enamel, fluoride does affect the caries process by modifying the bacterial attack itself. This occurs in two ways: by altering the ability of the organisms to produce acids, and by favouring the growth of some bacteria at the expense of others. Bacteria which take up fluoride do so predominantly in the form of undissociated hydrogen fluoride, present in acid conditions. The HF dissociates in the less acid environment inside the cell and the hydrogen ions so released lower the intracellular pH. This process may be associated with an outward movement of potassium ions. Ionised fluoride inhibits enolase, the enzyme which converts 2-phosphoglycerate to phosphoenol pyruvate in the glycolytic pathway. The amount of fluoride needed to produce a significant inhibition of glycolysis is as low as 6–12 μmol/mg in some streptococci; in most other species concentrations nearer ten times those in plaque fluid are required. Fluoride inhibits glucose transport by its effect on enolase because phosphoenol pyruvate is necessary for a phosphoenol pyruvate transferase system which enables the formation of glucose 1-phosphate. Transport of glucose is also linked to hydrogen ion gradients in some bacteria: an increase in intracellular hydrogen ion concentration inhibits movement of glucose via a glucose–hydrogen ion symport. Fluoride inhibits the membrane ATPase expelling hydrogen ions from bacterial cells by inhibiting glycolysis and decreasing the hydrogen ion gradient across the cell walls. The total effect of fluoride, then, is to inhibit acid production and to disrupt the general energy metabolism of the cells. As different bacteria show differing sensitivities to these fluoride effects, the ion exerts a selection mechanism within the oral flora which may reduce the proportion of cariogenic bacteria.

Toxic effects of fluoride

Harmful effects of fluoride on the teeth

The effects of fluoride on the teeth are not entirely beneficial. As the fluoride concentrations in drinking water increase, so does the incidence of tooth mottling. The recommended levels of fluoride for water fluoridation are based on observations of those which give the greatest reduction in dental caries whilst also being associated with the lowest incidence of tooth mottling. In the populations studied, there is a relatively high level of mottling of enamel observed at low water fluoride levels. This decreases as fluoride concentration rises to reach a minimum at between 0.05 and 0.1 mmol/l (1 and 2 ppm) and then increases again with higher fluoride levels. The mottling observed at low fluoride levels is thought to be due to the sequelae of caries of the deciduous teeth; abscess formation around the roots of the deciduous teeth may impair development of the enamel of the permanent successor. This type of idiopathic mottling therefore decreases as fluoride levels increase and caries experience in the deciduous teeth is reduced. However, above 0.1 mmol/l (2 ppm) fluoride in the water supply, the incidence of mottling due to fluoride itself increases (Fig. 10.1). At 0.3 mmol/l (6 ppm) the incidence of mottling reaches 100%. There are now reports that with the almost universal use of fluoride toothpastes in the Western world mottling of teeth is becoming increasingly common at water fluoride levels which were previously not associated with fluoride-induced mottling.

Enamel fluorosis manifests itself as localised increases in enamel porosity. In the least severe cases the teeth erupt with opaque white lines corresponding to the enamel perikymata. The porosity extends only a short distance into the enamel and as the tooth ages in the oral environment the lesions may be worn away and disappear, or they may take up stains and become brown and more visually prominent. In severe cases the whole of the erupting crown of the tooth may be chalky white and the porosity may extend through the full thickness of the enamel. Such enamel fractures and pits very easily because of its reduced strength and readily becomes stained. The balance of evidence favours the view that the main effect of fluoride on enamel development occurs at the maturation stage rather than during matrix formation or during the initial calcification process. Fluorosis in children has been linked with the administration of fluoride at the time of enamel maturation. Changes in ameloblast differentiation observed in animal experiments seem to occur only at high concentrations of fluoride. Although some inhibition of protein synthesis has been reported the numbers of proteins and their types are unaffected – the process in non-selective. Mineral deposition during the secretory stage of amelogenesis has been shown to be affected in vitro experiments with hypercalcification occurring at sites where calcification had already begun but with inhibition of calcification at other sites. In the normal maturation stage of enamel development there is removal of protein and increased mineralisation of the enamel, but in fluorosis neither of these events occur. Proline-rich material is retained in the enamel matrix and the degree of mineralisation is unchanged. The normal change in the amelobasts to a ruffle-ended appearance does not take place and proteolytic enzyme activity appears to be inhibited.

Fluoride causes enamel mottling by an adverse effect on amelogenin removal during enamel maturation

Toxic effects of high doses of fluoride

Both acute and chronic administration of high doses of fluoride is harmful

Chronic administration of higher doses of fluoride leads to more general symptoms of fluorosis. Systemic fluorosis is characterised by the development of exostoses on the long bones, and stiffness and pain in the joints, particularly in the spine. It would appear that fluoride stimulates bone growth and calcification. For this reason it has been used in relatively high doses in older patients to arrest the progress of osteoporosis.

The amounts of fluoride in toothpaste have been beneficial in reducing dental caries but may be sufficient to increase the possibility of dental fluorosis if there is a high intake of fluoride from other sources. Children must also be discouraged from eating toothpaste since this could present the problems of a large acute dose.

Acute doses of fluoride present a toxicological problem. From the dental point of view administration of single large doses in animals produces a transient increase in blood fluoride concentrations which result in the development of a calciotraumatic line in forming enamel and dentine. In enamel a hypercalcified line appears at first but this disappears in the fully mineralised tissue. With higher doses a hypomineralised zone develops outside the hypermineralised zone and this persists in the erupted tooth. In dentine the pattern is reversed in that a hypomineralised layer forms first and the hypermineralised zone is seen subsequently. Both these zones persist in the final dentine.

Doses of fluoride in excess of 20 mg/kg are probably lethal

Even a tube of toothpaste could cause severe effects in a small child

Doses in excess of 20 mg/kg in the human adult should be regarded as probably lethal. In accounts of deaths of adults from fluoride poisoning the doses ingested have been of the order of 30 mg/g, but data from cases where children have died after fluoride ingestion suggest that the probably toxic dose is nearer 5 mg/kg. This figure is not too far away from doses used therapeutically. A 5–6-year-old child weighs around 20 kg: a potentially toxic dose would be present in a 100-g tube of toothpaste, or in 8 ml of acid sodium fluoride gel used as a topical application to the teeth. The symptoms of acute fluoride poisoning are nausea, epigastric pain and vomiting. Limb spasms, tetany and convulsions may develop with high doses; blood pressure and pulse rate fall and respiration is depressed. Unconsciousness follows. Treatment is urgent: it consists of induction of vomiting if not already present, and then administration of 1% calcium gluconate or calcium chloride. Milk may be used if these are not available. Hospital treatment should be obtained: it should include maintenance of the airway, gastric lavage with calcium solutions, and intravenous administration of glucose, calcium salts and sodium bicarbonate. It may be necessary to provide artificial respiration and/or cardiac stimulation.

Further reading

Fluoride in Health and Disease, 3rd edition. Murray, J.J., Rugg-Gunn, A.J., Jenkins, G.N. Wright, Oxford, 1991

The Metabolism and Toxicity of Fluoride, 2nd edition. Whitford, G.M. Karger, Basel, 1996

Fluoride: Mechanisms of Action and Recommendations for USA. Special issue of the Journal of Dental Research 69: 1990

Fluoride in Dentistry. Ekstrand, J., Fejerskov, O., Silverstone, L. Munksgaard, Copenhagen, 1988

SECTION THREE

Oral sensation and activity; ageing

11 Oral sensation

The oral cavity is innervated by the maxillary and mandibular branches of the trigeminal nerve but also has an autonomic supply via the facial, glossopharyngeal and vagus nerves

Trigeminal nerve

The principal sensory nerve for the oral cavity is the trigeminal nerve, but only its maxillary and mandibular branches are involved. The trigeminal nerve is the fifth cranial nerve.

Nuclei of the trigeminal nerve

Unlike the other cranial nerves the trigeminal has several nuclei, one of which extends down into the upper segments of the spinal cord (Figs 11.1–11.3). The motor nucleus lies in the pons just below the superior cerebellar peduncle and lateral to the central tegmental tract and the nucleus of the locus coeruleus. It receives motor fibres from the pyramidal tract on the opposite side. The mesencephalic nucleus is immediately superior, almost in the peduncle.

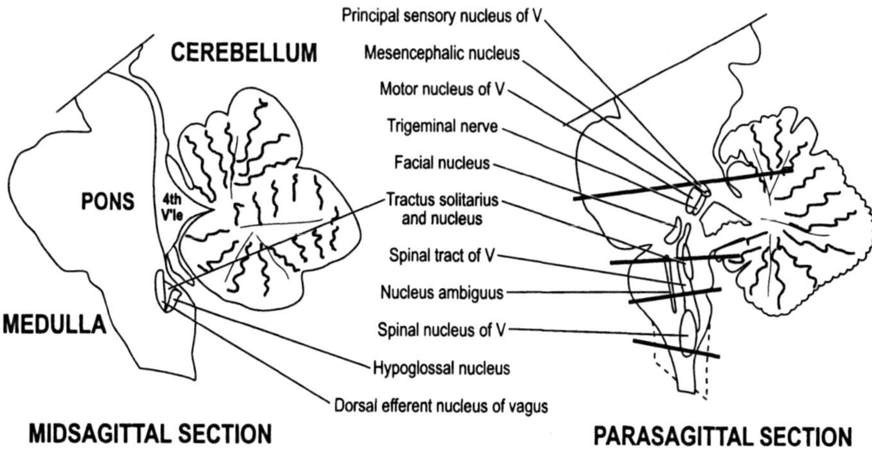

Fig. 11.1
Midsagittal and parasagittal sections through the brainstem to show the location of the trigeminal and other nerve nuclei associated with oral sensation. The coloured lines show the levels of the transverse sections in Fig. 11.2.

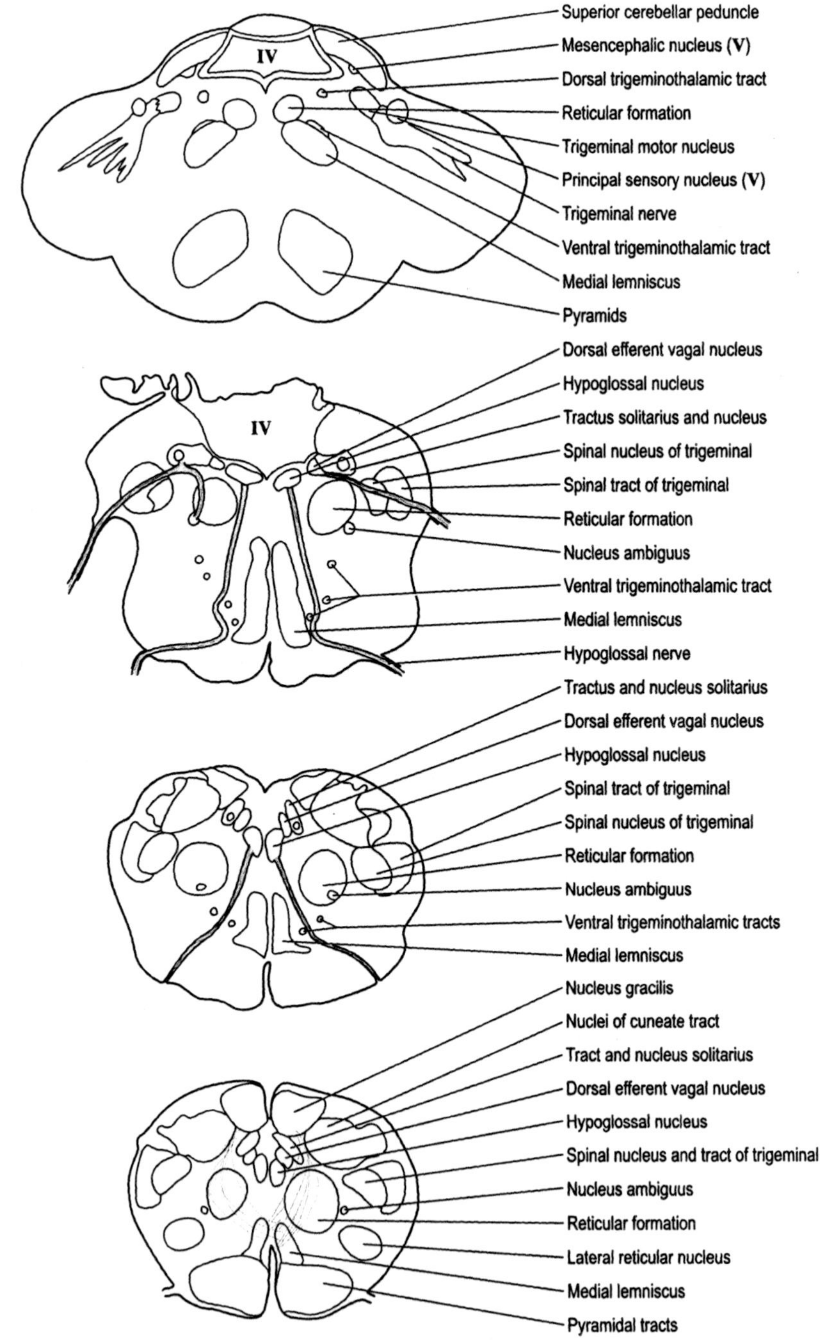

Transverse sections of the brainstem to show the nuclei of the trigeminal and other nerves associated with oral sensation. The upper section is at the level of the upper pons with the mesencephalic and motor nuclei of the trigeminal nerve, the next is in the lower pons at the level of the origins of the vagus and hypoglossal nerves, the next is in the upper medulla, and the lowest is at the level of the sensory decussation in the medulla.

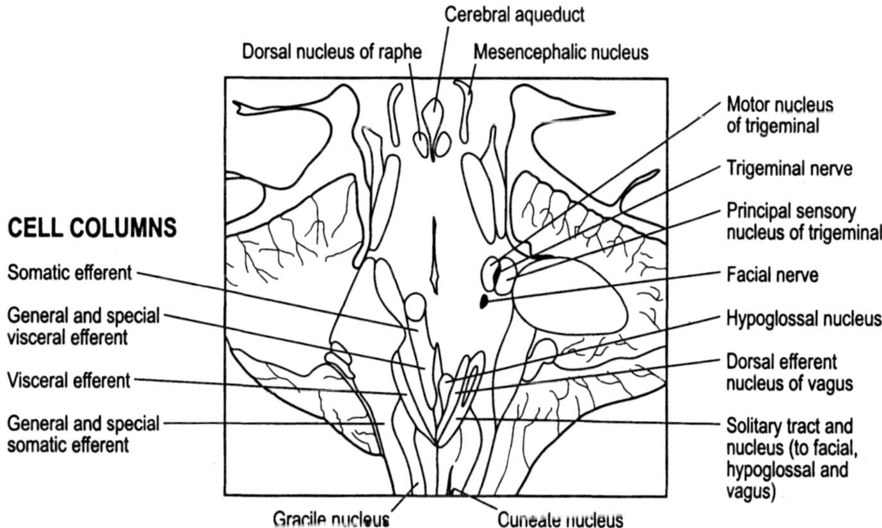

Fig. 11.3
A coronal or horizontal section through the brainstem showing the nuclei of the nerves involved in oral sensation as seen from the cerebellar aspect.

The trigeminal nerve has a mesencephalic nucleus, a principal sensory nucleus, and a threefold spinal nucleus

Lateral to the motor nucleus is the principal sensory nucleus, closely related posteriorly to the vestibular nuclei. From the principal sensory nucleus the spinal tract of the trigeminal sweeps downwards and backwards through the medulla oblongata into the third or fourth cervical segment of the spinal cord, forming three nuclei on its mesial side – the oralis, the central or interpolaris, and the caudalis.

The mesencephalic nucleus has one of the functions of the dorsal root ganglion of a spinal nerve: it contains the cell bodies of the nerves carrying proprioceptive information and sends fibres on into the motor nucleus, as well as to the sensory nuclei for onward transmission to the cerebellum and the cortex. The former pathway provides the route for the monosynaptic stretch reflexes of the muscles of mastication. The remainder of the trigeminal sensory nerve fibres have their cell bodies in the trigeminal ganglion (the Gasserian ganglion) which is analogous in this respect to a dorsal root ganglion. The fibres then enter the pons in the sensory root of the trigeminal and pass either upwards to the principal sensory nucleus (fibres carrying touch, pressure and some proprioceptive information) or downwards in the spinal tract to the sensory nuclei (fibres carrying pain and temperature information). The principal nucleus is analogous to the nuclei of the cuneate and gracilis tracts. The spinal tract is continuous with the substantia gelatinosa of the spinal cord. Fibres from the tract then pass into the various trigeminal sensory nuclei which contain the cell bodies of the secondary sensory neurones. These cross to the opposite side of the pons and ascend in the trigeminal lemniscus (the ventral trigeminothalamic tract) to transmit impulses to the thalamus – a route similar that taken by impulses in the tracts of the spinal cord. The sensory fibres from the mandibular division of the trigeminal nerve are in the dorsal part of the spinal tract and those from the maxillary lie ventral to them; both sets are confined to the upper part of the tract and do not extend below the level of the medulla oblongata.

The fibres of the trigeminal nerve leave the anterior surface of the pons above the level of the middle cerebellar peduncle, with the motor root medial and anterior to the much larger sensory root. The sensory root passes to the trigeminal ganglion which lies in a recess near the apex of the petrous part of the temporal bone close to the internal carotid artery and the cavernous sinus. From the trigeminal ganglion arise the three sensory divisions of the trigeminal nerve – the ophthalmic, the maxillary and the mandibular. Only the two last are considered here and then only in relation to their oral significance.

The maxillary nerve

The branches of the maxillary nerve supply sensory fibres to the oral region and act as the final pathway for some secretomotor fibres

The maxillary nerve (Fig. 11.4), after it leaves the skull via the foramen rotundum, reaches the pterygopalatine fossa and there gives off two branches to the sphenopalatine ganglion and, just before entering the infraorbital groove, three or four superior dental branches. One of these passes down the posterior surface of the maxilla to supply the posterior gingiva in that area and the adjoining cheek. The others pass into the maxilla to run in small canals in the wall of the maxillary sinus, supplying its mucous membrane and then forming a plexus above the dental arch from which fibres pass to the teeth and periodontal ligaments. The posterior superior dental nerve is distributed primarily to the molar region and the middle superior dental nerve to the premolar region. As the maxillary (or now infraorbital) nerve passes through the infraorbital canal it gives off the anterior superior branch which then runs in a canal in the anterior wall of the maxillary sinus. This supplies the incisor and canine regions and forms the anterior part of the superior dental plexus. The infraorbital nerve has a number of branches after leaving via the infraorbital foramen: a large and numerous group are termed the labial branches. They pass down the face behind the levator labii superioris muscle to supply the skin of upper parts of the cheeks and lips but also the mucous membranes of the upper parts of the vestibule and are secretomotor to the minor salivary glands in this region. It is likely that such secretomotor fibres are derived from the sphenopalatine ganglion and ultimately from the parasympathetic fibres of the facial nerve. The sphenopalatine ganglion also supplies sympathetic fibres although these are more likely to travel with the blood vessels than with branches of the maxillary nerve.

The mandibular nerve

Some branches of the mandibular nerve are motor to the muscles of mastication

The mandibular nerve (Fig. 11.5) is the largest division of the trigeminal nerve: it arises from the trigeminal ganglion, passes through the foramen ovale of the sphenoid bone and is immediately joined by the motor root of the trigeminal. It then lies between the tensor palati and lateral pterygoid muscles. It now gives off a branch to the medial pterygoid muscle which enters the posterior surface, but also sends some fibres through the otic ganglion, and finally emerges from the medial pterygoid muscle to supply the tensor tympani and

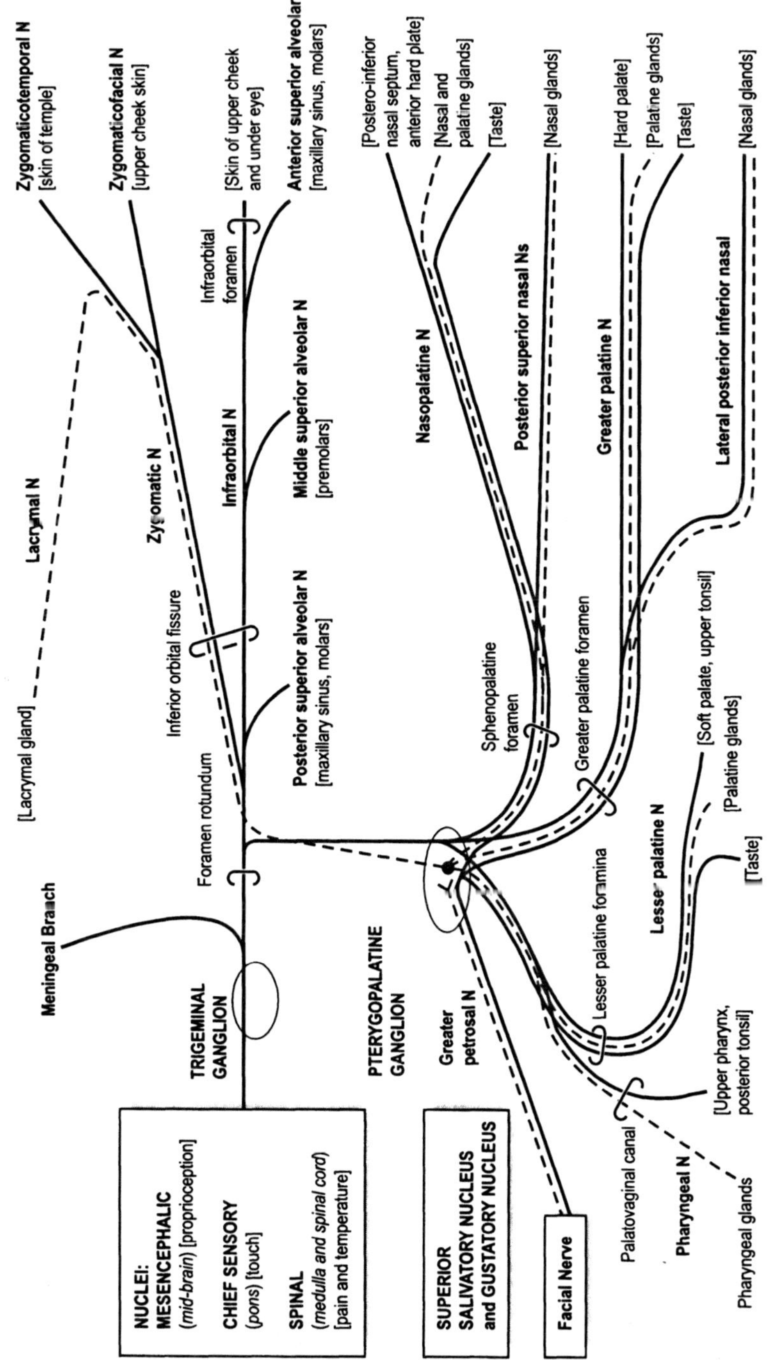

Fig. 11.4
The branches of the maxillary division of the trigeminal nerve. Somatosensory branches are shown as solid coloured lines and secretomotor branches as dashed black lines. The names of nerve branches are in bold type, ganglia are represented by ovals, and foramina or other passages through bone are indicated by broken loops.

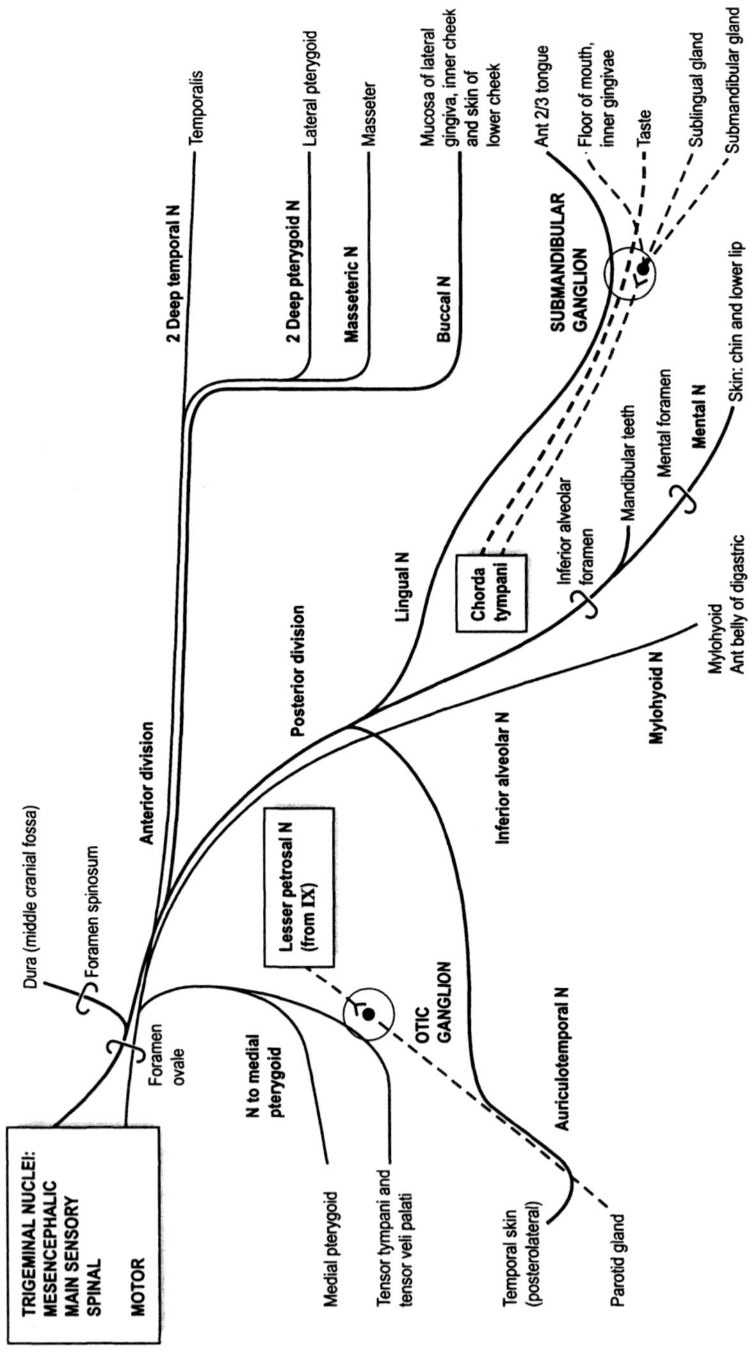

The branches of the mandibular division of the trigeminal nerve. Motor branches are shown as solid black lines, somatosensory branches as solid coloured lines, secretomotor branches as dashed black lines and autonomic sensory branches as coloured lines. The names of nerve branches are in bold type, ganglia are represented by circles, and foramina or other passages through bone are indicated by broken loops.

Other branches are sensory to the oral mucosa of the cheeks, floor of the mouth and lower jaw. They also carry autonomic secretomotor fibres and fibres carrying taste inputs

tensor palati muscles. Beyond the medial pterygoid branch the mandibular nerve divides into a small anterior trunk and a larger posterior trunk. The anterior trunk sends a predominantly sensory branch, the buccal nerve, between the two heads of the lateral pterygoid muscle and then downwards under the temporal muscle to reach the inner side of the ramus of the mandible close to the anterior border of the masseter muscle where it joins with the buccal branches of the facial nerve to supply sensation to the skin over the buccinator muscle, the mucous membrane of the inside of the cheek and the buccal surface of the posterior gingivae. It also sends fibres along its course to the lateral pterygoid, and possibly the temporalis muscle. The anterior trunk also gives rise to three or four motor nerves: the masseteric, passing above the lateral pterygoid muscle, between the temporomandibular joint and the tendon of the temporalis muscle to cross the mandibular notch and enter the deep aspect of the masseter muscle (with a branch to the joint itself); the deep temporal nerves which enter the deep surface of the temporalis muscle; and the nerve to lateral pterygoid which enters the deep surface of that muscle.

The posterior trunk is mainly sensory and has three major branches. The auriculotemporal nerve runs back between the lateral pterygoid and tensor palati muscles to pass between the sphenomandibular ligament and the neck of the mandible to reach the temporomandibular joint and the parotid gland, giving off articular and parotid branches as it does so. From there it ascends over the zygoma and breaks up into the superficial temporal branches to supply the skin in the temporal region. The parotid branch carries secretomotor fibres from the otic ganglion which ultimately derive from the facial nerve. The second division of the posterior trunk is the lingual nerve. As it lies between the tensor palati and the lateral pterygoid muscles it receives branches from the chorda tympani branch of the facial nerve and the inferior dental nerve. Leaving the lateral pterygoid muscle, the nerve passes downwards and forwards between the ramus of the mandible and the medial pterygoid muscle. It is anterior to the inferior dental nerve in this position. It then passes below the insertion of the superior pharyngeal constrictor muscle to the mandible and then lies on the lingual side of the mandibular third molar roots immediately beneath the mucosa. Taking a more medial direction it crosses over the styloglossus muscle to the side of the tongue and runs lateral to the hyoglossus muscle below the mylohyoid muscle and above the submandibular gland and the submandibular duct. After continuing forwards on the lateral aspect of hyoglossus and genioglossus muscles, in close relation to the submandibular duct first laterally and then medially, the nerve divides into its final branches under the mucosa of the tongue. The lingual nerve provides a sensory supply to the mucosa covering the lingual aspect of the mandibular arch, the floor of the mouth and the anterior two-thirds of the tongue. It carries secretomotor fibres to the submandibular and sublingual salivary glands which it acquires from the facial nerve via the chorda tympani, the submandibular ganglion and connecting branches from the ganglion, and it receives some fibres from a branch of the hypoglossal nerve to innervate the tip of the tongue.

The third branch of the posterior trunk of the mandibular nerve is the inferior dental nerve. This descends deep to the lateral pterygoid muscle and then passes between the sphenomandibular ligament and the ramus of the mandible. Just above the mandibular foramen the nerve gives off a branch which continues on down the ramus to reach the underside of the mylohyoid muscle and supply it and the anterior belly of the digastric muscle with motor fibres. The inferior dental nerve enters the mandibular foramen to pass in the mandibular canal below the molar and premolar teeth (although sometimes the roots of a molar may enclose the canal) until it reaches the mental foramen where it divides into an incisive branch which continues in the bone to form the incisive plexus with the contralateral nerve and supply sensation to the incisor and canine teeth, and a mental branch which leaves through the mental canal to supply the skin and mucous membrane of the lower lip. The molars and premolars, their periodontal ligaments and the buccal gingival tissue related to them are supplied from an inferior dental plexus derived from the inferior dental nerve as it passes through the mandibular canal.

Autonomic nerves

Autonomic fibres which are sensory in the mouth provide taste perception. They are mainly of parasympathetic origin and arise in the nuclei of the facial, glossopharyngeal and vagus nerves, although the facial nerve fibres ultimately reach the anterior part of the tongue via the lingual branch of the mandibular division of the trigeminal nerve.

The facial nerve

The facial nerve carries motor, secretomotor and taste fibres

The facial nerve (the seventh cranial nerve) (Fig. 11.6) supplies motor fibres to some of the muscles involved in mastication: it provides taste sensation from a large proportion of the taste receptors, and it carries secretomotor fibres for the salivary glands. Its motor nucleus is situated in the lower part of pons in the reticular formation, ventral and medial to the nucleus of the spinal tract of the trigeminal nerve. It receives descending fibres from the contralateral pyramidal tract. The motor axons pass first backwards and medially to run upwards superficially to the nucleus of the abducent nerve and then run downwards and forwards through the pons to emerge between the olive and the superior cerebellar peduncle as the motor root. The secretomotor fibres originate in the superior salivatory nucleus, close to the caudal end of the motor nucleus and they leave the pons in the sensory root. The sensory nucleus of the facial nerve is in the upper part of the nucleus of the tractus solitarius. Its efferent fibres pass through the thalamus to the hippocampal gyrus. The sensory root leaves the lower border of the pons close to the motor root and the auditory nerve and the three pass forwards and laterally to the opening of the internal auditory meatus where the facial nerve roots travel in a groove on the surface of the auditory nerve. There are some connections between the nerves. The facial nerve roots reach the bottom of the meatus and pass into the facial canal, where they run laterally to the medial wall of the epitympanic recess, bend backwards above the promontory, fusing and swelling to form the ganglion of the facial nerve, and then curving down in

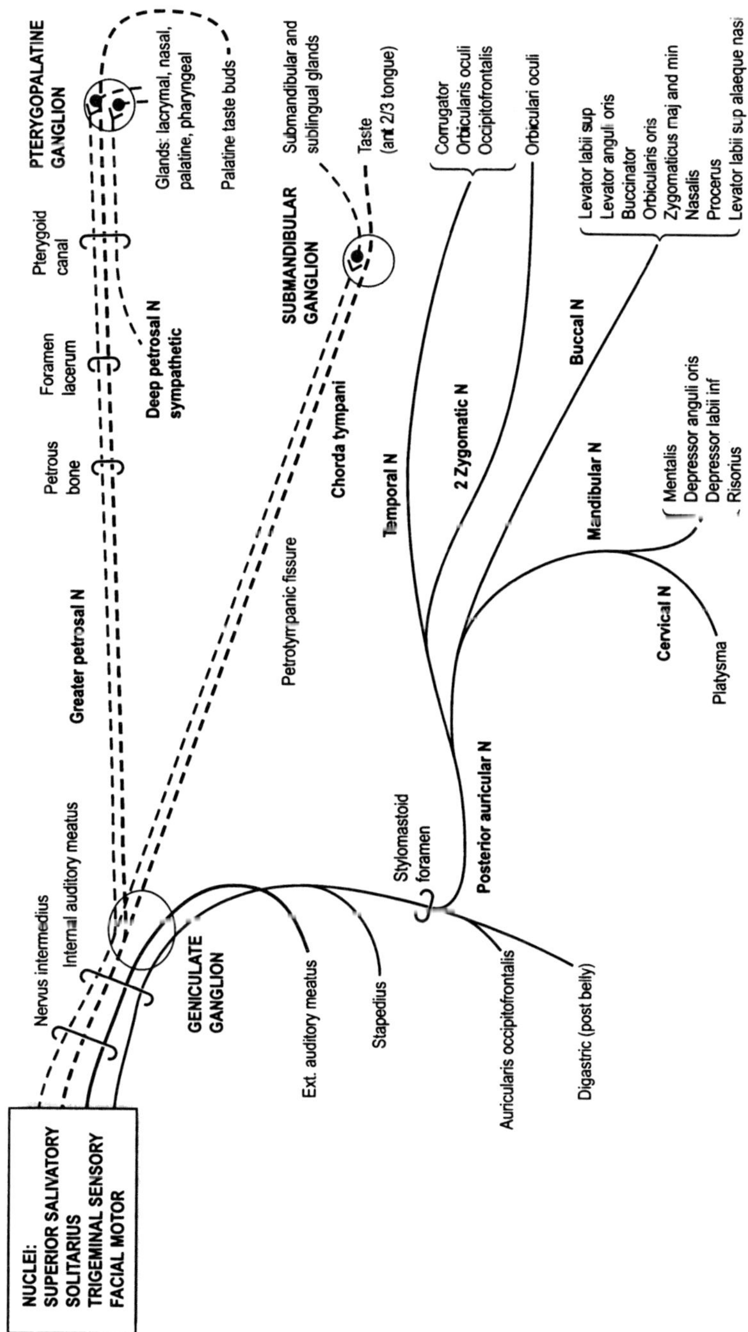

Fig. 11.6
The branches of the facial nerve. Motor branches are shown as solid black lines, somatosensory branches as solid coloured lines, secretomotor branches as dashed black lines and autonomic sensory branches as dashed coloured lines. The names of nerve branches are in bold type, ganglia are represented by circles, and foramina or other passages through bone are indicated by broken loops.

the wall of the aditus to reach the tympanic antrum as a single nerve trunk. The facial ganglion is an analogue of the dorsal root ganglia of spinal nerves and contains the cell bodies of the afferent nerves carrying taste sensation up to the nucleus of the tractus solitarius. It has connections with the sphenopalatine ganglion via the greater superficial petrosal nerve and with the otic ganglion via a branch which joins the lesser superficial petrosal nerve (a nerve which ultimately derives from the glossopharyngeal nerve) which carries secretomotor fibres destined for the parotid gland. The greater superficial petrosal nerve passes through a gap on the anterior surface of the petrous part of the temporal bone and continues in a groove on the bone to pass beneath the trigeminal ganglion to reach the foramen lacerum, where it is joined by the deep petrosal nerve to form the nerve of the pterygoid canal. This leaves the pterygoid canal to end in the sphenopalatine ganglion. The taste fibres pass through the ganglion to be distributed over the surface of the palate in the palatine nerves.

Within the facial canal the facial nerve has a connection to muscles in and around the ear but, more importantly from the present viewpoint, gives rise to the chorda tympani nerve. This runs upward and forward in a bony canal, perforates the wall of the tympanic cavity close to the edge of the medial surface of the tympanic membrane. It crosses forwards between the fibrous and mucous layers of the membrane to re-enter bone in the anterior canaliculus of the chorda tympani at the inner end of the petrotympanic fissure. It runs down the spine of the sphenoid bone and deep to the lateral pterygoid muscle and lateral to the tensor palati, passing close to the auriculotemporal and inferior dental nerves. It joins the lingual nerve to provide it with the taste fibres which are to supply the anterior two-thirds of the tongue and secretomotor fibres which pass to the submandibular ganglion. These are preganglionic parasympathetic fibres which synapse in the ganglion with the short postganglionic fibres which innervate the sublingual and submandibular glands.

After leaving the facial canal the facial nerve passes downwards to reach the stylomastoid foramen and runs forward in the substance of the parotid gland, whence it crosses the styloid process and the external carotid artery and divides behind the ramus of the mandible to form the parotid plexus from which the motor nerves to the muscles of facial expression arise. At the exit from the stylomastoid foramen the nerve has connections with the glossopharyngeal and vagus nerves and gives off motor branches to muscles around the ear and to the posterior belly of digastric and the stylohyoid muscle.

The glossopharyngeal nerve

The glossopharyngeal nerve carries secretomotor and sensory fibres, including those for taste sensation

The glossopharyngeal nerve (the ninth cranial nerve) (Fig. 11.7) carries fibres from four nuclei in the brainstem. There are motor fibres to the stylopharyngeus muscle which arise in the upper part of the nucleus ambiguous in the reticular formation of the medulla oblongata; this nucleus receives signals from the contralateral pyramidal tract.

Secretomotor fibres for the parotid gland arise from the inferior salivary nucleus, again in the medullary reticular formation. The sensory nuclei of the

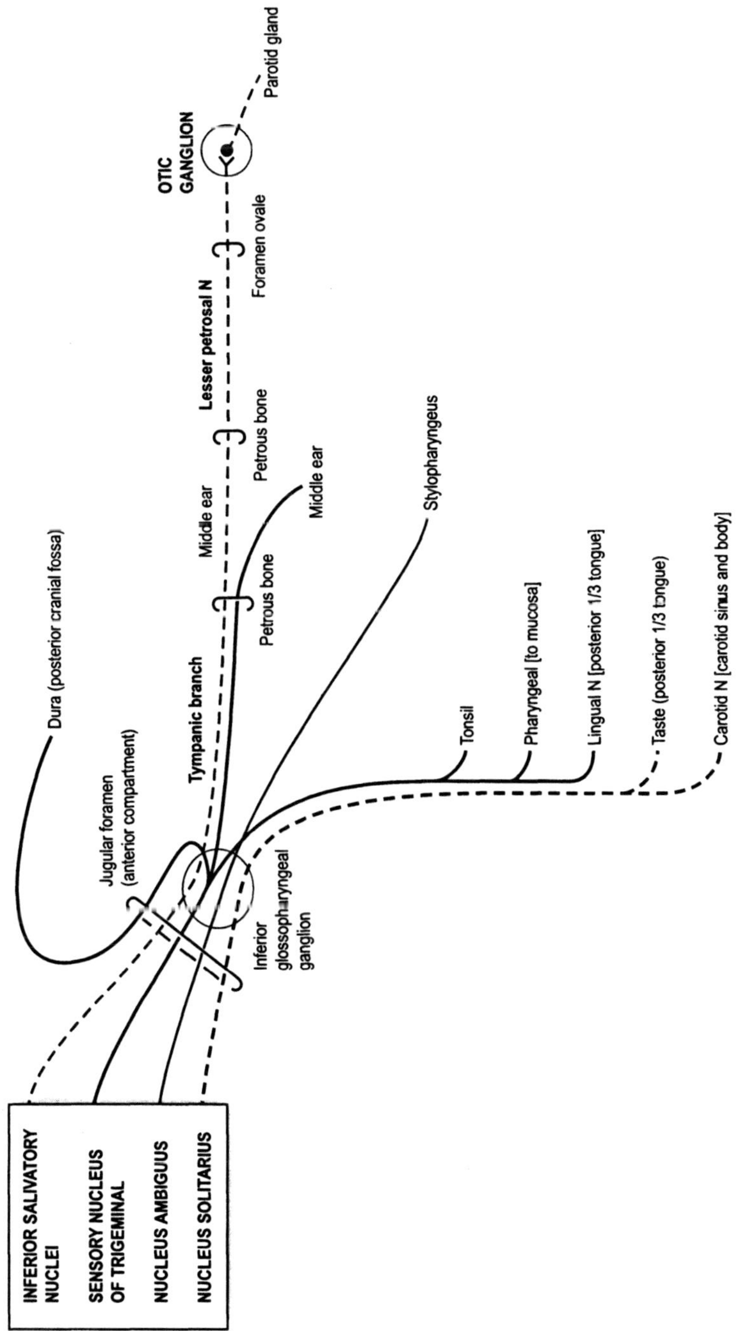

Fig. 11.7
The branches of the glossopharyngeal nerve. Motor branches are shown as solid black lines, somatosensory branches as solid coloured lines, secretomotor branches as dashed black lines and autonomic sensory branches as dashed coloured lines. The names of nerve branches are in bold type, ganglia are represented by circles, and foramina or other passages through bone are indicated by broken loops.

glossopharyngeal nerve are the dorsal nucleus of the vagus nerve for general sensation and the nucleus of the tractus solitarius for taste sensation. Both these receive afferent fibres from nerve cell bodies in the inferior ganglion of the glossopharyngeal nerve; the latter sends on information via the thalamus to the hippocampal gyrus. The nerve leaves the upper part of the medulla oblongata in the groove between the olive and the inferior cerebellar peduncle and passes forwards and laterally to the inferior surface of the petrous part of the temporal bone, reaches the jugular tubercle of the occipital bone and then bends sharply downwards through the jugular foramen to continue in company with the vagus and accessory nerves.

In the jugular foramen a small superior ganglion continues on into the inferior ganglion which lies in a notch in the lower border of the petrous part of the temporal bone. The superior ganglion appears to be merely a detached part of the inferior ganglion. From the inferior ganglion there are connections with the vagus and facial nerves and some six other branches. The tympanic nerve passes up through the inferior tympanic canaliculus to the tympanic cavity where it forms the tympanic plexus. This in turn gives off a branch to the greater superficial petrosal nerve, branches to supply the mucosa of the inner ear, and the lesser superficial petrosal nerve. The lesser superficial petrosal nerve leaves the tympanic cavity via a small canal, receives a filament from the ganglion of the facial nerve, and reaches the anterior surface of the temporal bone near the greater superficial petrosal nerve. Passing through the foramen ovale it reaches the otic ganglion, which lies medial to the trunk of the mandibular nerve and lateral to the tensor palati muscle. The preganglionic fibres of the lesser superficial petrosal nerve synapse in the otic ganglion with the postganglionic fibres which pass in a communicating branch to the auriculotemporal nerve and thence to the parotid gland to provide secretomotor signals.

The carotid branch forms the nerve of the carotid body and the carotid sinus. The remaining branches, apart from the motor branch to the stylopharyngeus muscle, carry afferent sensory fibres for general sensation and the special sense of taste. They are: the pharyngeal branches, which join with fibres from the vagus nerve to form the pharyngeal plexus and innervate the pharyngeal mucosa; the tonsillar branches, which supply the tonsil and form a plexus with the lesser palatine nerves which supplies the soft palate and the pharyngeal isthmus; and the two lingual branches, one supplying the vallate papillae and the mucosa along the sulcus terminalis of the tongue, and the other supplying the mucosa of the posterior third of the tongue.

The vagus nerve

The vagus nerve supplies some general and taste sensation in the oral cavity

The vagus nerve (the tenth cranial nerve) (Fig. 11.8) is also associated with taste and general sensation from the epiglottis and the upper part of the pharynx. Its central fibres connect with the nucleus of the tractus solitarius, the cell bodies being in the inferior ganglion of the nerve. The actual branch carrying the sensory fibres is the internal laryngeal nerve.

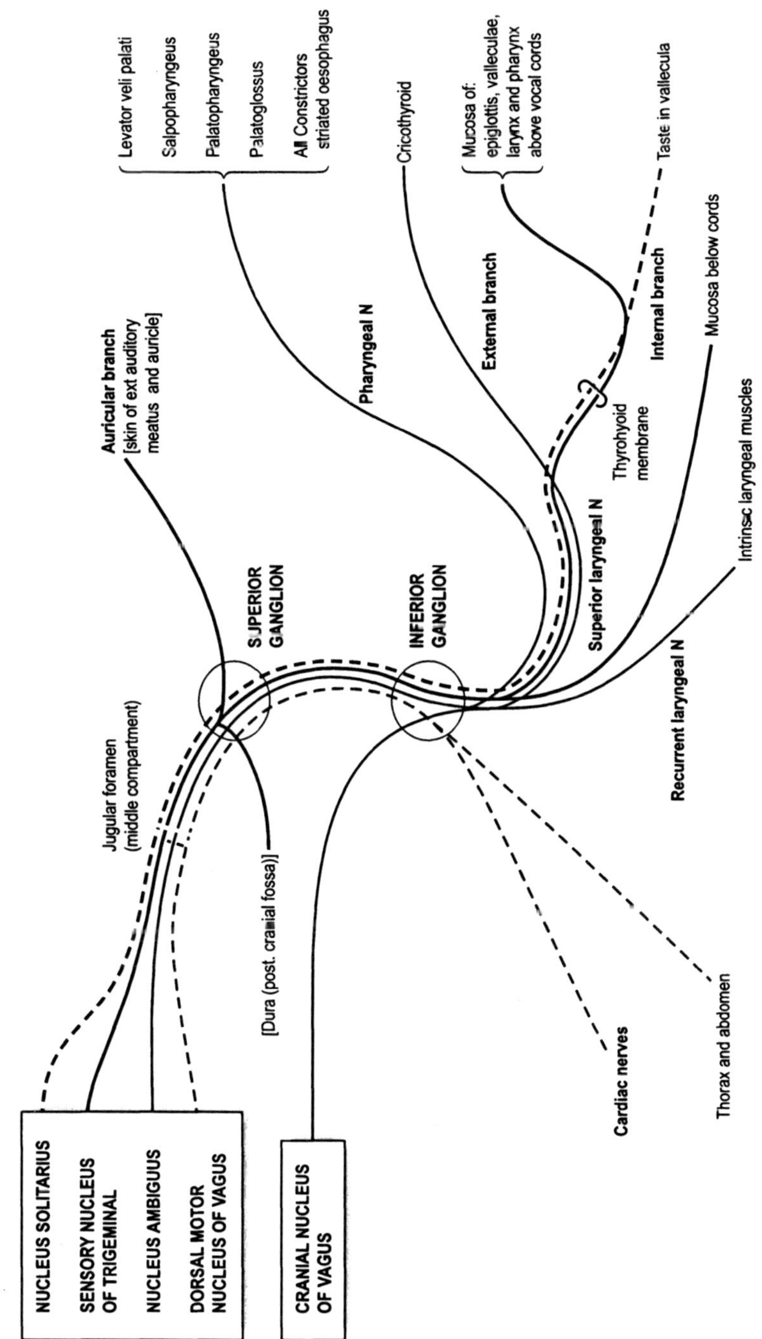

Fig. 11.8
The branches of the vagus nerve of oral significance. Motor branches are shown as solid black lines, somatosensory branches as solid coloured lines, autonomic motor branches as dashed black lines and autonomic sensory branches as dashed coloured lines. The names of nerve branches are in bold type, ganglia are represented by circles, and foramina or other passages through bone are indicated by broken loops.

General sensation in the oral cavity

The oral mucosa is sensitive to touch, pressure, temperature and pain. It can provide information on the shape of objects in the mouth

The oral mucosa is well supplied with sensory fibres of the trigeminal nerve. It is sensitive to the range of skin sensations – touch, pressure, temperature and pain – and also has a well-developed ability to detect the shape of objects, a property termed stereognosis. Despite this, there are few descriptions of specific end-organs or receptors in the oral mucosa except for those transducing the special sense of taste (considered later in this chapter). The signals giving rise to touch and pressure sensations travel in A beta and A delta fibres (group II and III sensory neurones) to their cell bodies in the trigeminal ganglion and then on to the sensory nuclei of the nerve. There interaction with other neurones can take place and secondary sensory neurones carry the signal to the other side of the brainstem before ascending to the thalamus. In the somatosensory cortex the area for the mouth is situated in the lower part of the postcentral gyrus and occupies a relatively large area – a physical demonstration of its high degree of sensitivity. Indeed, the lips are represented in an area totally disproportionate to their size and even larger than that for the thumb. Two-point discrimination is high on the lips and gingivae and on the tongue, slightly less so on the palate.

Temperature sensation

The mucous membranes of the mouth are also very sensitive to hot and cold. This is probably a protective mechanism to reduce the likelihood of taking into the mouth foods which may be hot enough to damage the oral tissues. The receptors are bare nerve endings and respond either to temperatures below a threshold (cold receptors) or to temperatures above a threshold (warm receptors). Skin temperature receptors appear to have a threshold close to the normal skin temperature of around 25°C and the same is true on the lips. The intraoral temperature receptors may have higher thresholds. The sensory fibres are A delta and C fibres (sensory groups III and IV) and therefore transmit information relatively slowly. There does not appear to be, as there is in the spinal cord, a separate pathway to the cortex for temperature and pain sensations, and the impulses probably reach the thalamus in the trigeminal lemniscus (the trigeminothalamic tract). The maximum tolerable temperature in the mouth is between 70 and 80°C; around this level the lips are unable to detect differences in temperature, and pain ensues – presumably due to cell damage. The tongue is slightly less sensitive than the lips at such high temperatures and the palate may blister at temperatures below this in susceptible individuals. Interestingly, the application of heat stimuli sufficiently hot to cause tissue damage on the tongue stimulates both cold and warmth receptors: this has not been reported elsewhere in the body.

The teeth are said to be sensitive to temperature

Although the statement is sometimes made that pain is the only sensation arising from the teeth themselves, there is evidence that heat may also be discriminated.

Pressure sensation

The periodontal ligament is sensitive to pressure on the teeth

The teeth appear to be sensitive to pressure whether applied axially or laterally but this is in fact a sensation arising from stimulation of receptors in the periodontal ligament. These have been identified as end-organs of the Ruffini type (Fig. 11.9). The nerve fibres are classified as A beta fibres. Although elsewhere pressure receptors of this type are slowly adapting, the response of these receptors varies according to their position in the

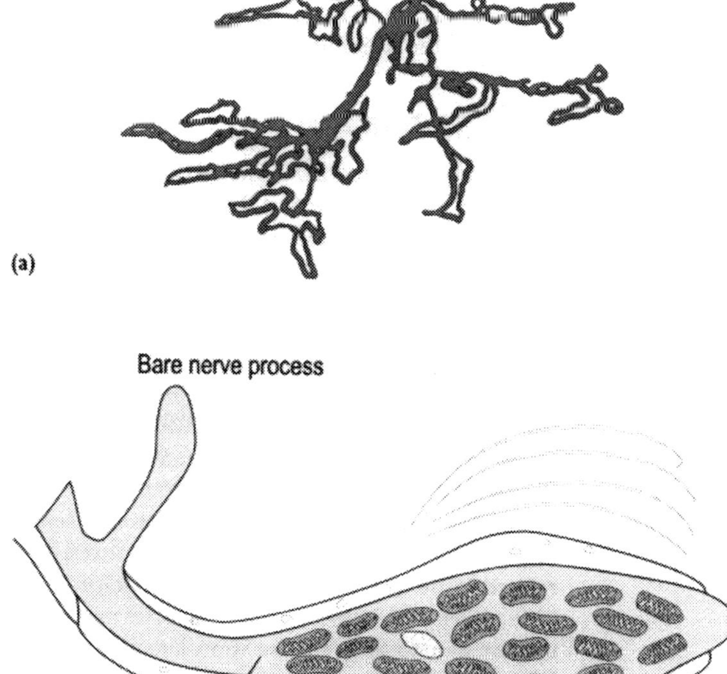

Fig. 11.9
Ruffini end-organs in the periodontal ligament: **a** as seen by light microscopy after using special stains, and **b** as seen by electron microscopy. The main terminal of the nerve is filled with mitochondria. The investing Schwann cell has many pinocytotic vesicles.

periodontal ligament. The teeth behave as if they have an axis of rotation in response to displacing forces and this is situated approximately two-thirds of the way down the root. The pressure receptors nearest to the axis of rotation of the tooth adapt rapidly whilst those furthest away adapt more slowly. This is thought to be due to the way in which pressure is transmitted through the ligament.

Proprioception

There are proprioceptive impulses from the muscles of the tongue and of mastication and from the temporomandibular joints. The tongue muscles and the mandibular elevators contain muscle spindles, but there are few if any in the depressor muscles. Joint receptors are present in the temporomandibular joints and several neuropeptides have been detected in the joint capsules and the synovial discs themselves, suggesting the presence of nerve fibres. The cell bodies of neurones carrying these sensations are situated in the mesencephalic nucleus of the trigeminal nerve and not in the trigeminal ganglion.

Pain sensation

Pain can be detected from any of the oral tissues, including the teeth, although enamel is not sensitive and there has to be direct stimulation of dentine or the pulp itself. Because pain is of such importance in dentistry, often the major cause of consultation, it is necessary to consider the sensation and its oral generation in some detail.

Pain sensations are usually responses to tissue damage and are termed nociceptive sensations

Pain receptors have no morphological distinguishing characteristics: they appear simply as naked nerve endings looking like those for touch or warmth or cold. There is no recognised definition of painful stimuli. It is clear that pain is not simply an excessive stimulation of some other sense such as pressure or temperature: it appears to be related to tissue damage at a cellular level. Physiologists studying animal responses to harmful stimuli do not use the word pain: the term refers to cognition of a sensation and includes an emotional component and so the term noxious is used for the stimuli and the receptors are termed nociceptors. It is helpful to use this terminology in humans also and reserve the term pain for the perceived sensation. Neurones involved in nociception are stimulated by products of inflammation or cell damage such as hydrogen ions, potassium ions, some prostaglandins, some polypeptides, histamine and serotonin (5-hydroxytryptamine). There is some evidence that aspirin may block the chemical receptors at nociceptive nerve terminals as well as having a central effect.

Pain is perceived via A delta and C fibres

Two types of nerve fibre are involved in transmitting signals that result in a perception of pain: the myelinated A delta, approximately 2.5 μm in diameter and conducting at 12–30 m/s, and the non-myelinated C fibres, 0.4–1.2 μm in diameter and conducting more slowly at 0.5–2 m/s. The C fibres have been described as polymodal and capable of transmitting a number of different stimuli, but it is thought that they may be purely nociceptive in humans. The A delta fibres may transmit information from nociceptors or from mechanoreceptors. Several neurotransmitters including substance P, glutamate and neurokin A have been identified at terminals of both A delta and C fibres in the spinal tract. The two types of fibre mediate different sensations of pain: the A delta fibres are associated with a sharp, localised sensation resulting from obvious mechanical damage, sometimes called first pain, and the C fibres with a more diffuse, dull pain that may follow the first pain or may arise independently from a variety of painful stimuli. The distinction is probably less clear, particularly for pain of dental origin. Repeated stimulation of A delta fibres, and probably of C fibres also, leads to hypersensitivity (hyperalgesia) in which even minimal stimulation causes pain in the area. The mechanism of this is not understood although it may be an example of facilitation – where there is upregulation of synaptic tranmission. In trigeminal neuralgia even the slightest stimulus in the trigger area causes intense and long-lasting pain which does not respond to conventional analgesic medication.

From nociceptive terminals the nerve fibres travel in branches of the trigeminal nerve, reach their cell bodies in the trigeminal ganglion, and then pass into the spinal tract of the trigeminal nerve and leave this medially for the nucleus of the spinal tract. No pain fibres pass any further down the tract than medullary level. The fibres from the mandibular nerve lie dorsomedial to those of the maxillary nerve, and those in turn are dorsomedial to the ophthalmic nerve fibres. The spinal tract of the trigeminal nerve is equivalent to the substantia gelatinosa of the spinal cord and is continuous with it. The grey matter of the medulla oblongata can be divided into zones analogous to those described by Rexel in the spinal cord and the functions of these in relation to transmission of pain information is similar (Fig. 11.10). The main fibres ending in layer I are those of the small non-myelinated C fibres with a few A delta and A beta. The C fibres are nociceptive; they are arranged somatotopically, particularly in the region of the nucleus caudalis, and they synapse with neurones passing to the spinal tract itself as well as on to the reticulothalamic tract and possibly the ventral trigeminothalamic tract (Fig. 11.11). Although most of these neurones are nociceptive, some may respond to very gross mechanical stimulation. All of them have small receptive fields. In the spinal cord this layer contains some endings of nerves from mechanoreceptors. Layers II and III are the substantia gelatinosa layers. They receive inputs from large myelinated fibres such as those from mechanoreceptors, touch and pressure endings, and from A delta fibres, again with small receptive fields. These layers, but particularly layer III, together with layer IV have many interneurones, some excitatory and some inhibitory. These interneurones, particularly the inhibitory ones, connect with all the other layers. Layers IV–VI also receive inputs from nociceptors, but these are predominantly those with large receptive fields. They include both A delta and C fibres. In addition, layer V receives inputs from touch and pressure receptors via A beta fibres, and from touch and temperature receptors via A delta fibres. In this layer many of the neurones have large receptive fields and there is considerable convergence so that localisation of the area stimulated is relatively imprecise. This leads to other effects: whilst single inputs of noxious heat stimuli are sensed as painful, repetitive stimulation of temperature receptors with less powerful stimuli may actually inhibit the passage of painful sensations. Layers V–VIII are part of the reticular activating system, whose sensory function is relatively non-specific and whose activity is

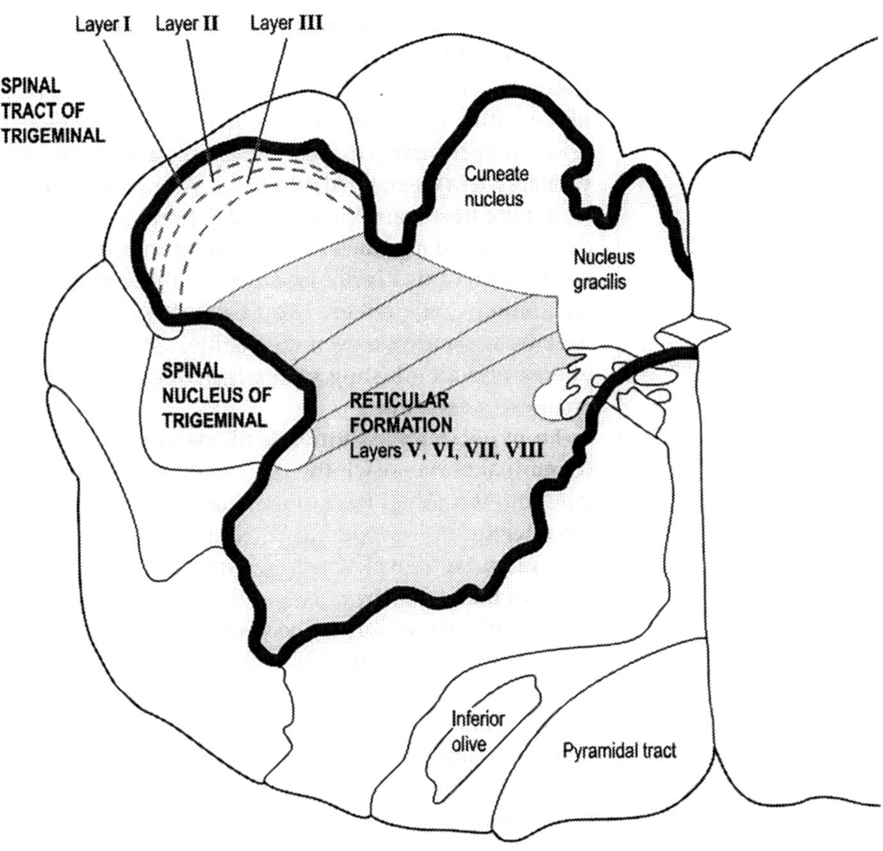

Fig. 11.10
The layers of the grey matter (enclosed by the heavy black line) in the medulla. The section is at a level approximately midway between the two lower sections of Fig. 11.2. The equivalents of the layers given numbers by Rexel are marked with layers I–III being in the spinal tract of the trigeminal nerve, and layers V–VIII being in the reticular formation. The reticular formation is shown coloured.

characterised by extensive interconnections between neurones. Although fibres from this area may project to the ventroposterior nucleus of the thalamus and to the somatosensory cortex, many are connected through the dorsobasal and other intralaminar nuclei of the thalamus to the more primitive parts of the cortex via the hypothalamus, and the perceived sensations may acquire emotional overtones. Layer IV cells in the spinal cord are thought to be the transmission cells postulated in the gate control theory of pain information transmission, but this function is almost certainly shared with the cells of layer V. The gate control theory was an attempt to explain why stimulation of other sensory receptors at the same time as the nociceptors can prevent the perception of pain. If the impulses in the nociceptor nerves could proceed up to the cortex, pain would be perceived – the 'pain gates' would be opened. If transmission at synapses in the substantia gelatinosa was blocked by inhibitory impulses in interneurones connected with large diameter sensory

Pain impulses are subject to modification by other ascending and descending pathways

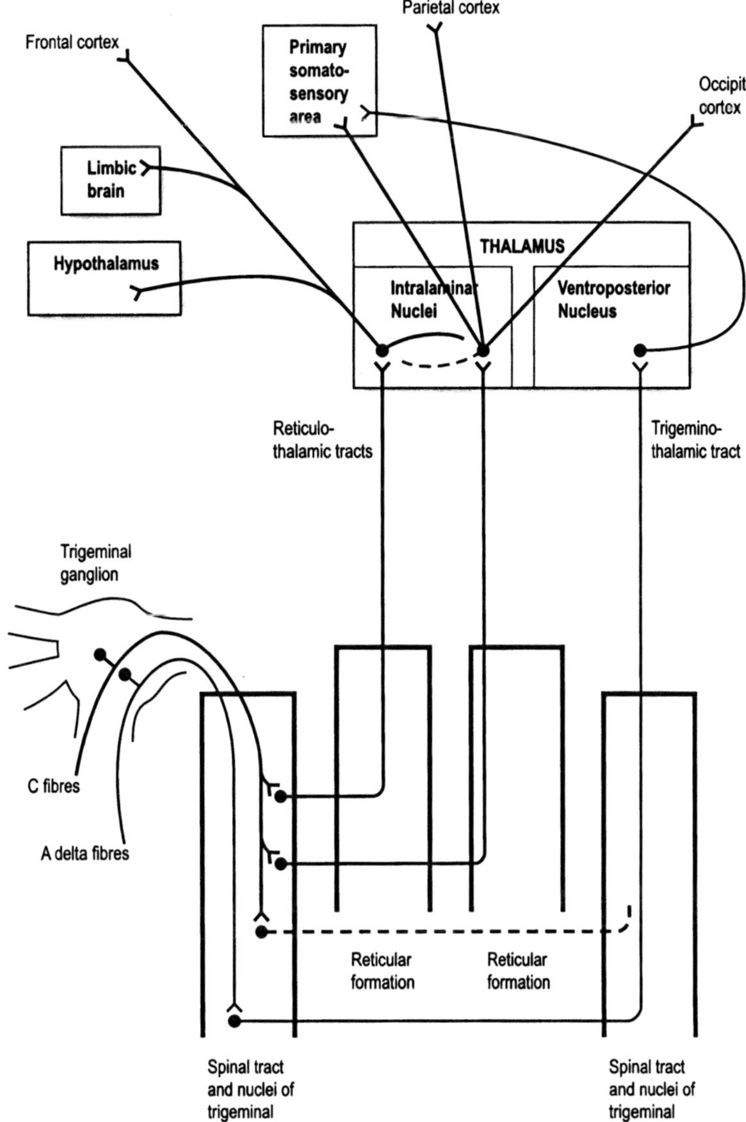

Pathways of nociceptive impulses arising from the area supplied by the trigeminal nerve. The intralaminar nuclei of the thalamus include the dorsomedial nucleus which has extensive connections with other thalamic nuclei, with the hypothalamus and with the limbic brain. The area of the somatosensory cortex associated with sensations from the facial area is at the lower end of the postcentral gyrus. The nociceptive fibres are shown entering only one root of the trigeminal ganglion since both maxillary and mandibular division fibres follow similar routes after entering the pons. The neothalamic pathway from the A delta fibres is shown in black, the archaeothalamic pathway from C fibres in colour. The dotted line from the C fibres to the trigeminothalamic tract is to show that some fibres do ascend in this tract. It is likely that there are also connections from the A delta pathways to the reticulothalamic tract.

afferent fibres, the 'gates' could be described as being closed as impulses from the C and A delta fibres would be unable to stimulate the postsynaptic neurones carrying impulses up to the thalamus. This explains theoretically why pressing on a painful area (sometimes even clenching on a painful tooth) can relieve the pain. Counter-irritants work in the same way, and the theory also provides a possible explanation for some acupuncture treatments. However, the theory tried to define the area of inhibition of pain sensation too closely: it is now clear that nociceptor fibres have synaptic connections at many levels and that inhibition occurs as a result of connections with neurones descending from other levels of the brain and brainstem, as well as with afferent fibres at the same level or in other nearby sensory nerves. Thus the connections to the hypothalamus and limbic brain pass in both directions, and there are inhibitory neurones arising in the thalamus and reticular formation as well as in lower parts of the pathways.

Endogenous morphine-like substances modify pain sensation

A further modification of ideas about pain sensation came when the endorphins and the related encephalins were discovered. The identification of receptors for morphine – a plant-derived inhibitor of pain sensations (an analgesic) – and the recognition that such receptors must have some natural ligand in the body, led to the discovery of a group of small peptides – the two endorphins – with 15 and 31 amino acids respectively, produced in the brain and the pituitary gland. Further work identified two smaller peptides with 5 amino acids (Fig. 11.12) as the active transmitters in the nervous system, and it became clear that these might be produced in a number of circumstances in which pain sensation was much less than might be expected from the strength of the stimulus. More recently another group of slightly longer but closely related peptides with similar properties – the dynorphins – has been identified.

Release of encephalins reduces or prevents the release of substance P, a neurotransmitter which is frequently associated with pain transmission pathways. The inhibition is a presynaptic inhibition. Some of the highest concentrations of substance P in the nervous system are found in the spinal nucleus of the trigeminal nerve. Experiments in animals with naloxone, which

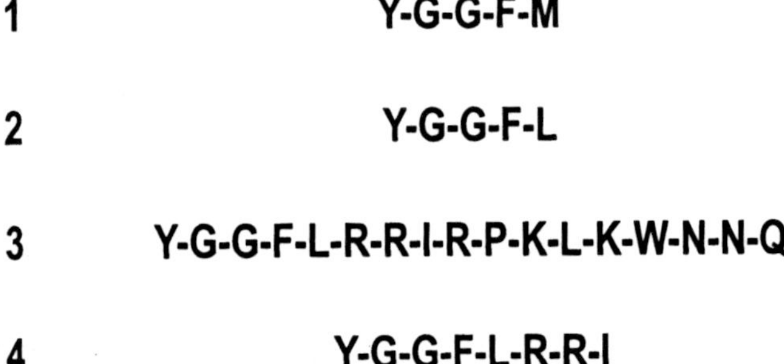

Peptide sequence of the encephalins and two of the endorphins: 1, met-encephalin; 2, leu-encephalin; 3, dynorphin; 4, dynorphin 1–8. One gene encodes for met-encephalin, and a second for leu-encephalin and the dynorphins.

blocks morphine receptors and hence abolishes the action of encephalins, show that the nucleus caudalis – where both substance P and encephalins have been demonstrated – transmits pain sensations more readily when naloxone is present. Naloxone has little effect on the nucleus oralis, which receives inputs mainly from fibres of general sensation with relatively few nociceptive fibres. On the other hand, encephalins inhibit transmission of nociceptive impulses in the substantia gelatinosa and spinal tract of the trigeminal nerve.

Electrical stimulation of the reticular system in the raphe nuclei – the nucleus raphe magnus and the inferior central raphe nucleus – and the peri-aqueductal grey matter causes analgesia widely in the trigeminal nerve distribution without affecting transmission from other afferent nerves, an effect related to the ability of these nuclei to secrete encephalins to influence neighbouring nerve cells. There are other connections between the nucleus raphe magnus and the trigeminal nerve fibres which use serotonin as a transmitter rather than an encephalin: these are not inhibitory.

The endorphins are products of a single gene. The encephalins, however, are coded by two genes: one for met-encephalin and one for leu-encephalin. The latter also codes for the dynorphins, another group of peptides with analgesic properties sharing the same pentapeptide terminal.

The encephalins have a very short half-life and so have not proved therapeutically useful; however, the idea of stimulating other sensory nerves to inhibit pain transmission has been taken up in the development of transepithelial electrical nerve stimulation (TENS) to produce analgesia in the oral region during dental procedures.

Whilst part of the perception of pain results from transmission of impulses to the somatosensory cortex, there is also a component due to impulses in fibres of the reticular system which pass to the hypothalamus and the limbic cortex, acquiring an emotional connotation – sometimes referred to as affect – and recognised as the unpleasant nature of pain. Pain differs from most other sensations in having this strong emotional component – which can be pleasurable as well as unpleasant. Patients may suck or wiggle a painful tooth and seem to derive some satisfaction from the stabs of bearable pain. In addition to the afferent pathways to the primitive limbic brain there are also efferent fibres which can inhibit nociceptor transmission: psychological factors affect perception of pain. Fear and worry lower the pain threshold; excitement and relaxation may both raise the threshold. Soothing music, or even the mixture of high sound frequencies known as white sound, is used in what is termed audioanalgesia.

Pain of dental origin

Dentine and the dental pulp are sensitive to painful stimuli

The distribution of nerves in the dental pulp has been described in Ch. 5. The pulp itself is normally enclosed in dentine, which is covered in the crown of the tooth by dental enamel and in the root by cementum. It is only when dental caries or the dental drill attacks the tooth or when the cementum layer at the neck of the tooth is worn away to expose dentine that pain is sensed. It would appear, therefore, that dentine is the sensitive tissue. All stimuli which produce any sensation through the dentine give a sensation of pain, although there is some evidence that heat, and possibly cold, may also be perceived as separate sensations.

The problem in considering dentine sensitivity, as discussed earlier, is in the identification of the sensory receptors. The most sensitive area in dentine, as judged by patients' responses, is at the amelodentinal junction. The cervical dentine when denuded of cementum can also be highly sensitive. The nerve supply to dentine is limited to the crowns of teeth; the nerve fibres are most numerous under the cusps but in any part of the dentine they do not extend into the tubules for more than a short distance from the pulp – between 0.1 and 0.2 mm. There is still argument over the extent to which the odontoblast processes penetrate dentine: on the one hand, there is a considerable body of evidence that the penetration is variable and probably no more than a third of the way into dentine; on the other hand, some recent reports suggest that they do extend virtually to the amelodentinal junction and could, therefore, in theory, function as receptors. Some workers have demonstrated that the odontoblast processes extend further into dentine in the region of the neck of the tooth. The nerves in dentine do not degenerate when the main nerve trunk to the tooth is cut, suggesting that these fibres are not somatosensory but may be autonomic. If this is the case, their proximity to the odontoblast processes and the presence of gap junctions may mean that they are in some way involved in control of odontoblast function. Although the odontoblasts are of neural crest origin they show little evidence of being neural in function. It is still possible that the odontoblast cell bodies, which appear to have occasional synapse-like junctions with the nerve fibres which pass between them from the subodontoblastic plexus, have some receptor function. However, when the stimuli to dentine which can cause pain are considered – heat, cold, touch and the application of osmotically active solutions – it is impossible to reconcile their variety with those of known receptor types. The only common feature to all these stimuli is that they could cause the fluid contents of the dentinal tubules to move in the tubules either towards or away from the odontoblast cell bodies. It is therefore thought that this must occur, and that such fluid movements are sensed either by the odontoblasts which then transmit some signal to the adjacent nerve fibrils, or to the nerve fibrils lying beneath the odontoblast layer and close to the subodontoblastic plexus. A further refinement of this idea is that the odontoblasts or their processes may be deformed by the fluid pressure and lose potassium through ion channels; the extracellular potassium could then affect the membrane potential of neighbouring nerve fibres. The hydrodynamic theory of dentine sensitivity is now generally accepted and explains the curious observation that the pain sensation is proportional to the osmotic activity of solutions applied; it also explains why substances which denature proteins or cause precipitation into the tubules will desensitise dentine. It is less clear why application of solution containing certain cations such as potassium or strontium, which could theoretically alter nerve conduction, are also able to desensitise dentine.

Movement of fluid in dentinal tubules when dentine is stimulated appears to be a factor in pain sensation from this tissue

Referred pain

One of the more curious aspects of pain sensation is that tissue damage in a deep organ may give rise to a sensation of pain peripherally in areas embryologically derived from the same somite. Thus pain of cardiac origin may be perceived in the left arm. Such pain must arise from convergence of somatic and visceral sensory impulses at one or more of three levels: prespinal, spinal or supraspinal. In the trigeminal area the equivalent levels would be prepontine, pontomedullary and suprapontine. There is little evidence that convergence occurs within the brain. Recordings from cells of dorsal root ganglia (equivalent to the trigeminal ganglion) have shown that nerve cells in the ganglion can have branches to both skin and viscera, so that convergence of impulses can occur at the prespinal or prepontine level. In addition, it has been demonstrated that there is convergence of visceral and cutaneous inputs on dorsal horn neurones in the spinal cord. In the trigeminal system this would represent convergence in the spinal nuclei of the trigeminal nerve. Pain in the oral cavity is therefore referred within the distribution of the specific division of the trigeminal nerve and does not cross the midline unless there is ramification of the nerve to the contralateral side as may occur in the incisor region.

There is evidence that migrainous headaches may be due to dental conditions, but this is not an example of referred pain. Such headaches are of vascular origin; research on transmission in central pathways of trigeminal origin has identified a vasodilator reaction to trigeminal stimuli, probably related to serotoninergic pathways. In some patients occlusal equilibration has reduced the incidence of tension headaches.

Taste

Taste sensation is a chemical sense transduced by parasympathetic nerve fibres from the oral cavity

This sensation is one of the four special sensations whose receptors are situated in the head, and one of the two chemoreceptor sensations perceived directly in the cortex. Nerve fibres subserving the function of taste are parasympathetic, although most of them travel with branches of the trigeminal nerve. Although taste receptors are predominantly located on the dorsum of the tongue, there are also taste receptors on the soft palate, the epiglottis, the pharyngeal wall and even some in the oesophagus (Fig. 11.13). The subject of taste is one of interest to most human beings – either for its value in survival or in the appreciation of food and drink – but is particularly important to the dentist. Taste is the main stimulant to saliva flow and the stimulation of saliva is important in oral health, taste often governs the use of aids to oral hygiene like toothpastes and mouthrinses, and taste governs food choice – so that the preference for sweet tastes generally leads to the selection of sucrose-rich foods which are the most cariogenic.

Taste buds

Most taste receptors are situated in groups of cells known as taste buds

The cells which act as taste receptors are found in small groups which are termed taste buds. These develop early in foetal life, those around the circumvallate papillae being fully formed by about 14 weeks intrauterine life. A young adult has a total of around 9000 taste buds, most of which are on the tongue and situated on the papillae on its dorsum. The tongue is

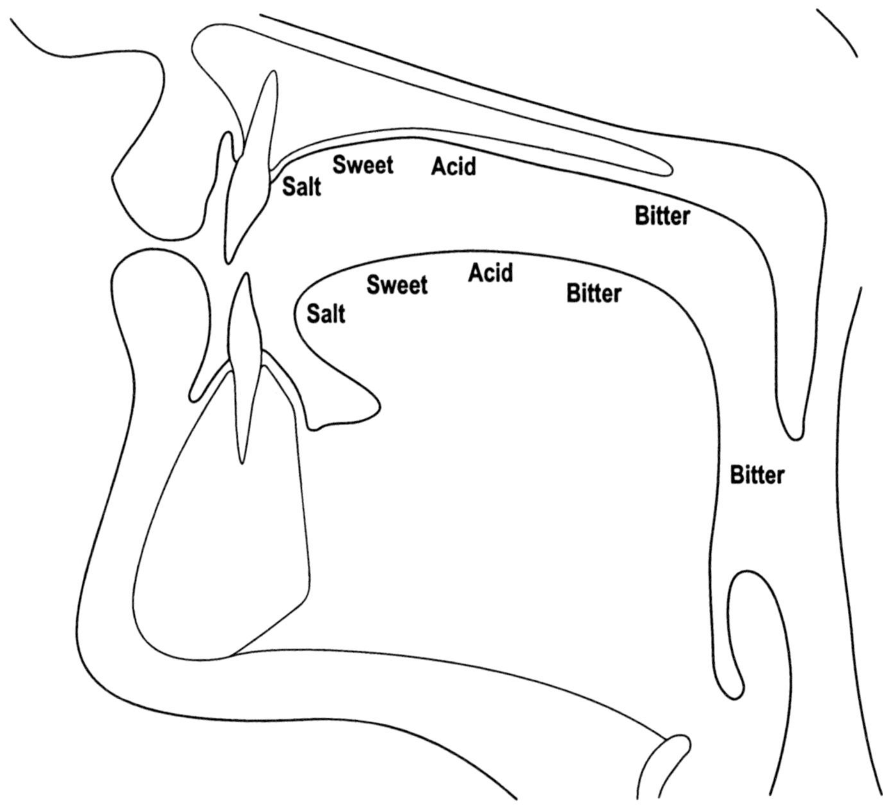

Fig. 11.13
Areas of the mouth where taste sensations have been reported. The nerve supplies to the different areas can be found in Figs 11.4–11.8.

embryologically derived from two branchial arches – the anterior two-thirds from the first branchial arch, and the posterior third from behind the sulcus terminalis with its backward pointing in a V-shape from the third arch – and the distribution of papillae and the nerve supply to them differs in the two areas of the tongue (see the account of oral innervation above). In the anterior part there are three types of papillae – the filiform, the foliate and the fungiform. The thin keratinised projections of the filiform papillae rarely have taste buds on them; the smooth, rounded projections of the fungiform papillae each have a few taste buds on their surface, but the foliate papillae, which are made up of a number of parallel ridges, may have five or more taste buds on each of the lateral walls of the ridges. The foliate papillae contribute up to 1500 taste buds in total. Anterior and adjacent to the sulcus terminalis are 8–12 large circumvallate papillae which can be seen with the naked eye. They consist of a central flat dome with a deep surrounding groove which gives them their name (Fig. 11.14). The central dome is keratinised, but the sides of the groove are non-keratinised and contain some 250–300 taste buds in each papilla, together with the orifices of the lingual glands of von Ebner, which produce a watery ('serous') secretion into the trough. The number of taste buds in the

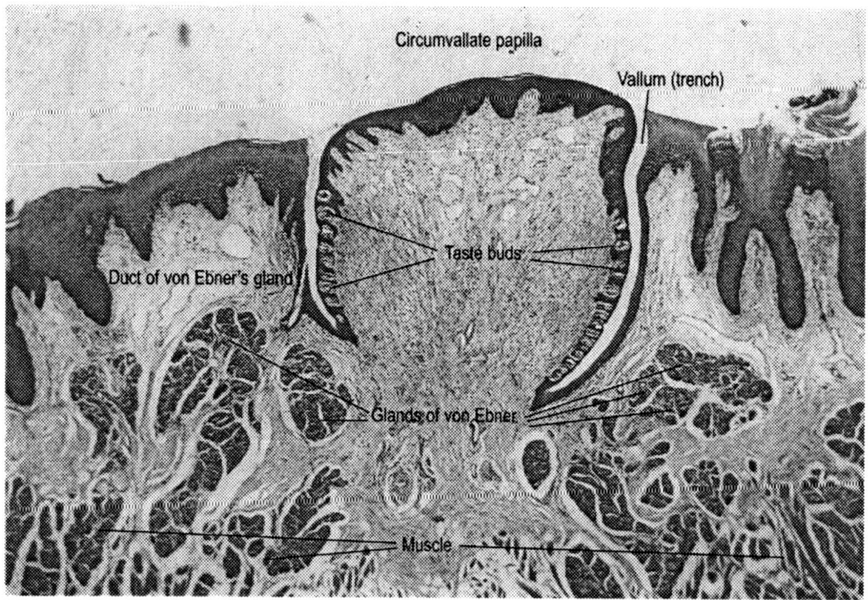

Fig. 11.14
A section through a circumvallate papilla from the sulcus terminalis of the tongue. The taste buds can be seen lining the inner wall of the vallum (ditch), and the duct of a gland of von Ebner can be seen entering the vallum on the right. The glands of von Ebner lie below the sides of the circumvallate papilla and may blend with the muscle of the tongue.

circumvallate papillae decreases with age, but still amounts to around 100 per papilla in subjects aged 70 years. Older people often complain of loss of taste sensitivity; this is unlikely to be due to the decrease in taste buds at this site as these taste buds are stimulated by substances with a bitter taste and it is other taste sensations which appear to be more affected. It is much more likely that these subjects, who are usually denture wearers, have lost some taste sensation from the receptors covered by an upper denture but, more significantly, have lost in the same way the ability of the palate to recognise the texture of foodstuffs.

A typical taste bud contains three main types of cell (Fig. 11.15) designated simply as types I–III, together with the basal progenitor cells (or type IV cells). Their tips extend up into a pit, or taste pore, which contains a gel-like material made up of glycosaminoglycans, ascorbic acid (vitamin C) and a number of enzymes. Round the periphery of the taste bud and between the other cells are the type I, or dark, cells. About two-thirds of the cells in a taste bud are type I cells. They have narrow, dense cell necks, with fibrillar or tubular elements and end in a flattened surface with about 40 short stubby microvilli. These are separated from the pit substance by a basement membrane which lines the inner surface of the pit. The presence of many characteristic apical granules which are chemically very similar to the pit substance suggests that their function is to secrete the pit substance. Their basal ends reach down to the

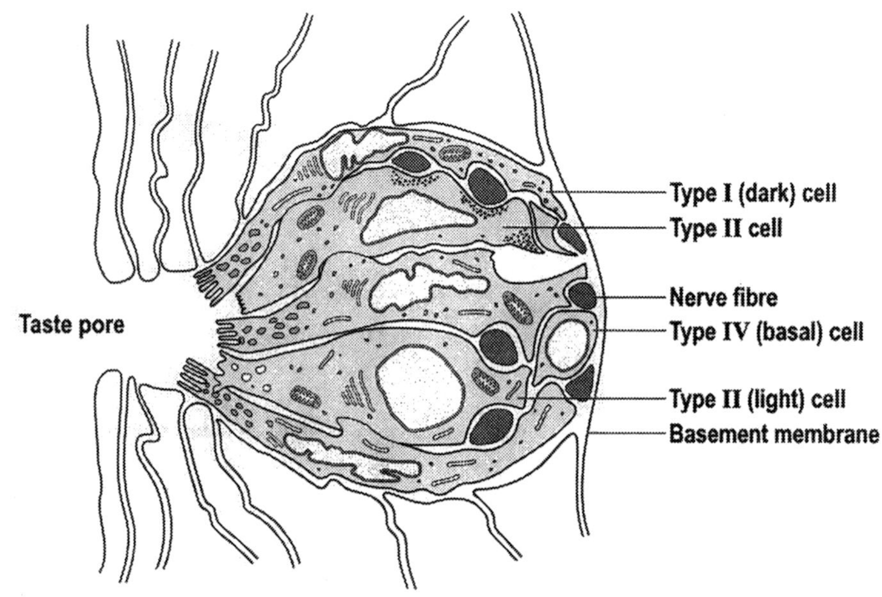

Diagram of the four types of cell to be seen in a taste bud. The type I cells are the most abundant; they are thought to secrete the pit substance. The function of the type II cells is not known. Type III cells synapse with the many nerve fibres entering the taste bud (grey), whilst the type IV cells are the precursor of the other types.

basement membrane. They have lateral extensions which extend across the other cells and nerve fibrils. In light microscopic descriptions these cells were termed sustentacular cells. None of the other cell types contains the granules seen in type I. Type II cells (light cells) have relatively thick microvilli projecting into the taste pit and have a number of vesicles immediately below these. Like the type I cells they have an apically situated nucleus but this is smooth-walled, unlike the invaginated nuclei of type I cells. They do not extend down to the basement membrane and they do not show any synapse-like features. About 20% of the cells in the taste bud are of type II, but there are also a small number of cells which appear to be midway between types I and II. The type III cells have slender peg-like tips with no microvilli. They contain vesicles which resemble the synaptic vesicles found in nerve fibres and they appear to synapse with adjacent nerve fibres. They are sometimes termed serotonergic cells because they react with anti-serotonin antibody reagents. In the base of the taste buds there are morphologically less well-defined cells (type IV cells) which are thought to be the progenitor cells for the other three types. Light microscopy shows taste hairs projecting into the pit substance but no similar appearance has been recorded by electron microscopy and these are thought to be artefacts of section preparation. All taste buds have similar structures and there does not appear to be a variation in taste sensitivity. They are epithelial cells and, like other epithelial cells, are subject to constant turnover – the life of a taste bud cell has been estimated at between 2 and 30 days. All taste buds contain nerve fibres; after entering the taste bud these lose their myelin sheaths and end closely adjacent to all the cell types. They are seen in invaginations in type I cells, coiled round type II cells, and forming synaptic connections with type III cells. The significance of these relationships between nerve fibres and taste bud cells has not been elucidated.

Sensory mechanisms of taste

Substances which stimulate taste receptors are referred to as sapid; the process involved in taste perception is termed gustation. In order to stimulate taste receptors, substances must be in solution, and if they are not ingested in solution they are solubilised in saliva or in the secretion of the von Ebner's glands. The sapid solution then reaches the taste pits where it may react with pit contents and finally the cells of the taste bud which are the taste receptors. Some earlier theories of taste perception considered that it was inhibition or potentiation of the enzymes – acid phosphatase, esterases, and ATPase – which had been detected in the pit substance which caused changes in the receptor cells. Modern investigations have not supported these theories and the function of the pit substance is now unclear. Most of the recent work has focused on changes in membrane permeability of the receptor cells – either cells of the taste bud or the nerve fibrils therein – as a result of binding of excitatory substances. Such changes in membrane permeability lead to generator potentials which can then trigger action potentials in the nerves or directly to potentials in the nerve fibres themselves. There is a linear relationship between the logarithm of the concentration of a sapid substance applied to the tongue and the frequency of action potentials in the gustatory nerve, a relationship which is similar to those exhibited by other sensory stimuli and sensory nerves as described in the Weber–Fechner 'Laws' (Fig. 11.16).

The nerve pathways which carry taste information from the tongue and other areas of the oral cavity (Fig. 11.17) have been described earlier in this chapter. They are all autonomic pathways and the signals are carried in small, myelinated, slowly conducting axons to reach the tractus solitarius and its nucleus, where they synapse. The secondary neurones cross the midline and travel in the medial lemniscus to the thalamus which then communicates with the lower part of the postcentral gyrus and the hippocampal gyrus. There are connections with the salivary nuclei to give a reflex pathway and there is almost certainly a link via reticular neurones to the hypothalamus and limbic cortex. The perception of different tastes depends upon the mixture of signals reaching the sensory cortex.

Taste sensations are arbitrarily described as having four modalities: acid, salt, sweet and bitter

The different tastes which human beings can perceive have been classified as sweet, bitter, salt and sour (or acid). This classification is somewhat arbitrary and its originator, Henning, did not in fact, talk about four modalities of taste, but of four extremes of taste type which he described as being the corners of a taste tetrahedron, with all tastes being at appropriate points on or in that tetrahedron. Other descriptors, such as alkaline and metallic, have subsequently been suggested but have not gained recognition as taste categories. Primitive languages classify tastes in different ways, confirming the arbitrary nature of taste descriptors. However, as it is possible to identify four substances which can clearly be defined as sweet, bitter, acid and salt, and

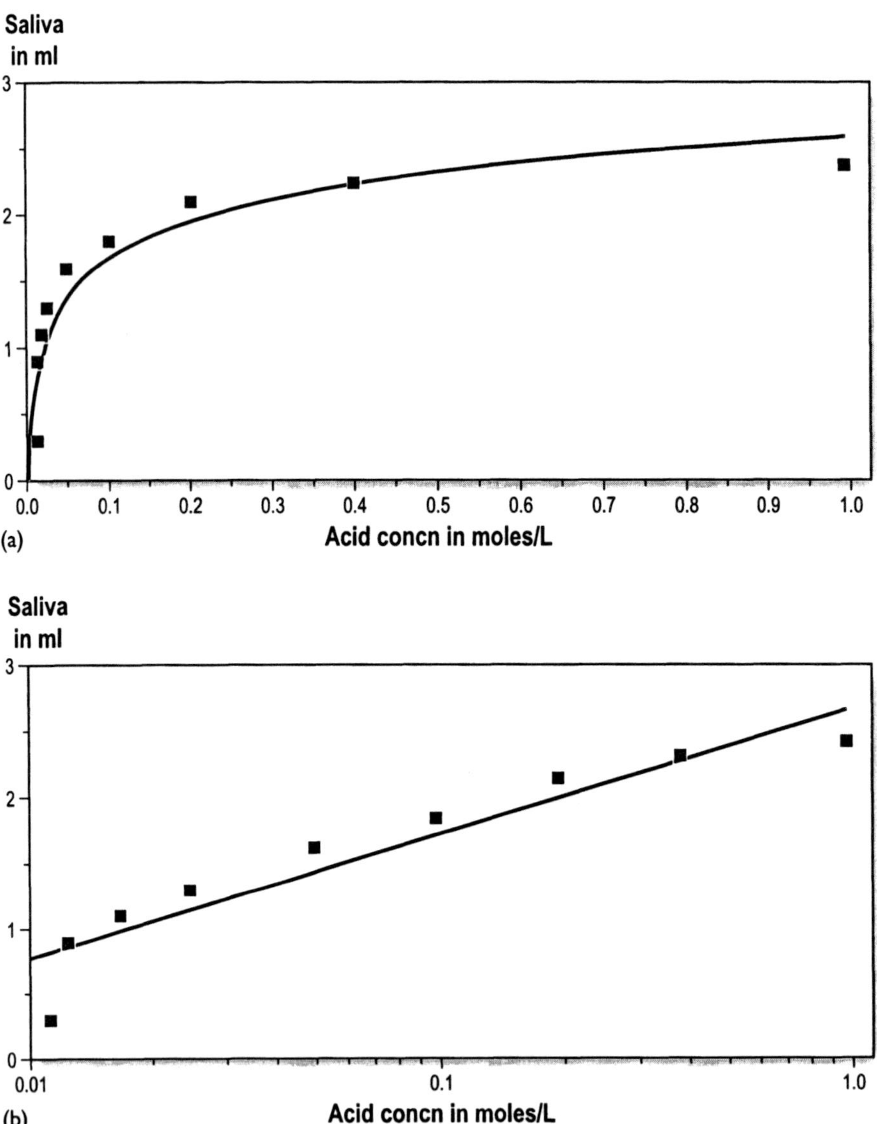

Fig. 11.16
Graphs of the response of a parotid gland to stimulation of the tongue with citric acid. In the upper graph the response is plotted on a linear scale and the increment in response can be seen to diminish as the citric acid concentration is increased. When plotted against a log concentration scale (lower graph), the curve approximates to a straight line. This illustrates the general relationship of perceived magnitude of stimulus to actual stimulus put forward by Weber and Fechner.

there does appear to be some degree of localisation of perception of the taste modalities on the tongue and in the mouth more generally (Fig. 11.18), the concept of four modalities has been retained and is used as a basis for testing taste sensitivity. The situation is more confusing at a neurophysiological level

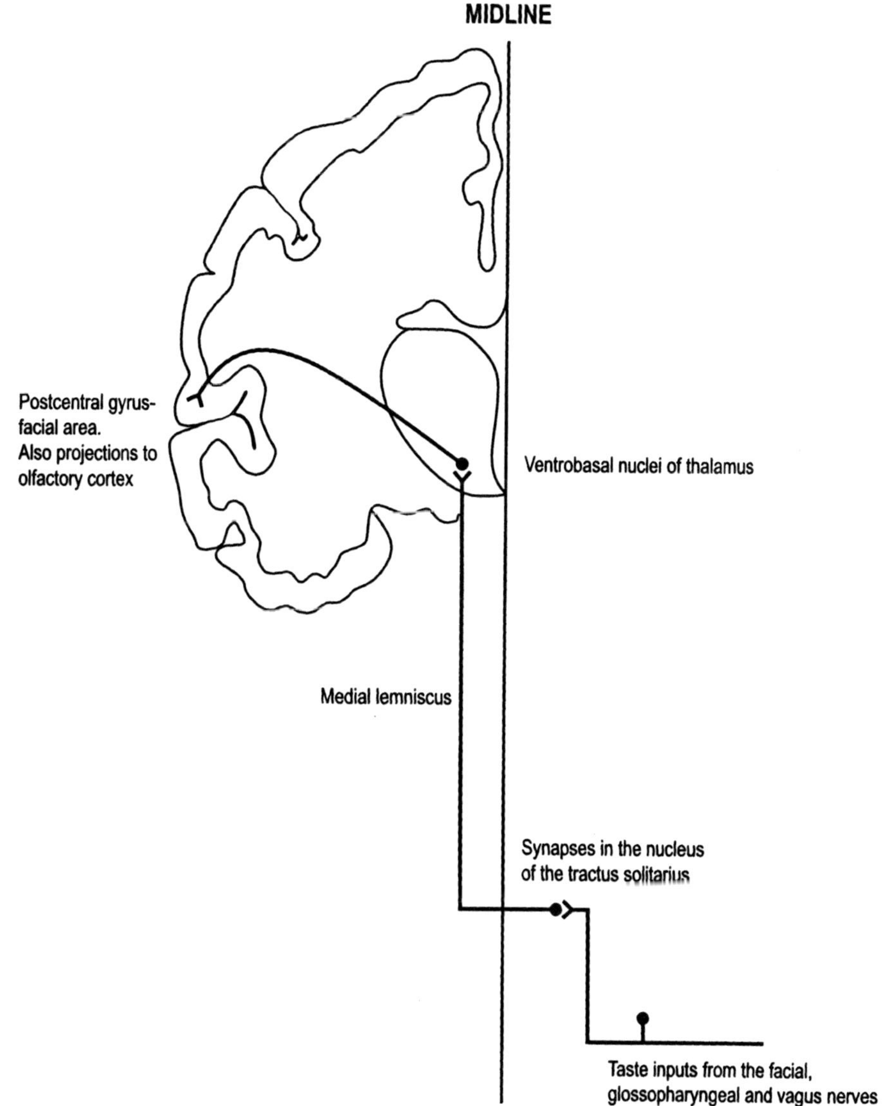

Fig. 11.17
The taste pathway. Although the pathway usually described passes to the lower part of the somatosensory cortex, there are also connections to the olfactory area, the hypothalamus and the limbic brain. There are also reflex connections to the salivatory centres in the brainstem.

Neither receptors nor nerves appear to be specific to one taste sensation

as up to five taste buds may receive branches of one taste fibre, and any one taste bud may receive branches from up to 50 nerve fibres. This can be demonstrated by cutting nerve fibres and observing the subsequent degeneration of taste buds innervated by that fibre. It can also be demonstrated by stimulating taste buds with different sapid stimuli and observing the action potentials in the nerve fibres leaving that area. This

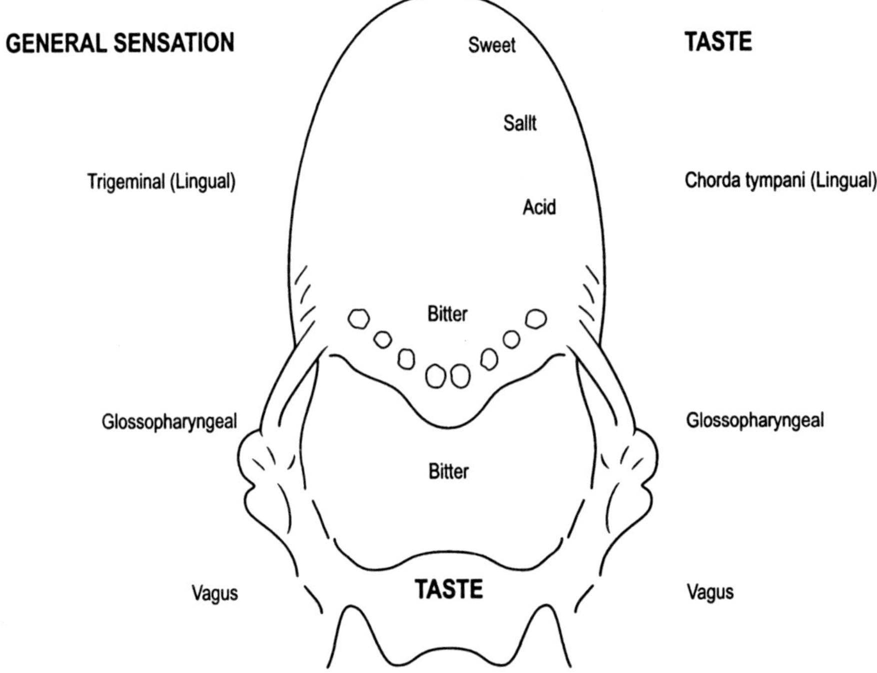

Localisation of taste sensation on the tongue. The nerves subserving both taste and general sensation in the different areas are indicated.

Hydrogen ions cause closure of potassium channels in receptor cells

further reveals that taste buds vary in sensitivity and, whilst a few respond to one taste modality only, most respond to more than one and some respond to all four. Usually, however, one modality is dominant. Research on the nature of the molecular structure of sapid substances, with a view to the synthesis of compounds with a particular taste, or to the identification of taste receptors at a cell membrane level, has been inconclusive. It is clear that the taste which is described as acid owes its sapid nature to its content of hydrogen ions. This has been confirmed by neurophysiological investigations which now show that hydrogen ions cause the closing of potassium channels in the cell membrane and the decreased permeability to potassium ions causes the membrane potential to move closer to zero – membrane depolarisation (as can be predicted from the Goldman equation). Despite this there is considerable variation in the taste of different acids depending upon the anion: inorganic acids tend to taste metallic, while organic acids tend to taste fruity. In general the degree of acidity seems to depend on the hydrogen ion concentration, although there is variation between acids and some organic acids taste more acid than hydrochloric acid at a similar hydrogen ion concentration. The usual test substances used to measure taste sensitivity to acid are hydrochloric acid and citric acid. Hydrochloric acid is usually detected at concentrations over 0.9 mmol/l, although the threshold for different individuals varies between 0.05 and 10 mmol/l.

The taste described as salt is less easily characterised. It arises from stimulation of receptors by cations and the type gustant is sodium chloride. However, there are differences in the taste perceived with different cations and these in turn are modified by the anion present. Sodium fluoride tastes slightly less salt than sodium chloride. In low concentrations some salt solutions actually taste sweet rather than salt – potassium chloride and potassium sulphate are good examples. Because of the variety of cations that might be tested, experiments on the mechanisms of action on the cell have been limited: it has been found that the diuretic amiloride abolishes sensitivity to sodium and lithium salts and this implies that stimulation with these salts causes the opening of sodium channels and consequent depolarisation of the cells. It is possible that the receptors for both acid and salt contain carboxyl groups as the active sites. Sodium as sodium chloride is usually detected by most people at concentrations in excess of 10 mmol/l; the threshold varies between 1 and 80 mmol/l.

The major difficulties arise when chemical similarities are sought for substances which taste sweet or for those which taste bitter. It has already been commented that dilute solution of potassium chloride and sulphate taste sweet: the same is true for similar salts of lithium. Lead acetate (sugar of lead) and some beryllium salts taste sweet. The type gustant for sweet is sucrose, but other organic substances of similar (most mono- or disaccharides and some substituted sugars) and very dissimilar structure, ranging from amino acids (glycine, glutamine and the synthetic sweetener aspartame – L-aspartyl-L-phenylalanine) to halogenated hydrocarbons (chloroform) and miscellaneous compounds such as saccharin and cyclamate, have a sweet taste. It has been argued that animals have developed a taste for sweet substances because these are usually nutritionally good, but many of the substances listed above are poisonous. There has been an intensive search for substitutes for sucrose because sweetness is an attractive flavour and yet sucrose is cariogenic in the mouth and excessive intakes are associated with fatness and obesity. Sugar alcohols such as sorbitol and xylitol have been used, but they can cause diarrhoea in quantity because they are not digested and the unabsorbed molecules raise the osmotic activity of the gut contents, preventing the absorption of water. The only common feature identified in most of the organic molecules which taste sweet is a group with a covalent hydrogen bond loosely attached either ionically or covalently to a second group giving a structure of the form A–H•••B. This conformation is thought to bind to a mirror image conformation on the receptor membrane. Whatever the form of the receptor molecule, binding of the sweet gustant stimulates the G-proteins to activate adenylyl cyclase and produce cyclic adenosine monophosphate (cAMP), which in turn causes the phosphorylation of potassium channels and their resultant closure. The decrease in permeability to potassium induces depolarisation. Sucrose is sensed at concentrations over 10 mmol/l by most subjects, although individual thresholds vary between 5 and 16 mmol/l.

Sweet-tasting substances stimulate G-proteins, raise cAMP levels and cause closing of potassium channels

The main G-proteins involved in gustatory sensation have been found to be similar to the G-protein in retinal cells known as transducin. Transducin itself has been found in taste cells, together with a similar protein which has been termed gustducin.

As with sweet substances, there is a variety of chemical compounds associated with bitter tastes. They include many alkaloids, and glycosides, and inorganic compounds such as picric acid, nitrous and sulphide groups, magnesium sulphate and calcium oxide. It has been postulated that bitter-tasting substances are often harmful or poisonous and that the taste is used as a warning by animals. The type gustant, however, is quinine – a substance of therapeutic value and one which is popular in providing a bitter taste in certain drinks. The molecular conformation which is associated with a bitter taste in most of the organic bitter gustants is similar to that associated with sweet tastes but has a shorter H•••B distance. There is as yet no neurophysiological evidence as to the cellular mechanism of stimulation leading to perception of a bitter taste, although G-proteins and calcium ions are thought to be involved. Quinine is a very powerful gustatory stimulant: the average threshold is around 8 µmol/l and the range of thresholds observed is from 0.4 to 11 µmol/l.

There appears to be some localisation of taste sensitivity in the mouth (Figs 11.13 and 11.18). The areas of the tongue innervated by the facial nerve fibres respond to sweet, salt and acid stimuli, and these traditionally are arranged progressively more posteriorly along the edge. The dorsum is more sensitive to acid and bitter stimuli. The areas of the mouth innervated by fibres of the glossopharyngeal nerve – the circumvallate papillae, the back of the tongue, and the palate – and by fibres of the vagus nerve – the tonsillar region, the epiglottis and the pharynx – respond to bitter gustants.

Flavour

Flavour is the total sensation from a foodstuff. It includes taste, touch, olfactory, and possibly pain, receptors in the mouth and nose

The term flavour is used to describe the total sensation induced when a particular foodstuff is introduced into the mouth. Taste is a major component of flavour, but flavour depends also on the possible simultaneous stimulation of olfactory receptors in the nasal cavity (which is continuous with the oral cavity through the nasopharynx), of touch receptors in the palate and other areas of mucosa, and reactions to irritant substances on the lingual surface in particular. Thus vanillin and citral (a component of lemon oil) cannot be tasted if access to olfactory receptors is blocked, and eating an apple while smelling an onion gives the apple a very curious taste. The flavour of a wine depends upon the acidity and sweetness but also upon the volatilisation of some of its components on the surface of the tongue. The texture of substances in the mouth is important: when patients complain of the taste of alginate impression materials, or children of the taste of vegetables, or pears, or peaches, it is often the texture to which they object. Irritants such as mustard, pepper, ginger and chillies stimulate nociceptor endings of the trigeminal nerve and give a hot taste. The final perception of the flavour of a food is a complex of all these types of sensation moderated by the limbic brain and the association cortex with an emotional or remembered context.

Factors affecting taste perception

Taste, like many other sensations, shows adaptation if the stimulation is continued. This is demonstrated by the decreased perception of sweetness in a food eaten after another obviously sweet food. A similar effect is seen at a more central level: individuals can accustom themselves to particular levels of, for example, sweetness or acidity in their food and these base levels influence their thresholds for that particular gustant. Thus a sweetened drink may be acceptable to a subject habitually consuming a relatively high sugar level, but intolerably sweet to another subject whose refined sugar intake is low. Some authors have suggested that sweetness, despite its classification as a taste modality, is actually an acquired taste, absent or only weakly present in infants, and that the preference for sweet-tasting substances is developed in the early years by adult conceptions of food pleasantness.

Temperature affects taste sensation

If taste perception is considered solely in terms of the four taste modalities, it can be affected by a number of local and systemic factors. Oral temperature is important: very cold foods such as ices and sorbets reduce the ability of the receptors and so higher concentrations of flavourings are required to maintain stimulation. The sucrose content of an ice cream has to be greater than that of room temperature or warm dessert to be acceptably sweet.

Taste sensations interact

Combination of gustants gives results on perception which are hard to explain on the four-modalities model of taste. Addition of sugar to acid foods does not alter the hydrogen ion concentration but suppresses the acid taste. This effect is not due to central processing of information because a similar effect can be seen when studying the gustatory–salivary reflex when acid and sugar stimuli do not produce an additive increase in salivary flow.

There are hormonal, genetic and ageing influences on taste thresholds

Hormonal influences on taste thresholds have been postulated, but the differences between males and females are within the range of individual variation and there is no significant difference on a population basis. Taste sensitivity declines with increasing age, but once again this is a trend rather than a statistically significant observation because of the large individual variation. There is a genetic variation in sensitivity to some bitter tastes: some 30% of a Caucasian population are unable to taste phenylthiocarbamide and 6-N-propylthiouracil.

Subjects deprived of salt exhibit a lower threshold for sodium chloride, whilst dehydrated subjects often have a raised threshold for this compound. This would seem a beneficial modification of taste sensitivity although it seems to be related more to saliva composition than to body needs. Thus rinsing with sodium-free water to clear the tongue surface of sodium chloride lowers the salt threshold as much as a hundred-fold. Obviously the taste of salt is always perceived against a background of the normal resting saliva concentrations.

Cigarette smoking is reported to diminish taste sensitivity in general but to increase sensitivity to bitter tastes. The data are not very consistent and it is only in subjects smoking more than 20 cigarettes a day that the differences become clear.

Taste is modified by tobacco usage and by many anaesthetic drugs

Local anaesthetics affect taste sensation: on the tongue salt and sweet stimulation is reduced, whilst on the palate acid and bitter are affected. Overall taste sensation is abolished first for bitter and then salt, acid and sweet in that order. Different anaesthetics give some differences in these effects. Gymnemic acid selectively reduces detection of sweet gustants. An extract of the African fruit, *Synsepalum dulcificium*, was named miraculin because of its ability to convert stimulation by any of the taste modalities into a sensation of sweetness. The relationship between concentration and strength of perception remains the same.

Further reading

Textbook of Pain, 3rd edition. Wall, P.D., Melzack, R. (editors). Churchill Livingstone, Edinburgh, 1994

Pain. Bond, M.R. Churchill Livingstone, Edinburgh, 1979

The Neurobiology of Pain. Holden, A.V., Winlow, W. (editors). Manchester University Press, Manchester, 1984

Neurophysiology of the Jaws and Teeth. Taylor, A. (editor). Macmillan, Basingstoke, 1990

Taste Perception. Lindemann, B. Physiological Reviews 76: 718–766; 1996

12 Mastication and deglutition

Ingestion of food involves incision, transport between teeth, mastication, transport prior to swallowing, and swallowing itself

In incision and mastication the mandible moves against the fixed maxilla

Eating consists of the taking of food into the mouth and the process of reducing it to a suitable consistency for the next stage of ingestion, that of deglutition or swallowing. The motor components can be divided into four phases: incision, transport to and between the molar and premolar teeth, mastication, and transport preparatory to swallowing (Fig. 12.1). The process of mastication has been extensively studied but the other phases are less well characterised.

Both incision and mastication are the fragmentation of food particles by the approximation, or occlusion, of the maxillary and mandibular teeth. In the partially or completely edentulous subject, approximation of the dentures or the gum pads will be substituted. The process involves movement of the mobile mandible against the fixed maxilla, the mandible rotating about the two articulating areas of the temporomandibular joints. It is appropriate, therefore, to consider first the temporomandibular joint, and then the muscles which move the mandible, the muscles of mastication.

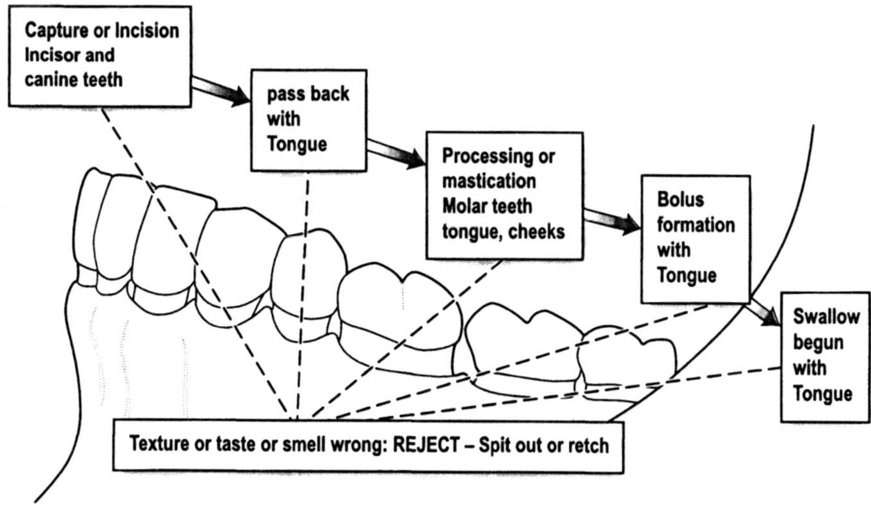

Fig. 12.1
The sequence of food intake and processing which leads to swallowing.

The temporomandibular joint

The temporomandibular joint is a synovial diarthrosis

Movements of the mandible against the maxilla are constrained by the nature of the articulating surfaces. The joint is a synovial diarthrosis and so has a mandibular joint surface, a temporal bone surface and a synovial disc between the two (Figs 12.2 and 12.3). The temporomandibular joint is peculiar to mammals but exhibits major differences in different mammals, having become specialised for its role in the mastication of specific foodstuffs. Thus in carnivorous animals the use of the teeth in food capture and aggression, and the reliance upon a digestive system capable of dealing with relatively large particles of muscle and fat, has resulted in a temporomandibular joint which operates as a bilateral hinge (a ginglymoid joint), whereas in the herbivores incision is less important and the reduction of plant foods with their thick cell walls to a paste which can be processed by the digestive enzymes has resulted in a flattened sliding joint which permits lateral grinding movements (an arthrodial joint). The human temporomandibular joint, like that of the pig, is adapted to an omnivorous diet, with the possibilities of both hinge and sliding movements.

The human temporomandibular joint is one appropriate to an omnivore

It is important to realise that the mandible in humans is a single bone which articulates on each side with a temporal bone. This means that movements of the mandible can be symmetrical and also asymmetrical, and forward movement of one condyle may be associated with a lesser forward

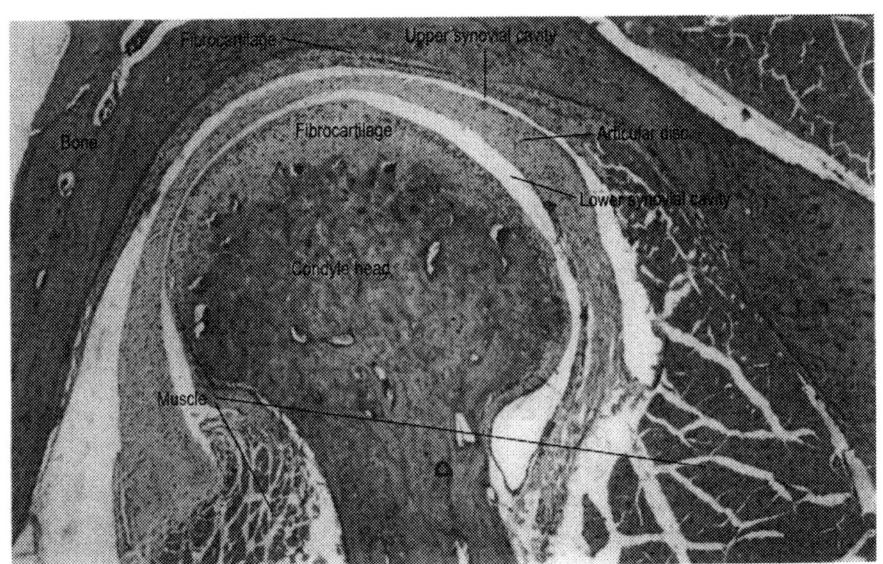

Section through the head of the mandibular condyle and the glenoid fossa to show the articulating surfaces, the articular disc and the synovial cavities above and below the disc. Note that the articulating surfaces are dense fibrous tissue over a fibrocartilage.

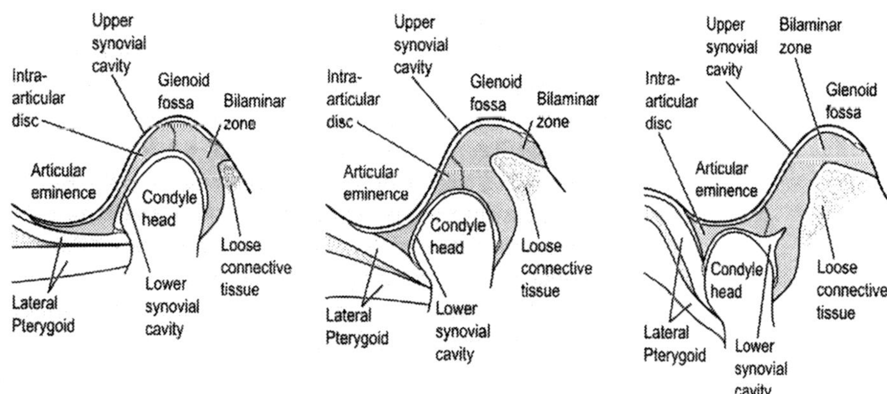

Fig. 12.3
Diagrams of the temporomandibular joint, showing how the articular disc moves as the mandibular condyle moves forward onto the articular eminence during separation of the jaws.

movement, no movement at all, or even a slight backward movement of the other condyle.

The articulating surface is fibrocartilage

The mandibular condyle broadens into the head which has an articulating surface oval in shape, about 18 mm by 10 mm, the long axes of the ovals being inclined mesially so that lines extended through them would meet at an angle of 150° in the region of the foramen magnum. In sagittal section the condylar head appears as a slight swelling above the neck of the condyle. The articular surface is not a hyaline cartilage as in the long bones, but a thin (less than 0.5 mm thick) layer of dense fibrocartilage covered by a layer of collagen. Between the collagen layer and the fibrocartilage is a proliferative zone which varies from a relatively broad zone in the growing child to virtually a single cell layer in the adult. It is this layer which can form more cartilage to allow remodelling of the joint surface. Remodelling is limited, and removal of cartilage occurs by the action of chondroclasts in this almost avascular area. The two heads of the lateral pterygoid muscle are inserted into the condyle immediately below the head, and the joint space is defined by the capsular ligaments which also insert below the head all round the joint. Anteriorly, the capsular ligament is continuous with the sheath of the lateral pterygoid, and in some 60% of subjects a few fibres of the muscle pass through to insert directly into the disc. The articulating surface of the temporal bone consists of the glenoid fossa and the articular eminence. The glenoid fossa is a depression in the surface of the temporal bone immediately anterior to the squamotympanic fissure. Like the condyle, the surface of the articular fossa and eminence are covered in dense fibrous tissue which extends out into the periosteum beyond the joint. The shape of the fossa and the eminence continuing anteriorly from it vary from mesial to lateral: in midsagittal section the fossa is deep and the slope to the eminence steep, whilst more laterally the S-shape is much flatter. Between the bony surfaces lies the interarticular disc. It fits over the head of the condyle and separates the joint cavity into two separate chambers. The disc is

An articular disc lies between the articulating surfaces

composed mainly of dense fibrous tissue with a small amount of elastic, particularly in the posterior region. It is thinner in the load-bearing zone anterosuperiorly and has thicker anterior and posterior bands. Anteriorly its fibres separate to insert into the articular eminence and the condylar head at the insertion of the lateral pterygoid, while posteriorly there is a bilaminar zone with a thin band of fibres passing over the head of the condyle to disappear into the periosteum and an upper lamina becoming loose connective tissue with collagenous and elastic fibres separated by blood vessels, nerves and adipose tissue. The description of the bilaminar posterior zone of the disc has recently been modified: the uppermost layer of the upper lamina has been found to be a narrow zone of dense fibroelastic tissue more like the lower lamina. The loose tissue in the posterior part of the disc allows both retrusion and protrusion of the head of the condyle during mastication. During normal movement in the healthy joint the disc moves with the head of the condyle (Fig. 12.3).

Surrounding the joint is the joint capsule: it is thickened laterally to form the lateral ligament which holds the condylar head in the glenoid fossa. No ligament is necessary mesially, partly because of the shape of the fossa, and partly because there are bilateral joints and movement inwards on one side of the head must result in movement outwards at the other. The inner layer of the joint capsule constitutes the synovial membrane and secretes the lubricant synovial fluid. There are no cells secreting synovial fluid on the surfaces of the joint or the interarticular disc. The capsule is made up of collagen fibres and contains both blood vessels and nerves. The inner layer consists of cells of varying morphology, but generally looking rather like large fibroblasts which stain readily with basophil dyes and contain many cytoplasmic vacuoles. There are two general types of cells which differ in the amount of Golgi apparatus and endoplasmic reticulum. The first type appear to function largely as macrophages; they have an abundant Golgi system, many pinocytotic vesicles, fine branched cytoplasmic filaments and they extend processes into the joint cavity. The second type have an abundant rough endoplasmic reticulum, less Golgi apparatus and fewer vesicles: they resemble matrix-secreting cells of cartilage and bone. Their main product is hyaluronate, the glycosaminoglycan which gives viscosity to the synovial fluid and enables it to lubricate the joint. There are no tight junctions between the synovial membrane cells and none of the characteristics of secretory epithelia: the process of secretion of hyaluronidate appears to draw water and salts into the cavity to give a typical extracellular fluid composition apart from the hyaluronidate. The fluid may be nutritive but the demands of the joint tissues are small. The fluid is reabsorbed by the macrophages and is also carried away by the lymphatics of the capsule. Synovial fluid usually contains some white blood cells, predominantly monocytes.

The joint is lubricated by a synovial fluid containing hyaluronate

Nerve supply to the temporomandibular joint

The main nerve supply to the joint is from the auriculotemporal nerve which supplies the posterior and posterolateral aspects of the capsule, and there are

The joint has nociceptor and proprioceptor nerve endings

also branches from the nerves supplying the mandibular elevator muscles, the masseter and temporalis, and the lateral pterygoid muscle. The joint receptors include corpuscular endings and non-corpuscular unmyelinated free nerve endings in the lateral ligament and a fine myelinated plexus throughout the capsule. The last are A delta fibres and the unmyelinated are C fibres: both these are concerned with nociceptive information. The corpuscular endings are of three types: globular or ovoid endings of the Ruffini or Meissner type, thickly laminated corpuscles like Pacinian corpuscles, and fusiform corpuscles of the Golgi type. The first are found scattered in the capsule, are low-threshold, slowly adapting mechanoreceptors, probably A beta fibres; the Pacinian corpuscles found in the deeper layer of the capsule and near blood vessels are low-threshold, rapidly adapting mechanoreceptors, still A beta; and the Golgi-type endings in the ligaments and tendons of the joint are high-threshold, very slowly adapting mechanoreceptors of A alpha fibres. These mechanoreceptors signal information on joint position and movement to the trigeminal nuclei and synapse with the trigeminal motorneurones.

The joint, unlike most synovial joints, is not loadbearing in its rest position, but it is subjected to load during mastication. The load is carried on the anterior surface of the condylar head as it meets the anterior surface of the glenoid fossa but is distributed by the intervening disc.

As the jaws are separated, the temporomandibular joint functions initially as a hinge joint, but at separations greater than 25 mm the condylar head moves from its position of retrusion in the glenoid fossa to slide downwards and forwards out of the fossa and on the eminence. At maximal separation, therefore, the condylar heads are rotated downwards and rest on the articular eminence. From that position approximation of the jaws takes place along a relatively smooth curve with the joint acting as a hinge. Just before the teeth come into occlusion, the condylar head slides back into the glenoid fossa and the hinge movement is completed in that position. The disc moves with the head of the condyle throughout: it is only in disturbances of temporomandibular function that the disc–condyle relationship is subject to variation.

The muscles of mastication

The major muscles of mastication are the jaw elevators; the infra- and suprahyoid muscles are important in depression

As both mastication and incision are primarily the breaking and crushing of food by movement of the tooth-bearing surface of the moveable mandible against that of the fixed maxilla, the muscles engaged in mastication are those attached to the mandible. However, those which are attached at their other ends to the hyoid bone – the depressor muscles – do not have a fixed attachment unless the hyoid itself is held stable by the infrahyoid muscles. These latter must therefore be included as masticatory muscles. A further group of muscles are essential for food transport, controlling the position of food in the mouth to permit mastication to take place. These are the muscles of the lips and cheeks – the perioral muscles, acting upon and from an insertion into the modiolus, and the buccinator – and the muscles of the tongue. In addition, other muscles of the head and neck may play an accessory role in mastication when greater forces are required, or during food capture and the cutting off of bite-sized portions which is termed incision.

Mandibular elevator muscles

The major masticatory muscles are the mandibular elevators (Fig. 12.4).

The masseter muscle

The masseter muscle is a quadrilateral muscle with two portions: the deep and the superficial. The superficial portion arises from the zygomatic process of the maxilla and anterior two-thirds of the lower border of the zygomatic arch, and it is inserted into the angle of the mandible and the lower half of the mandibular ramus (Fig. 12.4). The smaller deep portion arises from the medial surface of the zygomatic arch and the posterior third of its lower border and passes downwards to reach the lateral surface of the coronoid process and upper half of the ramus of the mandible.

The temporalis muscle

The temporalis is a large, flat fan-shaped muscle arising from the whole of the temporal fossa (Fig. 12.4). Its fibres converge into a tendon which is inserted

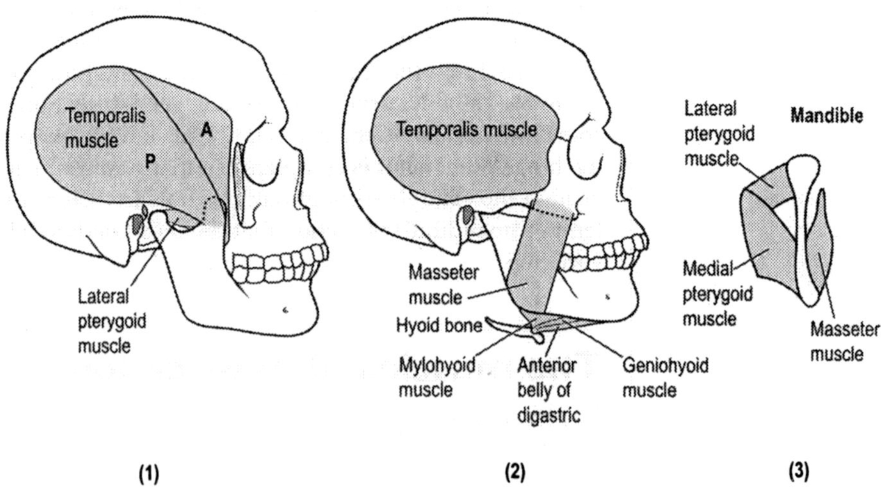

Fig. 12.4
Muscles involved in mastication: the elevator muscles of the mandible. The anterior and posterior parts of the temporalis muscle are designated A and P, respectively. The lateral pterygoid is shown in the mandibular notch in diagram 1, and the muscles attaching to the mandible and hyoid bone in diagram 2. Diagram 3 shows the ramus of the mandible from behind, demonstrating how the masseter and medial pterygoid muscles form a sling around its lower border and the lateral pterygoid passes from the condyle to the lateral pterygoid plate.

into the medial surface, the apex and the anterior border of the coronoid process and the anterior border of the ramus. The direction of the fibres means that this muscle can retrude the mandible.

The medial pterygoid muscle

The medial pterygoid muscle arises from the medial surface of the lateral pterygoid plate and from the tubercle of the palatal bone and is inserted into the lower and posterior portions of the medial surface of the ramus and angle of the mandible, forming with the masseter muscle a sling around the mandible (Fig. 12.5). All these muscles are supplied by the mandibular division of the trigeminal nerve.

The lateral pterygoid muscle

The lateral pterygoid muscle is not actually an elevator muscle even though it is attached to the mandible and to skull. Its direction of insertion makes it most important in lateral displacement and protrusion of the mandible, although it can be demonstrated to have some slight depressor activity. It is short and thick with two heads, one from the infratemporal surface and crest of the sphenoid bone and the other from the lateral surface of the lateral pterygoid plate (Fig. 12.4). The fibres are inserted into the neck of the mandible and a few into the articular disc.

Mandibular depressor muscles

The second group of masticatory muscles are the supra- and infrahyoid muscles.

The suprahyoid muscles

The digastric muscle can be used as a depressor of the mandible

The suprahyoid muscles act as mandibular depressors, provided the hyoid bone is stabilised at the same time by the infrahyoid group. The suprahyoid muscles are the digastric muscle with two bellies joined by a tendon, the

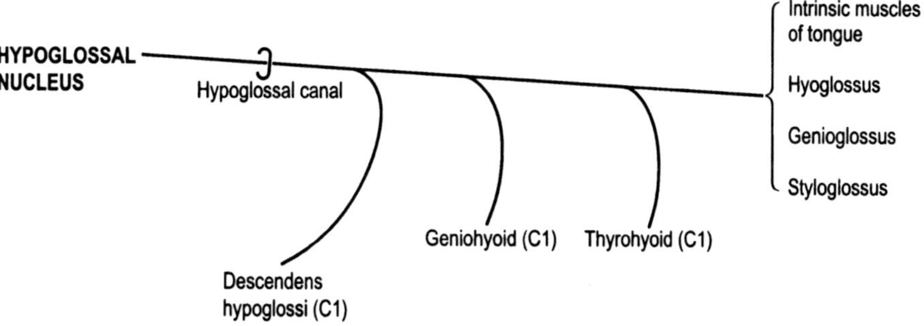

Fig. 12.5
The motor branches of the hypoglossal nerve in the oral region.

stylohyoid, the mylohyoid, and the geniohyoid muscles. The anterior belly of digastric is inserted into the digastric fossa on the base of the mandible near the midline and the posterior belly is attached to the mastoid notch of the temporal bone; the two meet in the digastric tendon which is held against the side of the body and greater cornu of the hyoid bone by a fibrous loop (Fig. 12.11). The anterior belly of digastric is the main depressor muscle of the mandible. The mylohyoid muscle forms the floor of the mouth. It arises from the mylohyoid line along the length of the medial surface of the body of the mandible and passes down to the front of the body of the hyoid bone, joining to its contralateral muscle in a fibrous raphe from the symphysis menti to the hyoid bone. Both these muscles are supplied by the mandibular division of the trigeminal nerve. The narrow geniohyoid muscles are attached to the genial tubercles on the medial surface of the body of the mandible: they run side by side down to the anterior surface of the body of the hyoid bone. This muscle receives motor fibres from the hypoglossal nerve. The remaining suprahyoid muscle, the styloglossus, is not attached to the mandible and its function relates more to the stabilisation of the hyoid bone: it arises from the styloid process and passes down to the body of the hyoid bone, actually being perforated at its insertion by the tendon of the digastric muscle. Its nerve supply is from the facial nerve.

The infrahyoid muscles

Infrahyoid muscles fix the hyoid bone and control movement of the floor of the mouth

The infrahyoid muscles are the sternohyoid, the thyrohyoid and the omohyoid muscles, together with the sternothyroid muscle; they are important in mastication only in fixing the hyoid bone so that the suprahyoid muscles can be used to depress the mandible. They also assist in allowing the upward movement of the floor of the mouth during swallowing and permitting the tongue movements during swallowing and speech. The most important of these muscles is the sternohyoid muscle, which arises from the medial end of the clavicle, the posterior sternoclavicular ligament and the upper and posterior part of the manubrium sterni and is inserted into the lower border of the body of the hyoid bone. The omohyoid muscle has two bellies, one arising from the upper border of the scapula and one from the lower border of the hyoid. The two meet at an angle in the intermediate tendon which is held in position by the deep cervical fascia. The other two muscles, the sternothyroid and thyrohyoid muscles, can be regarded as continuations of each other. The sternothyroid muscle runs from the manubrium sterni to the lamina of the thyroid cartilage and the thyrohyoid muscle from there to the lower border of the greater cornu of the hyoid bone. All the infrahyoid muscles are supplied by branches of the hypoglossal nerve (Fig. 12.5).

Directions of force exerted by muscles of mastication

Muscles of mastication have complex force vectors

Anatomical analysis of the elevator muscles shows them to be complex in their gross morphology, and consideration of the fibre directions indicates that different parts of a muscle may produce different movements of the mandible.

This is most obvious in the temporalis muscle where contraction of anterior or posterior fibres may produce vertical or horizontal movement, respectively. Fig. 12.6 gives a simple interpretation of the main lines of movement or force for each of the masticatory muscles. Further analysis of this, however, shows that each of the elevator muscles is capable of generating an angle of possible movements, and the actual observed movement of the mandible or direction of force is a result of the composite activity of a number of muscles (Fig. 12.6).

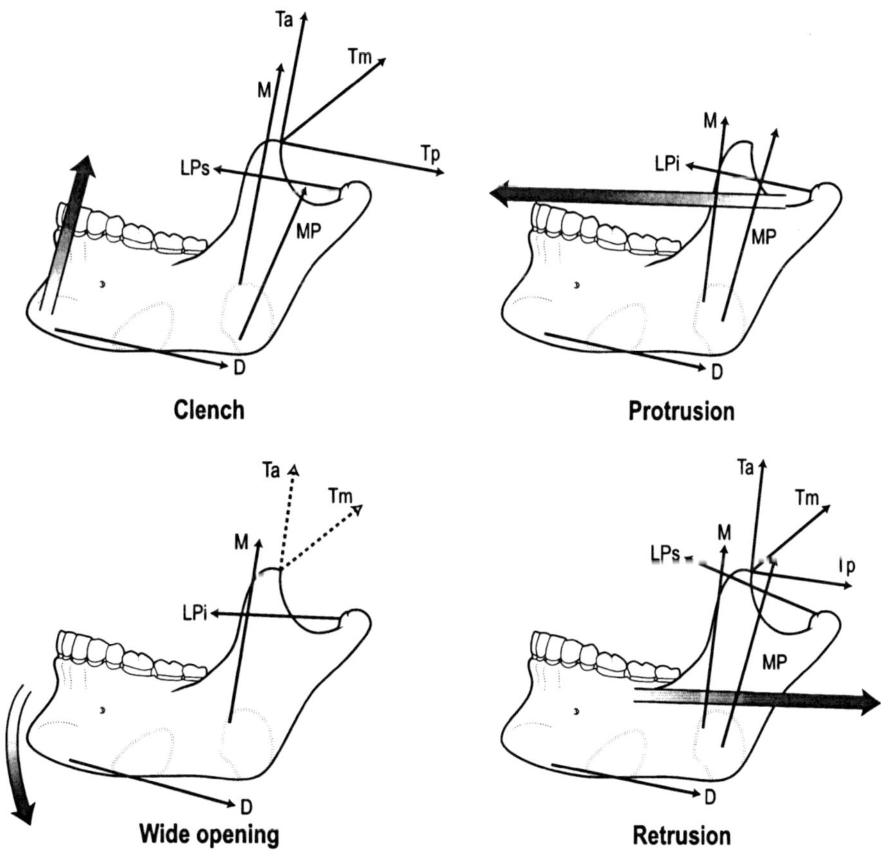

The muscles which have been demonstrated by electromyography to be involved in mandibular movements. They are labelled as follows: D, digastric; M, masseter; MP, medial pterygoid; LPi, inferior part of the lateral pterygoid; LPs, superior part of the lateral pterygoid; Ta, anterior temporalis; Tm, medial temporalis; Tp, posterior temporalis. The direction of force exerted by each muscle is shown by the thin arrow. Note that all movements involve multiple muscle action. The resultant of the muscle forces is shown by the heavy arrow. Mandibular movements are very carefully controlled and muscles may exert a braking action upon the movement; digastric activity is a good example but note that the masseter is active during wide opening for the same reason.

Histochemical characterisation of the muscles of mastication

Most of the major muscles of mastication have now been examined histochemically (Table 12.1) to determine from the pattern of enzyme types present what their working characteristics are likely to be. Most of the limb muscles in the body are made up of a mosaic of approximately equal proportions of type I and type II fibres. Type I fibres are the slow twitch, fatigue-resistant fibres which are used for long powerful contractions; type II fibres, the fast twitch fibres, are of at least three types (Table 12.2).

The fibres are grouped into motor units. In the masseter and temporalis muscles the low threshold slow motor units contain relatively few fibres – probably 100 or less – but as the number of fibres in the high threshold faster units is greater the average figure for masseter muscle is around 600 fibres per motor unit, and for temporalis muscle around 900. The range is estimated at between 60 and 960. These figures suggest a fairly precise level of control of

Table 12.1
Characteristics of the main skeletal muscle fibre groups

	Type I	Type IIA	Type IIB
Motor units	ST/SO	FOG/FR	FG/FF
Speed to peak tension	Slow	Fast, high threshold	Fast
Fatigue resistance	Resistant	Readily fatigued	Resistant
Myosin-ATPase	Slow	Fast	
Mitochondria	Many	Intermediate	Few
Glycogen	Little	Much	Much
Triglyceride	Much	Little	More

Types IM and IIAB (fast intermediate) are intermediate in properties between the three major groups. Type IIC is relatively infrequent.
FF, fast fatiguable; FG, fast glycolytic; FOG, fast oxidative glycolytic; FR, fatigue resistant; SO, slow oxidative; ST, slow twitch.

Table 12.2
Fibre characteristics of masticatory muscles

	Type I	Type IIA	Type IIB	Type IIC	Type IM
Masseter	70–86	0–7	6–20	<2	3–5
Temporalis	52–90		5–45	2.4	1–4
Medial pterygoid	50–78	1–5	15–41	2	5
Lateral pterygoid	81	0	8	3	8
Digastric	24–38	30–32	29–46		
Buccinator	52	47			
Orbicularis oris	25	74			

Fibre types are expressed as percentages.

the muscles. In masseter muscle actual motor unit territories are small and usually limited to one muscle compartment; a few extend over the whole cross-section of the muscle. The motor units with the lowest thresholds are found in the deep medial compartment.

The fibre types found in the muscles of mastication are appropriate for producing powerful forces without fatiguing

The distribution of fibre types implies that the masseter and medial pterygoid muscles are mainly power producers. The temporalis muscle probably acts as a stabiliser of mandibular position, enabling the masseter muscle to exert its force effectively, although the temporalis muscle itself can also produce force and movement. The lateral pterygoid muscle, with a very high proportion of type I fibres, seems appropriately constituted to perform a continuous workload at low forces without fatiguing. This again would be the kind of activity involved in stabilising the position of the temporomandibular joint elements. Both bellies of the digastric muscle have a similar fibre composition with an approximately equal distribution of types I, IIA and IIB fibres. This mixture therefore includes the slow fatigue-resistant fibres which are recruited early in contraction and may be used to brake the elevator activity as the teeth are brought together, and the IIA fibres with a high threshold which contract rapidly to provide bursts of intense activity, so that the depression of the mandible occurs more rapidly than the elevation. These fibres are resistant to fatigue. Limb muscles have a similar fibre distribution. The type I fibres of the buccinator muscle fit it for continuous contraction at low levels of work whilst the muscles of facial expression and speech, as exemplified by the orbicularis oris muscle, have a dominant type IIA component which makes for rapid responses and many small motor units which give precise control of muscle activity. The zygomatic muscles also have many type II fibres but they have large motor units and are therefore poorly adapted for fine graded movement.

Sensory receptors in the muscles of mastication

The elevator muscles but not the depressors have many proprioceptive nerve endings

The sensory receptors involved in control of muscle movement are unevenly distributed in the muscles of mastication. In general the elevator muscles are well supplied with muscle spindles whilst the depressor muscles and the zygomatic muscles have few if any. Spindles are an important feature of the tongue muscles. There are conflicting reports of whether the elevator muscles have Golgi tendon organs. It is, however, generally agreed that the role of the Golgi tendon organs in protecting against the overdevelopment of muscle tension is performed in the oral cavity by the periodontal ligament receptors which limit the force which can be applied in mastication.

Electromyography of the muscles of mastication

The elevator muscles have been extensively studied by electromyography

Superficial muscles such as the masseter, temporalis and digastric muscles can readily be studied by electromyography. The deeper muscles are more difficult in this respect but, nevertheless, the patterns of activity within all the masticatory muscles have been observed both during specific manoeuvres and during normal mastication and swallowing. In general the results are as would be predicted from the anatomical arrangement of the muscles, but the patterns during specific movements show complex combinations of activation to achieve the objectives. Thus although masseter, medial pterygoid and temporalis muscles are all elevator muscles they are activated in sequence during the approximation of mandible and maxilla (Fig. 12.7). The digastric muscle, as well as operating during mandibular depression, shows bursts of activity during mandibular elevation, presumably to brake the rate and force as the teeth come together. It is noticeable that activity of the masseter muscle begins relatively late during elevation and ceases before the stroke is completed. Electrodes placed on other muscles in the region have shown that the sternocleidomastoid muscle is active during hard clenching of the teeth.

Occlusion and rest position of the mandible

Normally at rest the teeth are slightly separated; there may be several slightly different positions of occlusion in the same subject

The relationship between the mandible and maxilla is obviously variable over what is usually termed the envelope of motion of the mandible, but a few positions can be defined. The position in which the teeth are in contact is termed occlusion. The individual habitual position in which the teeth are in light contact is termed centric occlusion, or the intercuspal position (Figs 12.8 and 12.9). It may differ slightly from the clench position and it does not necessarily mean that the midlines of upper and lower arch will coincide, although in the ideal situation they will. Both intercuspal and intercuspal clench positions are static: the term 'median occlusal position' is sometimes used to denote the light tooth contact position which is briefly reached in a normal chewing cycle. Usually this is very close to the centric occlusion. At rest the teeth are held slightly separated in the 'rest position': the mandible is then held in position by the sling formed principally by the masseter and medial pterygoid muscles and the temporomandibular joint is not loaded. Electromyographic analysis of muscle activity has given conflicting evidence as to whether there is contraction of the masseter muscle in the rest position. The space between the teeth in the rest position is usually termed the freeway space, but is also known as the interdental space or speech space (because speech becomes possible at this tooth separation). In centric occlusion the head of the mandibular condyle lies somewhere between the most posterior position possible in the glenoid fossa and the position in which it is contacting the anterior wall of the fossa with the disc between not being compressed. In determining the optimal position for intercuspation of dentures the mandible is manipulated into its most retruded position; this again may or may not be the position the patient had previously adopted when teeth were still present.

There are two reproducible other clench positions of the mandible which can be studied and have relevance to mastication and to analysis of jaw function: the incisal clench such as is seen in incision of food, and the lateral clench with the canines in tip-to-tip occlusion which represents the extreme of lateral movement normally attained. Although the mandible is fixed to the maxilla only at the two temporomandibular joints, the jaws are in contact

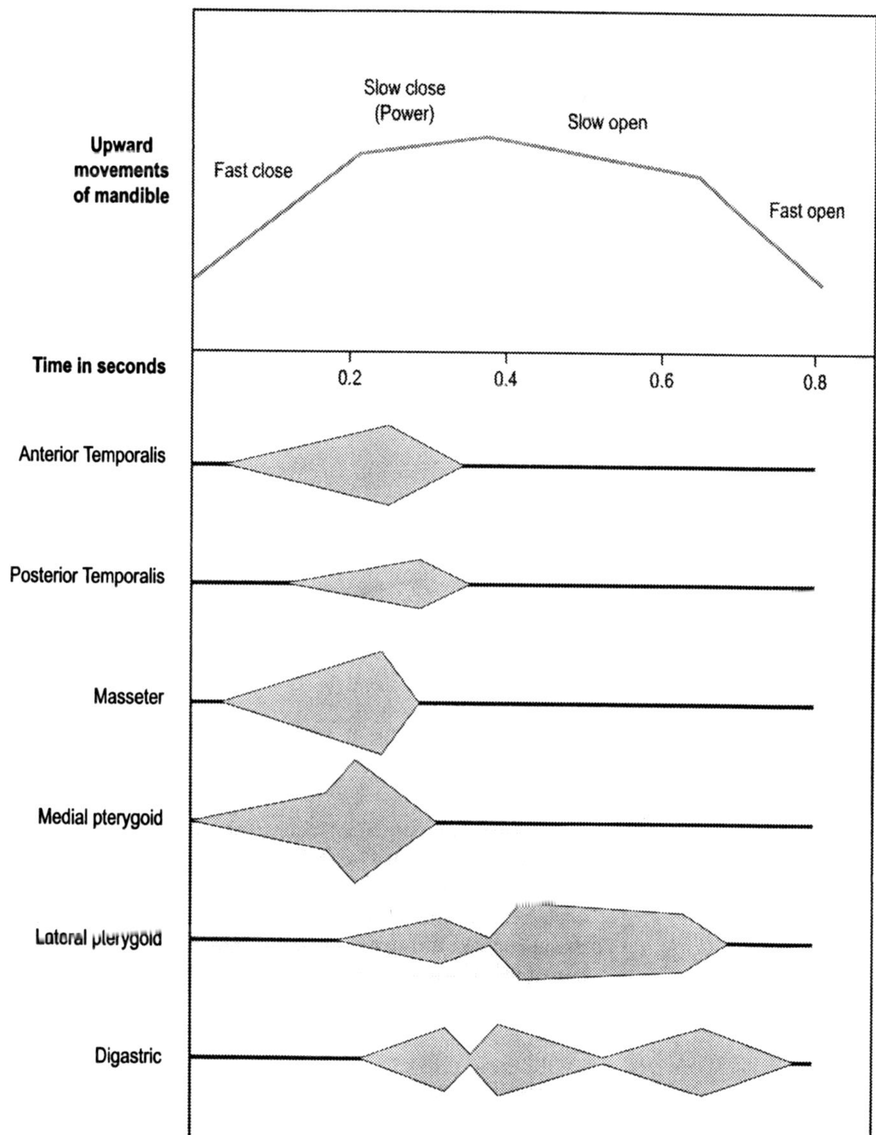

Fig. 12.7
Electromyography of the muscles of mastication during the conventional phases of a chewing cycle. Observations of this kind have usually been made on subjects told to chew, with or without a bolus of specific material: recent observations of natural chewing with common foodstuffs do not show such well-defined phases and the sequence depends to a large extent on whether the food is hard or soft or if it is brittle. Note, however, the braking activity of the digastric and lateral pterygoid towards the end of the power stroke.

through the teeth during occlusion. The contact of the teeth is therefore termed articulation. This also means that the periodontal ligament receptors function as articular receptors and monitor the load upon the articulating

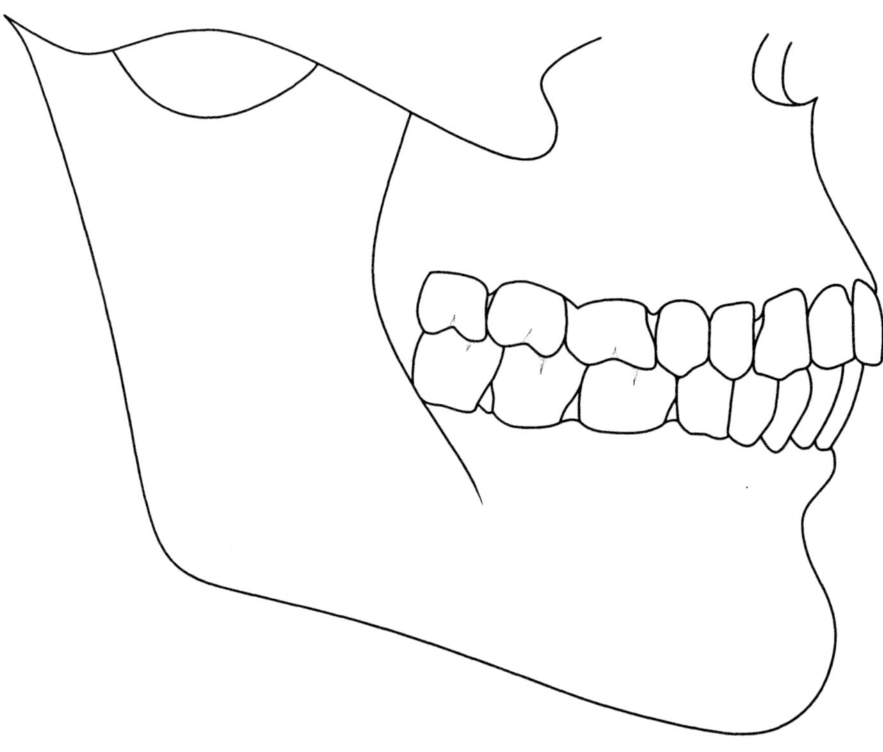

Fig. 12.8
The normal intercuspal position or occlusion of the teeth: Angle's orthodontic class I. The lower incisors are positioned inside the arch of the upper incisors and in light contact with their palatal surfaces, whilst the mesial cusp of the lower first molars occludes with the distal slope of the upper second premolar and the mesial slope of the upper first molar. Although this intercuspal position is described as normal it is not necessarily the normal occlusion in non-Caucasian races.

surfaces. The main pressure receptors of the periodontal ligament are found in the apical third of the ligament where the articular pressure will be most readily apparent, and they are similar to Ruffini endings (Fig. 11.9). Functionally they are equivalent to Golgi tendon organs. Their sensitivity to tooth contact is high and they communicate with cells in the cerebellum directly – i.e. without any synapse or interneurone. This gives them a very rapid and powerful role in the control of masticatory neurones.

Incision

Incision begins with mandibular protrusion and ends with a movement from

Incision consists of a protrusive movement of the mandible, with the condylar heads sliding forwards and downwards onto the articular eminence, depression of the mandible in the protruded position, and then a hinge movement to elevate the anterior part of the body and bring the incisors into

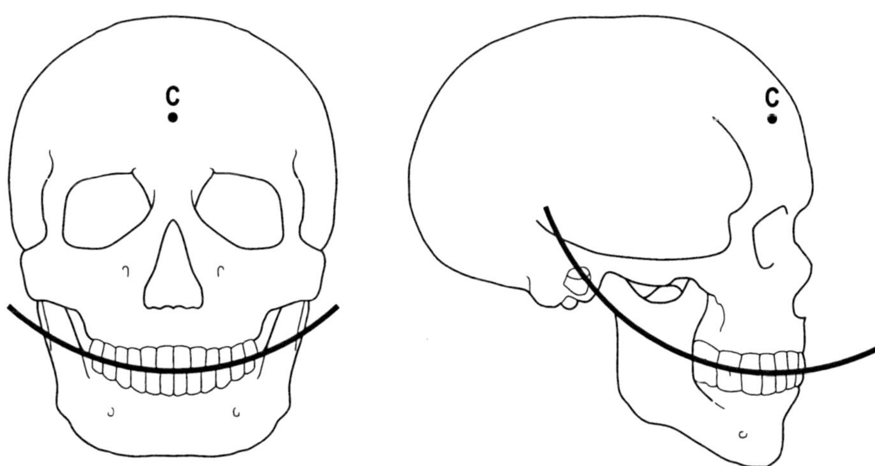

Fig. 12.9
The occluding surfaces of the teeth are described as lying on the surface of a hypothetical sphere with its centre in the midline above the nose and having a radius of approximately 10 cm. This has been variously described from different angles of view as the curves of Monson, Spee and Villain, although all these writers postulated that the curves passed through the anterior border of the mandibular condyle – which is clearly not the case.

edge-to-edge contact of the incisors towards normal occlusion

an edge-to-edge position. The mandible remains in protrusion. The movement is achieved in the first part largely by the action of the lateral pterygoid muscles and the final elevation involves medial pterygoid and masseter muscles. The maximum extent of jaw separation is normally about 3 cm, but the movement is usually only that necessary to allow the food to be placed between the teeth.

Experimental studies show that perception of the distance between the upper and lower incisors is remarkably good. Clinically the maximum separation attainable by patients with limited jaw movement is usually assessed by finger-widths. Dislocation of the temporomandibular joint can occur if excessive jaw separation is attempted: this is more likely to occur during the yawning reflex than during incision. Such dislocation is caused by the condyle moving forward beyond the highest point of the articular eminence and so the correction requires a downward as well as a backward pressure in the third molar region on both sides.

The events following the moment at which the upper and lower incisor teeth make contact with the food depend upon the consistency of the food (Fig. 12.10). With highly resistant foods the mandible begins to retrude but stops as resistance is felt. The teeth are pressed into the food and a side-to-side oscillating retrusive slide begins. The head and shoulders are held rigid and pulled backwards as the hand and arm twist downwards. When the food portion separates the mandible drops slightly to release the particle and the lips guide it towards the tongue and cheeks. The tongue then transports the food towards the posterior teeth. With moderately resistant foods the

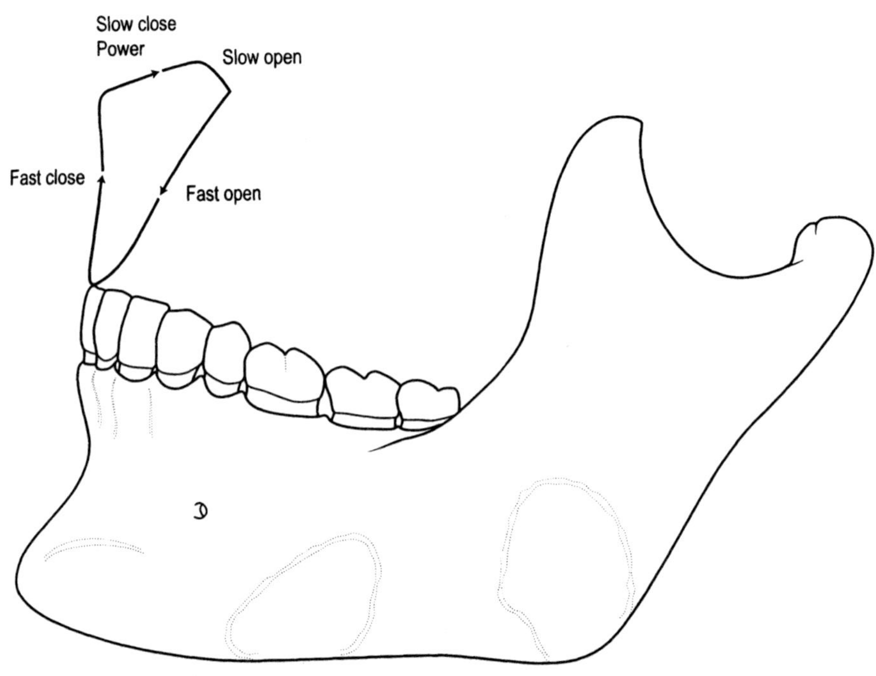

The masticatory cycle. The cycle of jaw separation plotted against time can also be seen as the movement of the jaws as seen in sagittal section. The curve approximates to the inclines of the molar cusps in the slow close and slow open phases.

mandible slides back towards the intercuspal position of the teeth and the food portion separates in the scissor-blade movement. Soft foods are sheared by the incisors but not actually cut through: the food thins and then parts. The bringing together of the upper and lower incisor teeth is usually sufficient to cut through the food, but lateral movement in the protruded position may be used to add a sawing motion to assist in cutting tougher materials. Sometimes the incisors are used to grip food held by the hands and fracture is achieved by a downward jerk of the head. Such tugging may be amplified by lateral head movements. These head movements are similar to those seen in carnivores who grip a piece of meat between upper and lower incisors and canines (or even carnassial teeth) to tear off a portion for transport into the mouth.

The muscles involved in incision are the medial and lateral pterygoid muscles on each side for protrusion and the digastric and suprahyoid muscles for mandibular depression, followed by the medial pterygoid and masseter muscles for mandibular elevation.

Estimates of a 'mouthful' vary from 12 ml to over 20 ml

The maximum volume which can be taken into the mouth varies between 20 and 50 ml, but the actual size of a mouthful is only some 20% of the maximum. There have been attempts to measure the volume of fluid which can be taken into the mouth; one small study of six people reported nearly 30 ml for men and nearly 16 ml for women. In another study of 41 subjects, both males and females took a mouthful of fluid measuring about 12.5 ml. Dawes estimated that swallowing was initiated when a volume of 4 ml was present in the mouth. There are few data on the size of a solid food mouthful, although it has been reported recently that the mean portion bitten off a banana was 12.5 g (12.5 ml), 7.5 g (about 10 ml) off an apple and 2.5 g (about 7 ml) off a biscuit.

Food transport muscles

The muscles of tongue and cheeks are used in food transport between the teeth and preparatory to swallowing

In addition to the muscles which control the movements of the mandible, there are muscles involved in moving the tongue and the lips and cheeks, to pass the food back and forth between the teeth and to take part in the process of swallowing. The tongue is made up of the terminal parts of the extrinsic muscles, which anchor it to the bony structures of the mandible, the hyoid bone and the styloid process and hence control its overall position and movements in the mouth and the intrinsic muscles which govern its shape (Fig. 12.11).

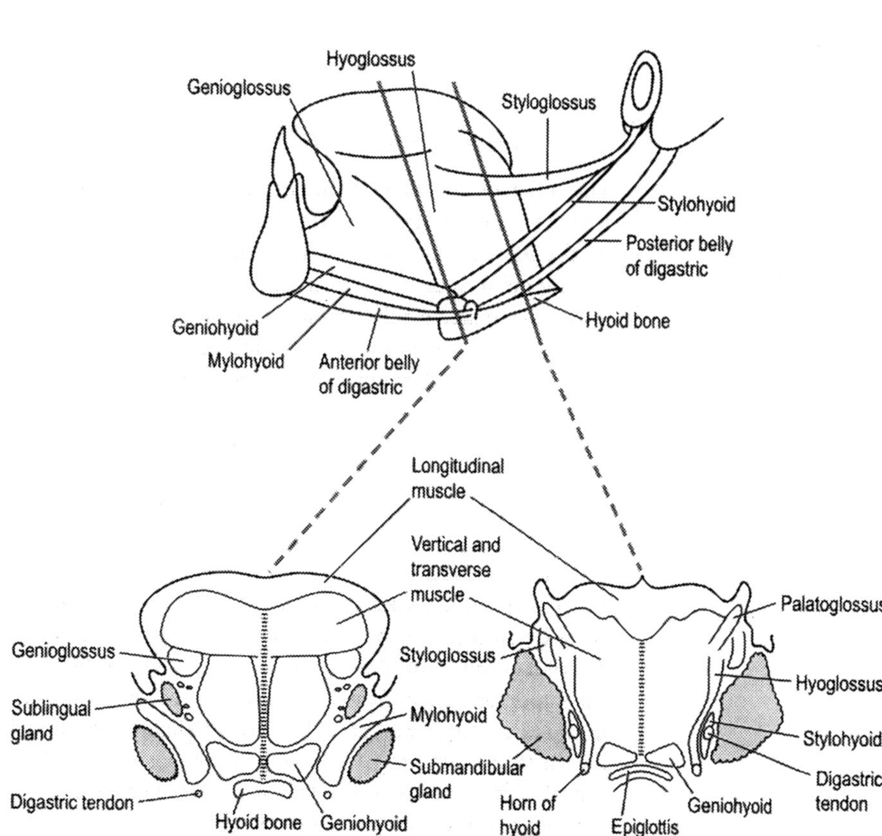

Fig. 12.11
The extrinsic and intrinsic muscles of the tongue.

Extrinsic muscles of the tongue

The extrinsic muscles are: the genioglossus, arising from the genial tubercles on the inner surface of the symphysis menti, which passes into the whole length of the lower surface of the tongue, but also attaches to the upper surface of the anterior part of the body of the hyoid bone; the hyoglossus, arising from the whole length of the greater horn of the hyoid which enters the side of the tongue; the chondroglossus, arising from the lesser cornu of the hyoid and inserted into the tongue in similar fashion to the hyoglossus; and the styloglossus, arising from the styloid process and passing almost horizontally into the side of the tongue (Fig. 12.11). These muscles are supplied by the hypoglossal nerve (Fig. 12.5). The genioglossus muscle pulls the tongue forward and can cause it to protrude from the mouth. It also makes the tongue surface concave when the muscles on both sides act together. The hyoglossus and the chondroglossus muscles depress the tongue, whilst the styloglossus muscle draws it upwards and backwards. A further extrinsic muscle, the palatoglossus, arises from the aponeurosis down the centre of the soft palate and passes downwards and forwards in front of the tonsil to enter the side of the tongue and spread over the dorsum. It pulls up the root of the tongue and, with its partner on the other side, reduces the size of the oropharyngeal opening.

Intrinsic muscles of the tongue

The intrinsic muscles of the tongue are the superior and inferior longitudinal muscles, the longitudinal muscle and the transverse muscle. They are supplied by the hypoglossal nerve. The longitudinal muscles shorten the tongue and the superior longitudinal in addition turns the tip and sides up to form a concave surface whilst the inferior pulls the tip down and makes the surface convex. The transverse muscle narrows and elongates the tongue while the vertical muscle flattens and broadens it.

Facial muscles involved in food transport

Of the facial muscles, the one most concerned with mastication is the buccinator, the muscle which forms the cheek itself. This is a thin muscle, roughly quadrilateral in shape, which is inserted superiorly into the alveolar process of the maxilla in the region of the molar teeth, and inferiorly into the alveolar process of the mandible in a similar position. Posteriorly it arises from the pterygomandibular ligament, which separates it from the anterior fibres of the superior constrictor of the pharynx. The facial nerve provides motor fibres to the buccinator muscle. The muscle pushes food back between the masticatory surfaces of the teeth, in opposition to the outward pressures of the tongue, and so aids in the transverse movements of food during mastication. Although it forms the outer wall of the buccal pouch in which food can accumulate – or even be 'stored' – during mastication, this function is relatively less important in humans than in many animals. The anterior fibres of the masseter muscle separate to sweep above and below the lips, intermingling as they do so with the fibres of the perioral muscles –

principally the orbicularis oris. The lips are closed and then protruded by the actions of the orbicularis oris muscle; opening is achieved by its relaxation and the actions of the muscles of facial expression around the mouth – the levator labii superioris, the levator anguli oris, the two zygomatic muscles, the depressor labii inferioris and depressor anguli oris. The elevator muscles arise from the maxilla and the depressor from the mandible; all are innervated by branches of the facial nerve. The mentalis muscle, arising from the incisive fossa of the mandible, raises and protrudes the lower lip. All these lip muscles, but particularly the orbicularis oris muscle, help to retain food in the mouth and perform a similar function in relation to the oral vestibule to that of the buccinator muscle in relation to the buccal pouch.

Mastication

Mastication consists of a number of chewing cycles which result in the production of a soft bolus of food

Mastication is a complex process involving movements of the body of the mandible in a vertical plane, but usually also laterally in a horizontal plane, so that the teeth are alternately separated and approximated, together with movements of the tongue, lips and cheeks to control the position and form of the food (Figs 12.1 and 12.7). Food particles are progressively reduced in size and mixed with saliva to form a softened mass which is termed the bolus. Although the breakage of food particles occurs primarily between the occluding surfaces of the posterior teeth, there is also some comminution and moulding of the food bolus by the tongue acting against the surface of the hard palate. The precision with which the whole process is carried out is demonstrated by the way in which foods of different consistencies are handled and the rarity of biting one's own tongue, cheeks or lips during the process.

The process of mastication has been studied in humans, monkeys and other animals. Although recent studies of human mastication have suggested that there is considerable variation in chewing patterns, it has been customary to describe each masticatory stroke, or chewing cycle, as being composed of three phases. There is a phase during which increasing separation of the occlusal surfaces of the teeth occurs, usually termed the jaw opening phase, a phase in which the occlusal surfaces are brought together, termed the jaw closing or rapid closing phase, and a phase in which the food particles are crushed between the occlusal surfaces, termed the slow jaw closing phase. This last is also known as the tooth contact phase or the power phase.

Jaw opening phase

There is an opening phase, a rapid closing phase and a slow closing or tooth contact stage

In the chewing cycle there is first a bilateral activation of the mylohyoid muscle, then the anterior belly of the digastric, and finally the inferior head of the lateral pterygoid muscle (Fig. 12.7). Contraction of the anterior belly of the digastric would be ineffective were there not simultaneous fixation of the hyoid bone by the infra- and suprahyoid muscles. The degree of separation of the occluding surfaces is variable even in one person because it depends on the size and consistency of the food in the mouth, but normally the lower incisors move downwards by between 10 and 15 mm from their position in centric occlusion. This movement is sufficient to require some forward sliding of the condylar heads down the anterior surfaces of the glenoid fossae. It may take place at a relatively constant speed over some 150 ms or it may be split into two phases: a slow opening followed by a rapid opening (Figs 12.7 and 12.10).

Rapid jaw closing phase

The rate of mandibular depression becomes zero and a closing stroke begins. Activity in the inferior lateral pterygoid muscles ceases and the medial pterygoid muscles become active. The majority of human subjects have a preferred chewing side and it is towards this side that the chewing stroke will usually swing. In many cases it is easy to determine from the subject that the preference was established because of pain in eating on one side, or because of permanent or temporary disturbance of the occlusion on one side, but often no clear reason for the side preference can be found. The fast close phase is achieved by contraction of the masseter, medial pterygoid and temporalis muscles, the lateral component being provided by the lower fibres of the temporalis and lateral pterygoid muscles. In addition, the activity in the medial pterygoid muscles varies on the two sides, the contralateral muscle contracting before the ipsilateral. The condyle on the working side moves back almost horizontally, swinging to that side; the condyle on the balancing side moves upwards and backwards following in reverse the path traversed during opening but swings towards the working side as it does so. The terminal position before a slow close begins is with both condyles displaced laterally but with the working side condyle about 0.25 mm below its original starting position. The sequence of muscle activity on the working side is the lower head of the lateral pterygoid, anterior and posterior temporalis, and deep masseter muscle, followed by medial pterygoid and deep masseter muscles; on the balancing side activity begins with contraction of the medial pterygoid muscle, followed by contraction of the deep masseter muscle.

Slow jaw closing phase

The fast closure phase ends when resistance is detected between the teeth; thereafter a slow closure follows which may result in tooth-to-tooth contact. If this occurs, the path of mandibular closure will be determined by the slide of the mandibular teeth along the cuspal inclines of the maxillary teeth (Fig. 12.10). There are three possible outcomes of the slow closure stroke: failure to penetrate the intervening food particle even after a power stroke which aims to crush it: slow penetration of the food particle and tooth contact; or a sudden breakage of the food particle leading to the unloading reflex and separation of the occluding surfaces. In all these outcomes it is the stimulation of periodontal receptors that helps initiate the next cycle. During the slow closure and particularly during the power stroke there is increasing force of contraction in all the elevator muscles on both sides – anterior and posterior temporalis, superficial and deep masseter muscles, the medial pterygoid, and upper and lower heads of the lateral pterygoid muscles. The power stroke returns the condylar head on the working side to its starting position with both medial and upward movement whilst the balancing condyle, already at the original higher position on the anterior slope of the fossa, now regains its original more lateral position. Activity in the elevator muscles cuts off rapidly some 20–30 ms before contact of the teeth in centric occlusion. When the fast closure phase is observed from the front, the midline of the lower incisors is observed to veer towards the working side and then return to the midline during the slow closing phase.

Control of mastication

After voluntary initiation of mastication, the process is continued under the control of a central rhythm generator in the pons

Mastication can be initiated voluntarily: this is usually the case but there follows an involuntary period of apparently reflex activity subject to the possibility of overriding voluntary control. Stimulation of the anterior sensorimotor cortex will also initiate masticatory movements. The automatic rhythmic activity was at one time thought to result from an alternation of elevator and depressor reflexes stimulated perhaps by stretch receptors and by intraoral touch or pressure receptors. By the 1970s a central rhythm generator was being postulated, analogous in operation to the respiratory pattern generator, and evidence was adduced of a possible generator near the motor nucleus of the trigeminal nerve. Such rhythm generators are thought to operate by neurones stimulating elevator muscles simultaneously inhibiting tonically active depressor muscles but also inhibiting their own activity via a longer pathway. Current thinking still envisages a pattern generator but sees its activity largely modified by sensory inputs from intraoral, muscle and joint receptors (Figs 12.12 and 12.13).

Information from local receptors modifies the masticatory rhythm and the food movement in the mouth

The process of mastication is better considered as the first part of the transport of food material in the processes of ingestion and digestion. The control of the process, then, is a control of food handling in the mouth and its onward passage in swallowing. This may be summarised in a flow diagram such as Fig. 12.1. Once food has been taken into the mouth, or incision has occurred, the rhythmic pattern of mastication is initiated. Receptors in the periodontal ligaments, the muscles and the joints and the touch and pressure receptors of the tongue and palate monitor the hardness and the degree of comminution of the food and adjust the activity of the muscles by feedback to the motor neurones, to the rhythm generator and to the cerebellum. Thus soft foods are chewed faster than hard foods. The masticatory cycle is longer at the beginning of ingestion of a given food as the jaws are brought together with a slower, more powerful, stroke, even though the food may not be penetrated completely at this stage. Different types of food will fragment or soften in different ways and this will affect the subsequent strokes. When the food bolus is judged by the oral receptors to be appropriate the complex of actions which constitute swallowing is initiated. Both the masticatory sequence and the initiation of the swallowing sequence are subject to voluntary control from the motor cortex. The amount of chewing before swallowing is largely a characteristic of the individual, although it is influenced by the nature of the food. Thus the number of chewing strokes before swallowing – despite popular advice – is greater for men than for women, and greater for women than for children. It is not markedly influenced by the state of the dentition although the efficiency of food comminution is.

The consistency of the bolus governs the initiation of swallowing

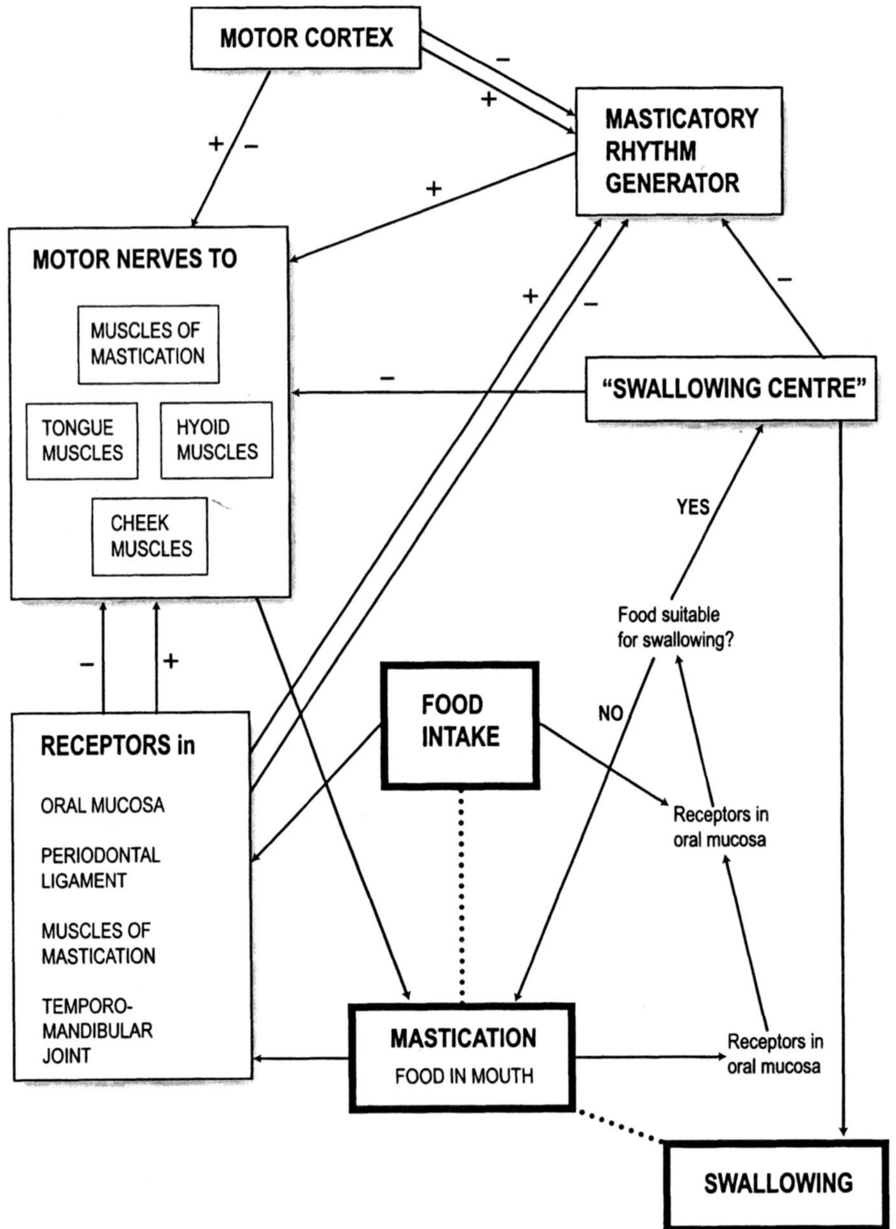

Fig. 12.12
The control of mastication. Mastication may be controlled entirely voluntarily by the motor cortex. However, it is thought to be controlled automatically by a rhythm generator in the pons. This is subject to modifying influences from sensory receptors in the oral mucosa, the muscles of mastication, the periodontal ligaments of the teeth and the temporomandibular joints. When the food bolus is perceived to be of an appropriate consistency the swallowing centre is activated and this takes over control of the food transport process.

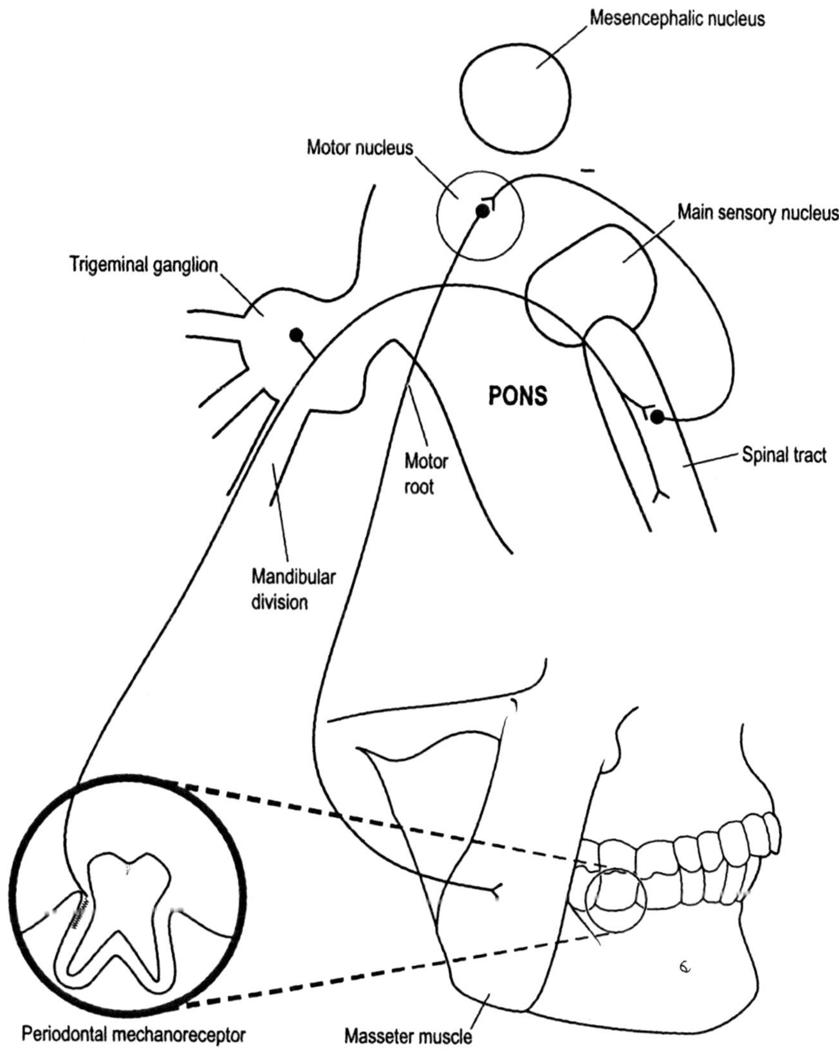

Fig. 12.13
The control of masticatory force by periodontal ligament receptors. In addition to inhibiting neurones in the motor nucleus of the trigeminal nerve via inhibitory interneurones, the receptor nerves also communicate with the rhythm generator.

Bite force

The maximum force exerted during the bite when typical Western foods are being eaten is around 80 N; full denture wearers who are imposing a force across the whole surface of the alveolar mucosa with its greater sensitivity to pressure and pain, can usually produce forces of around 64 N. These forces are well below the forces which can be generated by the powerful muscles of mastication: there are moments when acrobats and trapeze artists support the weight of the body by the muscles attached to the jaws. An instrument which

Bite forces can be as high as 500 N, but Western diets require less than a tenth of this

measures maximal bite forces on an electrical or mechanical transducer is called a gnathodynamometer, and such instruments show that static forces of around 440 N can be produced in the molar region, declining to around 150 N in the canine region. Males generate greater forces – around 520 N; females lesser forces – around 340 N. The conventional Western diet requires little chewing and so these forces are well in excess of what is needed for its digestion. Swallowing of pieces of food in cloth bags and analysis of the contents of the bags when collected from the faeces demonstrates that foods such as fish, eggs, rice and bread are completely digested without chewing. Chicken and stewed meats leave little undigested residue, but other meats and vegetables such as potatoes, peas and carrots do require chewing. Despite this apparent lack of importance of the masticatory process in food ingestion, chewing does fulfil a number of important functions. The controlled process of mastication, leading on to initiation of swallowing when the receptors in tongue and palate indicate that the bolus consistency is appropriate, reduces the possibility that, on the one hand, large particles will reach and damage the oesophageal or even the gastric mucosa, and on the other hand that food is so finely ground that it passes too rapidly through the gut for adequate digestion. The stimulation provided by mastication to the mucosal circulation and to keratinisation of the mucosal surface is important in maintaining the health of the mucosa. Chewing also has some psychological value: the rhythmic movement of the jaws seems to answer some emotional need. This is apparent in gum and possibly tobacco chewers but may also be part of the drive to eat in people who have given up some activity. The satisfaction or calming effect induced by chewing are probably examples of the primitive emotional responses to oral stimulation.

If regular chewing of hard objects is carried out over a period of time there is training of the masticatory musculature and the maximal forces developed can readily be increased by about a third. An extreme instance of training over a long period is provided by studies of Eskimo women in their original primitive lifestyle. The women traditionally chewed sealskins to make them soft enough to use as clothing: their maximal bite forces were between 1450 and 1700 N.

The limit on bite force is the force exerted within the periodontal ligaments of the occluding teeth. Low biting forces on the teeth compress the periodontal ligament, but even at levels achieved during normal mastication the bone of the jaws may flex and when even greater forces are reached pain receptors in the periodontal ligament are stimulated. The varying figures reported in the literature for axial tooth movement under occlusal loads arise from the different methodologies employed, but it is clear that the rapid movement resulting from initial compression of the periodontal ligament gives way to a much slower movement at forces which are less than 10 N.

Masticatory reflexes

Masticatory reflexes include the jaw jerk, the jaw opening reflex and

A number of reflexes involving the masticatory muscles can be demonstrated in isolation, and these presumably may contribute to the modification of the central rhythm. Thus the jaw jerk reflex is a good example of a muscle stretch

the unloading reflex. They are probably of little importance in normal mastication

reflex. Its significance in ordinary mastication arises because it forms part of a servo control. There is co-activation of alpha and gamma neurones in the masseter muscle and so any state of muscle contraction in which stretch is signalled in the contracted muscle spindles will result in further activation of the extrafusal fibres. The unloading reflex which results when the teeth close on a resistant object consists in the human of a reduction in masseteric activity and produces digastric, or depressor muscle, activity only if the loading continues for some time. The human reflex does not usually result in mouth opening; it is simply a cessation of the tooth approximation activity.

The process of mastication is controlled by a central pattern generator; nonetheless, specific reflexes of the masticatory muscles can be demonstrated and some of these may have a role in the control process. The length of a muscle must obviously be closely controlled during any activity and this is achieved by adjusting the degree of contraction by signals from muscle spindles which monitor the stretch within a muscle either directly or in comparison to a set length defined by the contraction of the spindle's intrafusal fibres, and from tendon organs which monitor the tension exerted by the muscle. In the masticatory muscles there are muscle spindles in the elevator muscles and there are tendon receptors at the origins and insertions of the muscles. Additionally, there are periodontal ligament receptors which can be regarded as the equivalent of tendon receptors at the articulation of the teeth. Three muscle reflexes have been identified in the masticatory apparatus: the jaw jerk, the jaw opening reflex and the unloading reflex.

The jaw jerk

The jaw jerk is a stretch reflex similar to the knee jerk reflex. A sharp downward tap on the chin when the mandible is held loosely in the rest position results in contraction of the masseter muscle to bring the teeth into occlusion. The pathway for this reflex is shown in Fig. 12.14. It is a monosynaptic reflex generated by stretching muscle spindles in the masseter muscle (and other elevator muscles) and it has the short latency of a monosynaptic reflex – some 7–12 ms. After the contraction of masseter muscle there is a so-called silent period during which no electromyographic signals can be detected from the muscle. This can be explained as an effect of spindle unloading. The reflex can be amplified by causing the subject to bite on an object between the teeth, and reduced by contracting the jaw depressor muscles to force against an upward pressure under the chin. Monitoring of depressor muscle activity shows that they relax during the jaw jerk; however, there is no depressor muscle equivalent to the jaw jerk because of the scarcity or absence of muscle spindles in the depressor muscles.

The jaw opening reflex

The jaw opening reflex occurs as a result of mechanical or electrical stimulation of the lips, oral mucosa or teeth (indirectly the periodontal ligament). In humans it manifests as an inhibition of activity in the mandibular elevators without simultaneous contraction of the depressors. A similar effect is seen when the teeth come into contact or when a hard particle stops

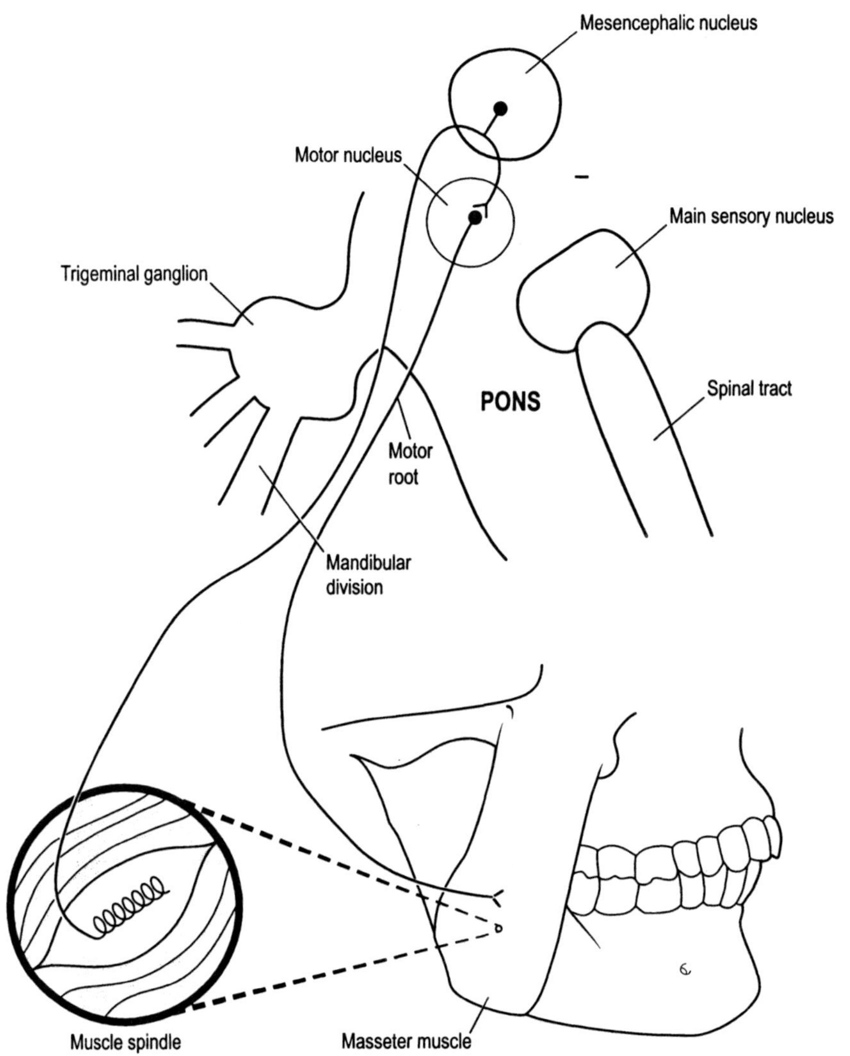

Fig. 12.14
The jaw jerk reflex or masseteric reflex. This is a monosynaptic stretch reflex.

mandibular movement. In animals other than man there is contraction of the depressor muscles.

The unloading reflex

The unloading reflex is important in the control of mastication. When there is a sudden reduction in the resistance of a food particle being chewed, the teeth are protected against the sudden occlusal load by an immediate halt in mandibular closure by a decrease in masseteric activity and a simultaneous increase in digastric activity. This is facilitated by the digastric activity already present during the power stroke (Fig. 12.7). The halt in masseter muscle activity is probably due to the sudden inactivation of the muscle spindles.

Swallowing

Swallowing is a complex group of reactions to move food onwards in the digestive tract while preserving the airway

The final stage in the mouth of transfer of food material onwards in the digestive system is the preparation of the bolus for swallowing and the swallowing process itself. Swallowing is a complex of reflex actions which are true reflexes; they are present in the foetus so are not a learned behaviour and they are present in all normal members of the species. The complicated nature of the swallowing act results from the dual function of the pharynx as part of the digestive tract and part of the route by which air passes in and out of the lungs. The reflex activities are therefore of two kinds: the major reflex of food transfer to the oesophagus must also involve reflex protection of the airways. A purely protective reflex which prevents access of possibly harmful material to either trachea or oesophagus is that of gagging or retching. This will be described later. When several possible reflexes may be stimulated they will be activated according to their priority in survival so that protective reflexes will always take precedence over others, and reflexes maintaining respiration will take precedence over those involved in food transfer. Such prioritising of reflexes takes place within the reticular system where the co-ordinating centres for these reflexes are situated. Although the term swallowing describes all modes of transport of material from the mouth to the oesophagus, there are differences between the process in the infant when suckling and, after weaning, in the way liquids and solids may be handled.

Suckling

In the infant, suckling is the earliest means of food transport

Suckling is a very primitive reflex which can be demonstrated as early as 20 weeks in utero but is not fully developed until just before birth. It provides a useful test of progress of premature babies for this reason. In breast feeding the baby pulls and sucks the nipple into the mouth. Part of the areola is also held in the mouth and so the nipple is held as far back as the junction of hard and soft palates. The tooth pads are not approximated – indeed they cannot be anteriorly if the nipple is between them. The whole of the lower jaw is raised and lowered alternately with a rocking motion. The tongue is protruded and remains in contact with the lower lip throughout. As the jaw is lowered the body of the tongue moves downwards and forwards. This produces a low or negative pressure in the oral cavity which facilitates the passage of milk from the nipple, although the oxytocin-induced milk let-down reflex triggered by touch receptors in and around the nipple is sufficient to give a flow of milk. The upward movement of the mandible with upward and backward movement of the body of the tongue increases pressure in the oral cavity and forces the contents into the upper part of the pharynx, initiating relaxation and then contraction of the pharyngeal constrictors. Mandibular position is held by the masseter muscle and the medial pterygoid muscles; the tongue movements are a combination of intrinsic muscle contraction to change the shape of the tongue with the geniohyoid and genioglossus muscles controlling its general position.

The airway is maintained during suckling.

Bottle feeding differs from suckling in that there is no let-down reflex and the child has to exert positive pressure on the teat with the tongue against the upper tooth pad. Backward movement of the body of the tongue can then squeeze the milk along and out of the teat.

In both suckling and bottle feeding the lips and the tooth pads are separated and the tongue can extend forwards to touch the lower lip. Once the teeth have erupted this situation is changed.

Sucking and drinking

Food transport for fluids to the oesophagus is achieved by sucking and drinking

It is possible to ingest fluids without any oral activity. If the head is tipped back so that the oral cavity and the oesophagus present a straight pathway, fluid may be poured down this. Sword swallowers and persons drinking a yard of ale make use of this anatomical disposition. The so-called cricopharyngeal sphincter at the upper end of the oesophagus is a functional rather than anatomical sphincter, and it normally relaxes in response to stimulation of the posterior pharyngeal wall except in the gagging reflex. Despite the absence of swallowing activity the tongue makes wave-like movements as if to assist the fluid passage.

More usually the ingestion of fluids proceeds in two stages: an accumulation of fluid in the anterior part of the oral cavity with the tongue hollowed at the tip but raised posteriorly, and then a raising of the tip of the tongue to touch the palate behind the upper incisors and a wave of contraction to bring the body of the tongue progressively back along the palate while the posterior portion drops down. The fluid may be taken into the mouth by sucking – pursing the lips to form a narrow opening, bringing the tip of the tongue over the lower incisors to touch the lower lip and then depressing the dorsum of the tongue to increase the volume of, and hence decrease the pressure in, the oral cavity. The posterior part of the tongue remains in light contact with the palate. A similar situation is seen when a drinking tube or straw is used, except that the lips are sealed round the tube. When the anterior chamber of the mouth holds an appropriate volume of fluid – somewhere between 5 and 20 ml, depending on the individual – the tongue movement to force it back and initiate the pharyngeal phase of swallowing begins. This part of the process is under voluntary control. The pharyngeal phase is broadly similar to the pharyngeal phase of swallowing the semisolid bolus produced by mastication to be described below, but for fluids it involves the sealing of the nasopharynx by raising the soft palate to contact the pharyngeal wall and the adenoidal pad. The larynx is raised and the fluid is deflected away from it by flowing on either side of the epiglottis. When the drinker is in an upright position the fluid can pass down the oesophagus under the influence of gravity, but even then there is contraction of the superior pharyngeal constrictor and initiation of peristaltic waves in the oesophagus. It is still possible to drink fluids standing on one's head – demonstrating that the transport process is an active one.

Drinking from a cup or other vessel modifies the above sequence only in that the fluid is part poured and part sucked into the anterior part of the oral cavity. Once the characteristic volume of fluid is in the mouth the vessel is moved away from the lips, and the lips and teeth can be brought together in the pattern of activity described below.

Swallowing of the food bolus

Swallowing of solid foods which have been converted into a bolus begins with an oral phase in which the bolus is transported towards the pharynx

The process of swallowing is described as having three phases – an oral phase, a pharyngeal phase and an oesophageal phase. The oral phase begins with bolus formation and ends as the bolus is passed back in the mouth. It lasts about 1 s and is voluntary in that it can be stopped or started voluntarily. The pharyngeal and oesophageal phases are entirely reflex; the pharyngeal phase lasts about 0.1 s.

Oral phase of swallowing

The oral phase itself consists of two phases: the moulding of the food and saliva into a ball or bolus, and the forcing of the bolus back in the mouth to contact the posterior pharyngeal wall and the palatoglossal arches.

When the oral receptors signal to the masticatory pattern generator that the particle size and consistency of the food is now suitable for swallowing, the rhythmic movement of the mandible is reduced and the food is gathered into a bolus by actions of the cheeks and tongue. Receptors in the cheeks are activated by contact with the food and send impulses via the mandibular nerve to the trigeminal spinal nucleus. Second-order neurones then pass to the trigeminal motor nucleus, adjusting activity of the muscles of mastication, and to the facial motor nucleus to send impulses via the gamma efferents to the intrafusal fibres of the muscle spindles of the buccinator muscles. This results in adjustment of the buccinator muscle activity. Sensory impulses from the tongue pass in the lingual branch of the mandibular nerve and the glossopharyngeal nerve to the hypoglossal motor nucleus which then sends motor signals to the muscle spindles and extrafusal fibres of the intrinsic muscles of the tongue. The bolus is finally formed in a hollow between the depressed dorsal surface of the tongue and the hard palate. The moulded bolus is now moved backwards in the oral cavity. In infants this is achieved by bringing the tip of the tongue up against the hard palate and producing a wave of contraction against the hard palate which carries the bolus back. In adults, larger and denser boluses have to be swallowed; the mouth is a much larger cavity and transport of the bolus requires greater forces. The pressure necessary to move the bolus can be generated most efficiently by bringing the teeth into centric occlusion and developing a lip seal by contraction of the orbicularis oris; if the tip of the tongue can thrust against the anterior teeth, a pressure of up to 10 kPa can be generated in the midline of the tongue. As the body of the tongue drops back from the palate and the pharyngeal musculature relaxes, a negative pressure is induced at the back of the mouth and the bolus moves down the pressure gradient. The forces between the teeth are said to be small, but with a voluntary forced swallow they may rise to as high as 300 N. The frequent act of swallowing saliva throughout the day brings the teeth into centric occlusion sufficiently often to stabilise the occlusal position; this is one of the factors that make it necessary to have a period of retention of a new occlusal position after orthodontic treatment. If the lip seal is inadequate to counter the forces exerted by the tongue against the teeth, protrusion of the teeth will occur. Similarly, in patients with a tooth-apart swallow, the orbicularis oris and buccinator muscles have to contract more forcibly to contain the pressures developed. The main muscle involved in generating the tongue pressure and in flattening the tongue against the hard palate is the mylohyoid muscle. During this stage of swallowing the hyoid bone moves upwards and the infrahyoid muscles have to contract to stabilise it and allow the mylohyoid muscle to generate force within the oral cavity.

Inflammation of the tongue from any cause may interfere with this phase of swallowing: such difficulties are referred to as oral dysphagias.

Pharyngeal phase

Stimulation of the posterior part of the oral cavity initiates the reflex stage of transport and the protective reflexes for the airway

Stimulation of the posterior part of the mouth and pharyngeal wall, but particularly the anterior pillars of the fauces (the palatoglossal arches) and the uvula, initiates the pharyngeal phase. It has also been suggested that when the bolus is particularly fluid it may flow round the tongue and stimulate the epiglottis. The nerve fibres carrying impulses as a result of these stimuli are in the glossopharyngeal nerve and the lesser palatine branches of the mandibular nerve, possibly also with some vagal fibres from the pharynx. Pressure in the pharynx rises as the bolus moves back to around 4 kPa; this is only about two-thirds of the mean pressure previously in the anterior chamber of the mouth because there is at first a loss of pressure into the nasopharynx. The afferent signals set in motion a pattern of activity preset within a swallowing centre in the reticular formation. This pattern of activity protects the airway and prevents diversion of the bolus away from the digestive tube. It lasts only about 100 ms but comprises several almost simultaneous responses. Respiration is inhibited – inspiration being most affected, although the inhibition of respiration may occur in any part of the respiratory cycle – and the airway is closed by approximation of both true and false vocal cords. The forward movement of the tongue during its elevation reveals a depression anterior to the epiglottis called the vallecula. In many animals this is an important storage site for food as it is passed back in the mouth; in humans its relatively small volume reduces its importance, but food reaching the vallecula spills over on either side of the epiglottis (the pyriform fossae) to be deflected away from the central laryngeal opening. Contraction of the stylopharyngeus, the salpopharyngeus and the palatopharyngeus muscles causes elevation of the larynx and pharynx and in so doing raises the epiglottis. During rapid sequences of swallowing the epiglottis remains in a raised position, but towards the end of a single swallow the thyrohyoid muscle contracts and the epiglottis falls back as a passive cap over the larynx. It is important to realise that throughout most of the pharyngeal phase of swallowing the protective function of the epiglottis is in the deflection of the food flow. The nasal cavity is sealed off from the mouth by elevation of the soft palate as a result of contraction of the tensor and levator palati muscles and by contraction of the superior constrictor to narrow the intervening space. In terms of neural activity, this is a complex group of actions: whilst the tensor palati is innervated by the trigeminal nerve, the levator palati receives motor fibres from the accessory nerve via the vagus and the pharyngeal plexus and the superior constrictor motor supply comes from the vagus and accessory nerves through the pharyngeal plexus.

Swallowing problems arise when the nasal cavity cannot be sealed off from the oropharynx: patients with palatal clefts and patients with paralysis of the soft palate such as may occur in myasthenia gravis can force food and liquids into the nasal cavity when trying to swallow.

Oesophageal phase

The superior constrictor conveys the bolus on to the oesophageal transporter

The cricopharyngeal muscle normally exhibits sufficient tone to prevent the ingress of air into the oesophagus during inspiration: stimulation of the posterior wall of the pharynx causes it to relax and the pressure in the oropharynx helps to move the bolus down into the oesophagus where the pressure is lower. A peristaltic wave begins with the sequential contraction of the superior constrictor of the pharynx, followed in turn by the middle and inferior constrictors and then by the striated muscle in the upper third of the oesophagus. The process is controlled at first by the vagus nerve carrying fibres from the nucleus ambiguus, but once food enters the oesophagus local receptors are stimulated and modify the pattern of muscular activity. Swallowing of liquids when the body is in an upright posture does not lead to oesophageal peristalsis as gravity is sufficient to allow their passage; the drier the bolus the harder it is to swallow and the more oesophageal activity is required to transport it. As the bolus or fluid enters the oesophagus respiration is re-established with an inspiration. The waves of contraction reach down to the smooth muscle of the lower third of the oesophagus and continue under control of the myenteric plexus supplied by the vagus nerve. Between food intakes the oesophagus is normally relaxed, except for a sphincter-like lower zone preventing reflux of the gastric contents. Relaxation of this zone allows the bolus to pass into the stomach which also undergoes a reflex relaxation (the so-called receptive relaxation). As the bolus reaches the stomach the sphincteric zone contracts again. The oesophageal phase takes a few seconds to complete.

Frequency and volume of swallows

Only one-quarter of the average 600 swallows a day relate to food ingestion; the remainder are to swallow saliva

Although a typical subject has been observed to swallow around 600 times in 24 h, only about a quarter of the swallowing actions occur during food ingestion. The remainder are necessary to swallow the saliva which is constantly being secreted by the unstimulated submandibular, sublingual and accessory glands; during sleep when salivary flow diminishes the swallowing frequency drops to about 6 an hour. The volume of a swallow in drinking, and probably in bolus transport, varies from 5 ml in a small child to 10–14 ml in women and 15–20 ml in men. This gives a useful indication of the volume that is appropriate for mouthwashes. When saliva is being swallowed the volume is much less, and there is evidence that accumulation of less than 5 ml of saliva in the mouth triggers a swallowing reflex.

As swallowing is such a frequent activity it plays an important role in maintaining or altering the position of the teeth. Patients with a tooth-apart swallow will exert a different balance of forces particularly on the anterior teeth because the tongue thrust to raise intraoral pressure is then against the cheeks and lips. The orbicularis oris has to contract vigorously but is less powerful than the tongue, and the upper incisors incline forward to a zone where the forces are balanced. The tooth-apart swallow is often seen in subjects who have had an extended thumb- or finger-sucking habit.

Gagging or retching

Irritation or noxious stimulation of the posterior of the oral cavity results in the gagging or retching response which transports the irritant away from the pharyngeal area

When the posterior part of the mouth is stimulated, a swallowing pattern of reflexes is set up. In some circumstances irritation or noxious stimulation can actually lead to a vomiting reflex. However, if the swallowing reflex pattern is inhibited, the mouth is held open, the cricopharyngeal sphincter and the nasopharynx are closed and attempts are made to expel the stimulating material from the mouth by movements of the tongue which start at the back of the mouth and move forward. This is termed gagging or retching. The materials used in taking impressions for denture construction, particularly in the upper jaw, can stimulate the back of the mouth and cause a gagging reflex. Very sensitive patients may require anaesthesia of the oral mucosa before denture impressions can be taken. The retching reaction is the first stage of reflex protection of the digestive tube; it gives way to the more powerful protective reflex pattern of vomiting if the irritant material cannot be removed by retching.

Further reading

Craniomandibular Muscles: Their Role in Form and Function. Miller, A.J. CRC Press, Boca Raton, 1991

Occlusion: Principles and Assessment. Klineberg, I. Butterworth Heinemann (Wright), Oxford, 1991

Occlusion, 2nd edition. Thomson, H. Butterworth Heinemann (Wright), London, 1990

Mastication and Swallowing: An Overview. Thexton, A.J. British Dental Journal 173: 197–206; 1992

Deglutition. Miller, A.J. Physiological Reviews 62: 129–184; 1982

13 Speech

Although the oral cavity is in continuity with nose and upper airways, it is not habitually used for breathing in most individuals. It can be used to increase air intake when nasal flow is insufficient, although the mouth lacks the protective hairs and cilia of the nose and has a very different secretion pattern. However, the mouth can control and modify air flow through itself and this provides the means of altering expiration of air to produce a variety of sounds which can then be used for communication between individuals.

The generation of sound frequencies

Speech is produced by modifying the expiration of air. The tension and separation of the vocal cords allows them to impart a vibration to the air passing between them

Sound results when molecules vibrate longitudinally and rhythmically in a direction radial to the vibrating source. This produces alternate increase and decrease of pressure at a receiver such as the human ear or a microphone: the frequency of the pressure changes gives the pitch of the sound and the amplitude of forward and backward movement gives its pressure change or loudness. A graph of pressure changes against time has a sinusoidal form and so the sequence of pressure changes induced by the vibrating source is termed a sound wave. In humans sounds of a carefully controlled kind are produced as a means of communication. Such sounds are known as speech: the ability of human beings to work together and to advance their experience and knowledge has only been possible because of the development of a precise means of communication in speech and the further elaboration of that into written symbols which can endure for long periods of time and can be decoded by others. The production of intelligible speech sounds is a modification of expiration by forcing the outflowing air through a narrow gap bounded by structures of variable and controllable elasticity. These structures are the vocal cords (Figs 13.1–13.3). They are caused to vibrate, and hence to impart vibration to the air passing through them, by their own elastic resistance to the airflow (myoelastic theory), or by the combination of movement and recoil induced in them by the vortices generated on the side away from flow as the airflow adjusts to the wider pipe it reaches on the side of the cords (aerodynamic theory). The airflow is actually partially occluded by the vocal flaps and it is the thickened edges of these which form the vocal cords. The vocal folds are made up of fibroelastic connective tissue and contain two muscles, the lateral crico-arytenoid and thyro-arytenoid (Fig. 13.3).

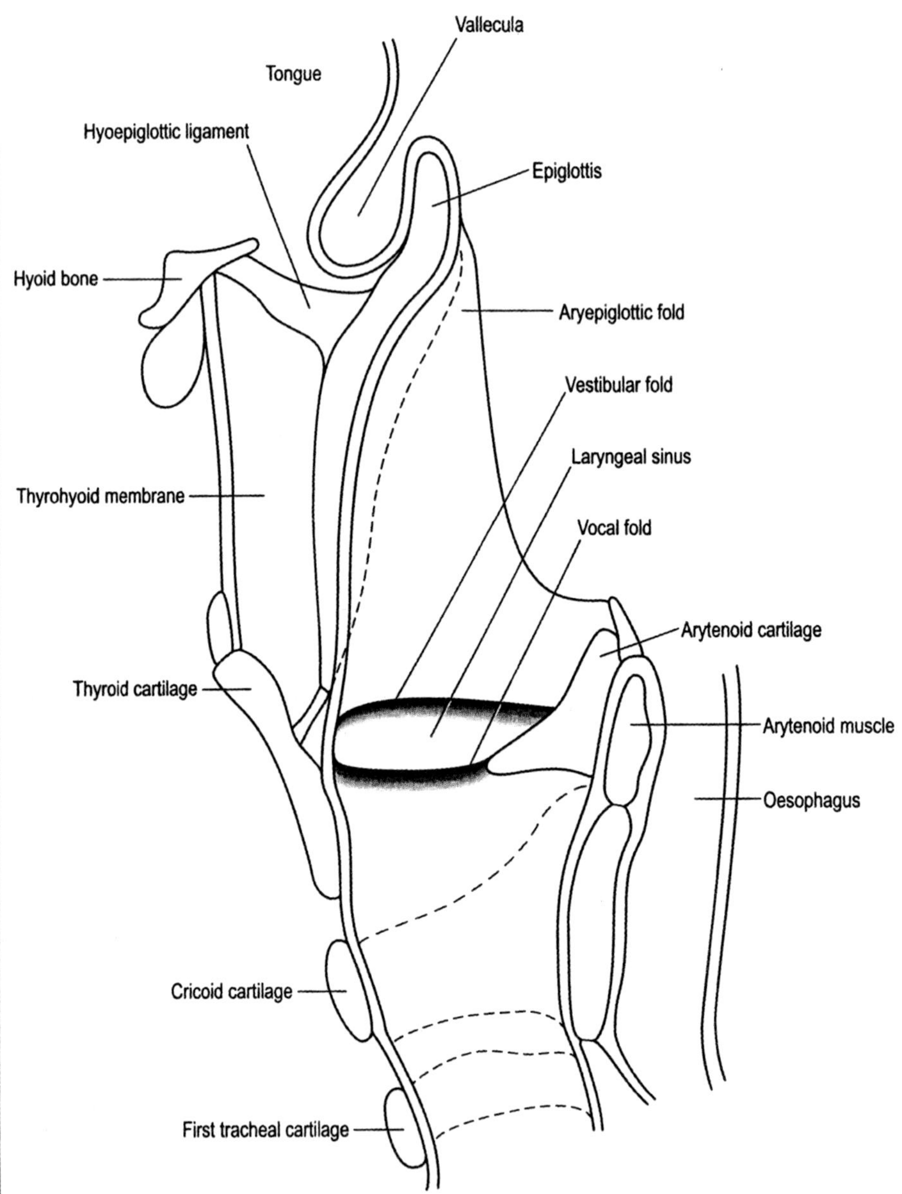

The anatomy of the larynx to show the position of the vocal ligaments or folds (or vocal cords) and the vestibular folds or false cords.

A strand of this latter lies near the thickened edge and has an important role in controlling the tension of the cord; it is sometimes termed the vocalis muscle. The cords themselves are largely elastic tissue. In normal respiration the vocal folds give very little restriction to airflow: the triangular space between them -

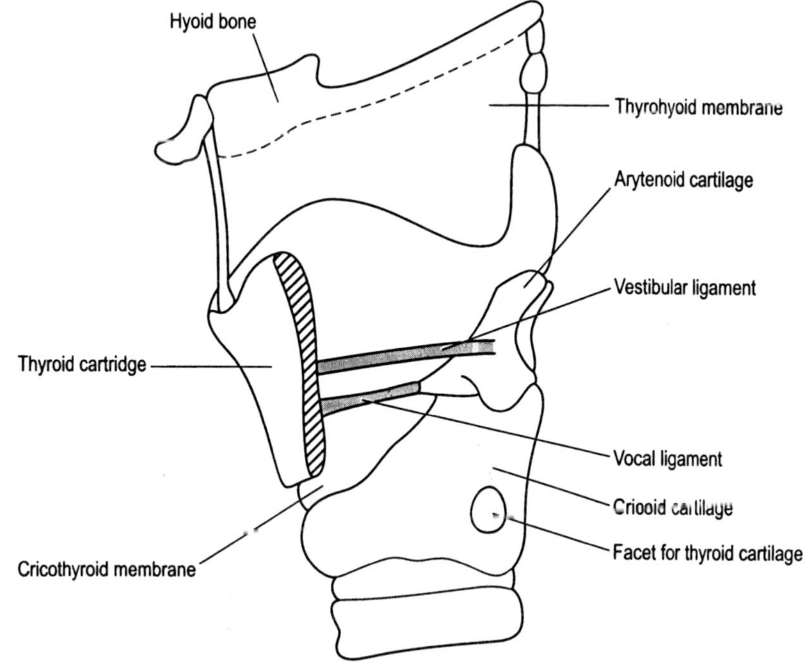

Fig. 13.2
The cartilages and ligaments of the larynx.

the rima glottidis – is sufficiently wide to allow air to pass easily. As part of a general pattern of reflex activity, as for example, in swallowing or vomiting, the lateral crico-arytenoid muscles and the thyro-arytenoid muscles cause the cricoid cartilages to rotate and their anterior arms to move together; simultaneously the transverse and oblique arytenoid muscles move the pivot points of the cartilages together. This combination of activities closes the glottis and stops air flow, protecting the respiratory tract. In order to generate sounds the glottis must be closed but only to such a degree that it can be forced open by the airflow. A tightly closed glottis is associated with louder sounds because a greater air pressure is needed to open it: when the cords are only lightly approximated the expiratory pressure can be small and the sound quiet. In whispering only the anterior part of the rima is closed and the cords are separated posteriorly. The pitch or frequency of the sounds is controlled by thelength and tension of the vibrating cords and to some extent by their thickness and shape. Whilst closing the cords together induces tension in them, the tension can be increased by moving the cartilaginous insertions of the muscles farther apart. Thus the thyroid cartilage can be held in position by the infrahyoid muscles, and the position of the arytenoid cartilages depends upon the contraction of the cricothyroid and posterior crico-arytenoid muscles (Fig. 13.3). The position of the cricoid cartilage itself is governed mainly by the cricothyroid muscle which pulls it upward but whose posterior fibres pull the cartilage backwards. Because of their elasticity, relaxation of muscles tensing the cords is sufficient to reduce

Loudness is controlled by airflow

The initial mix of frequencies is given by the length and tension of the vocal folds or cords

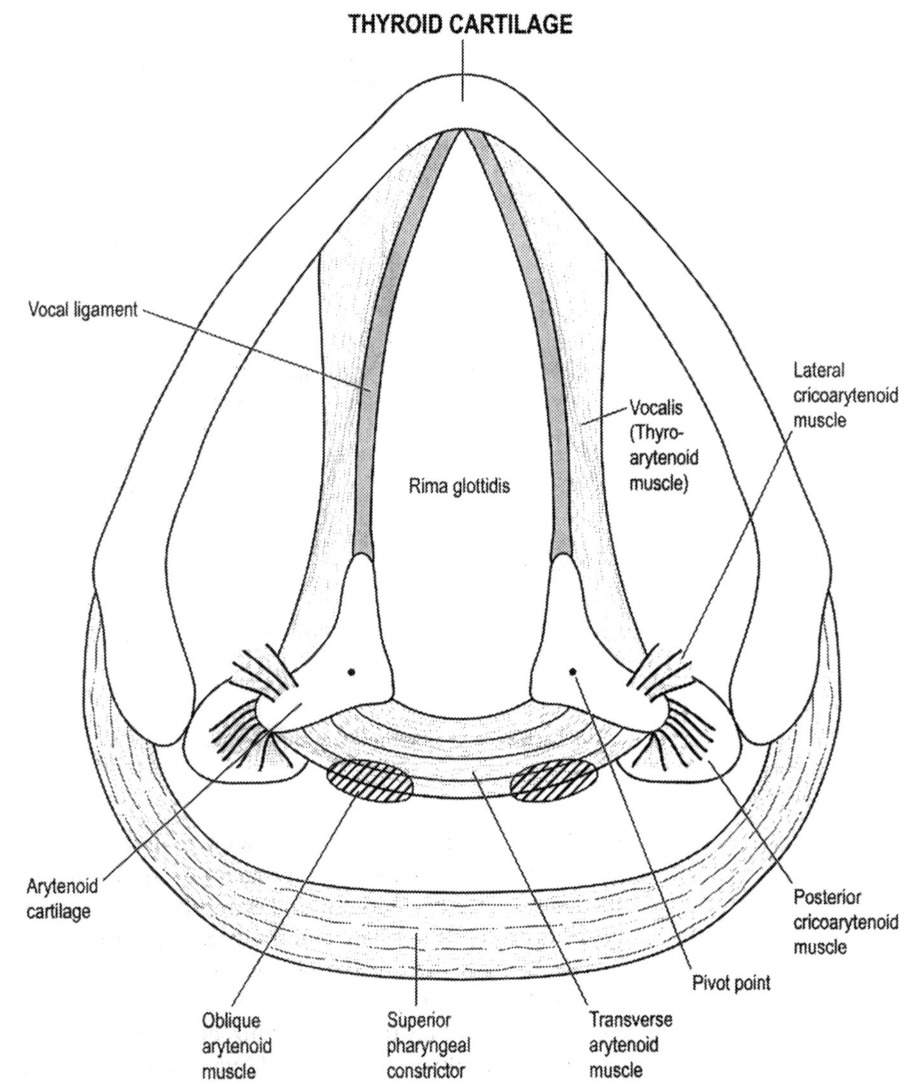

The vocal ligaments (vocal folds or vocal cords), their attachments and associated cartilages and muscles.

their tension. A further mechanism for altering the characteristics of the vocal cords is thought to be provided by the false cords, a second pair of folds which lie above the true cords. If they touch the vocal cords they effectively shorten their effective vibrating length and thus enable a higher sound frequency to be attained. The false cords contain mucus-secreting cells and may also be necessary to lubricate the cords themselves. The frequency of vibrations of the cords can be adjusted at low frequencies simply by altering tension in the cords in their resting approximated condition and by altering their thickness

Control is exerted by Broca's area in the cerebral cortex, although impulses to the muscles are generated in the motor cortex

or cross-sectional shape. As the frequency to be produced becomes higher, the cords are first stretched by tilting the thyroid and cricoid cartilages, and then their tension is increased by muscle contraction without change in length, and finally the false cords shorten the vibrating length. Increase in airflow – which increases loudness – also tends to increase the frequency of the sound.

The neural control of the sound frequencies generated at the cords is via the vagus nerve, principally through the recurrent laryngeal nerve. The only muscle involved in vocalisation not innervated by the recurrent laryngeal is the cricothyroid muscle which is innervated by the external laryngeal nerve.

The ultimate control of vocalisation, however, is from the cerebral cortex, in an area just anterior to the motor cortex, immediately above the Sylvian fissure. This is Broca's area (Fig. 13.4), and it controls actual word formation and the necessary adjustments to respiration by activating appropriate muscle signals in the motor cortex. Broca's area in turn is under the control of Wernicke's area in the superior temporal gyrus to which it is linked by the arcuate fasciculus. Wernicke's area is concerned both with the understanding of language – spoken or written – and with the generation of intelligible speech. Thus, lesions of Wernicke's area or of the connecting fasciculus result in a condition termed fluent aphasia, in which the patient can generate a mixture of recognisable and nonsense words which do not link together into intelligible speech. Lesions of Broca's area result in errors of articulation. Speech production is controlled from the categorical hemisphere; lesions on the representational side have no effect on speech.

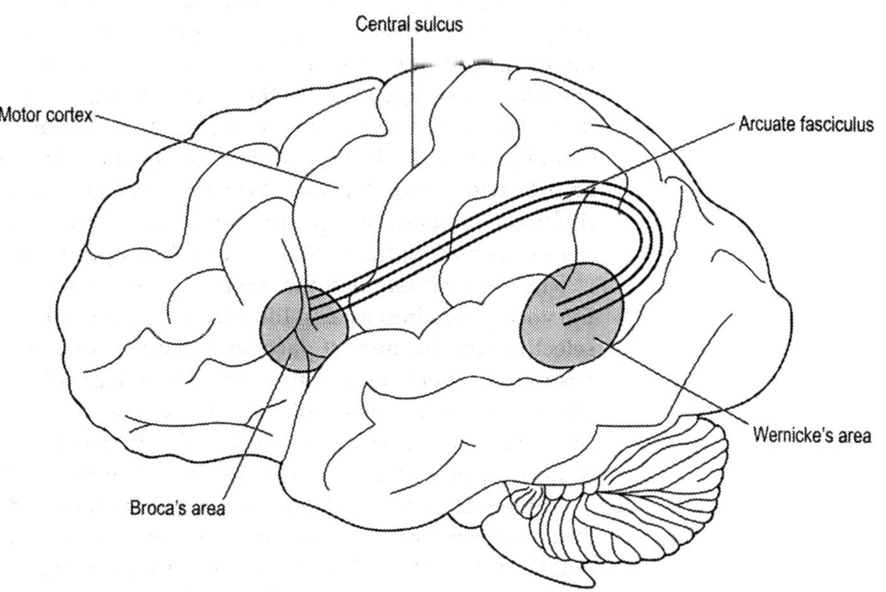

Fig. 13.4
The location of brain areas involved in the production of speech sounds.

The length of the vocal cords dictates the lowest frequency possible for an individual. Women reach puberty earlier and have shorter cords and hence higher voice frequencies

Although it might be assumed from the above that production of speech sounds depends solely upon control of expiration (and inspiration, of course), the process of sound production at the vocal cords merely generates a mixture of sound frequencies and it is the subsequent modification of this mixture by stoppage or airflow and amplification of certain frequencies that turns sound into speech. These modifications are made to the greatest effect by muscular activity in and around the mouth.

The mixture of sound frequencies will consist of one or more basic frequencies directly related to the length and tension of the cords and a number of harmonics of these. The later puberty of the male gives more time for growth of the laryngeal cartilages and as a result the vocal cords of the male double in length to about 15 mm during the pubertal growth spurt. This drops the male voice frequency by approximately an octave in comparison with the two to three tone drop in the female voice frequency during puberty as the cords grow from around 7–8 mm to around 11 mm. In normal speech, therefore, the male voice uses frequencies between 100 and 150 Hz and the female voice the higher frequency of 200–300 Hz. The human ear is highly sensitive to sound at these frequencies although its greatest sensitivity is in the range 1000–4000 Hz. Singers can be trained to produce notes as low as 50 Hz easily, but 27 Hz is now considered the lower limit and the former upper limit of just over 2000 Hz has been extended another octave up to 4000 Hz! Loudness of the sound depends primarily on the force of expiration; measurement of the loudness achieved by shouting gives figures up to 110 dB.

Control of sound production is adjusted by the sounds heard by bony conduction

The control of the muscles in and around the vocal cords is very precise in order to achieve changes of length of around 1 μm for each step change in frequency. This level of control is exerted first by matching the muscle forces to some internal standard of frequency – a standard highly developed in singers described as having perfect pitch – and then by the usual controls of muscle activity, the muscle spindles and joint receptors. There is a simultaneous comparison of the sound intended with that produced and then heard by the ears to give the final tuning. A complication here is that the sound produced is heard by bony conduction, whereas in the matching with an externally generated sound the latter is heard by airborne conduction. This difference explains why people find it difficult to recognise their own recorded voices even when the quality of recording approaches perfection.

The mixture of frequencies is modified by resonating chambers to give the vowel sounds and by stoppage of airflow to give consonants

The transformation of the mixture of frequencies generated by airflow past the vocal cords into intelligible speech is achieved by two processes: the selective amplification of particular frequencies by variation of the size of resonating chambers, and the controlled release of the expired air. The term phonation is used to describe the production and selection of frequencies, and the term articulation is used to describe the patterning of the air release. Some writers include frequency selection in articulation rather than in phonation.

Frequencies are selected by the use of Helmholtz resonators. In a tube, frequencies whose wavelength is the same as the length of the tube, or the length of the tube divided by a whole number, are transmitted but other frequencies are suppressed. This arrangement is a pipe resonator. In the airways there are a number of pipe resonators: the larynx, the pharynx and the nose can be considered as such (Fig. 13.5). They give an individual the characteristic voice sound and when they are blocked or damaged that

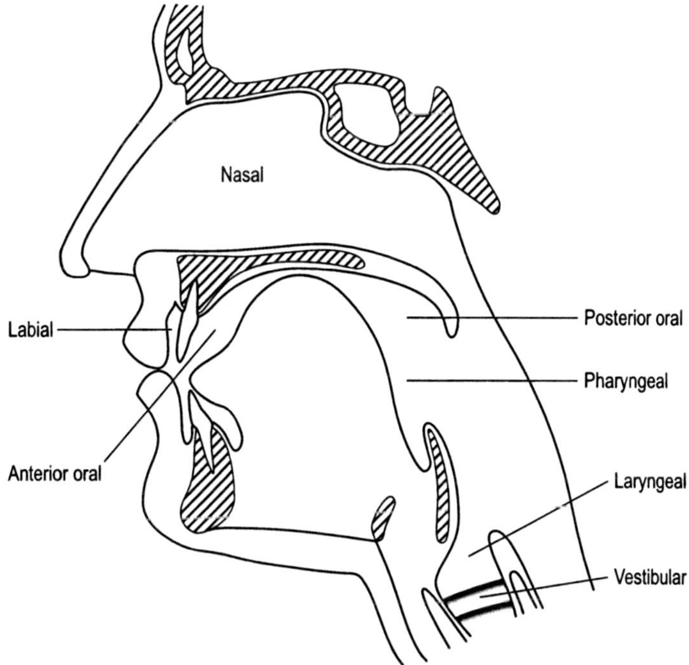

Fig. 13.5
The vocal resonators. The resonator chamber labelled as vestibular is more properly termed as that of the laryngeal sinus since the term vestibule is usually given to the chamber labelled here as laryngeal. Note how the tongue can be raised to provide anterior and posterior oral chambers. However, it can also be held in a low position for the so-called back vowels.

recognisable voice will be altered. Upper respiratory tract infections like the common cold, and abnormalities of the pipe such as a cleft palate giving communication between the oral and nasal cavities, will produce predictable changes in the sound of the voice. A Helmholtz resonator is a box with an opening for air entry and a narrow exit opening. The volume of the box defines the frequencies which will be retained and amplified. The different parts of the sound production pathway can all function as resonators of this kind but only a few of them are adjustable to give speech sounds rather than voice sounds. Thus the vestibular resonator between the true and false vocal cords, the laryngeal and pharyngeal resonators are relatively fixed in form. The nasal and paranasal sinus resonators are similarly fixed in form but variation in sound can be achieved according to whether they are used or not: if air is directed only through the mouth these resonators are not used. The labial or vestibular resonator between lips and teeth is relatively unimportant, but the oral resonator itself is the main site at which frequency selection for speech production takes place. This is because the oral resonator is readily divided into two resonators – the anterior and posterior – which are separated by the tongue. The position of the tongue in relation to the palate can be varied and thus the relative sizes of the these two resonating chambers can also be varied (Fig. 13.5). The two frequencies selected in this way are known as format frequencies and they give the characteristic sound of vowels.

Vowel sounds

All vowel sounds are composed of two formant frequencies produced by the chambers anterior and posterior to the raised dorsum of the tongue

It is perhaps an oversimplification to define the anterior and posterior oral resonators as being entirely within the oral cavity with the dental arch as a boundary, because the separation of the teeth enables the labial resonator to be added to the anterior and the posterior is in fact continuous with the pharyngeal resonator. In the English language, as in many others, the soft palate seals off the nasal cavity during vowel production, but in French the nasal cavity remains in communication with the pharynx for certain vowel sounds. This again changes the volume of the posterior chamber. The two main formant frequencies for a vowel are a lower frequency amplified by the posterior chamber and a higher frequency amplified by the anterior chamber (Table 13.1). A third formant frequency has been described for vowel sounds but this is relatively constant for most sounds in the English language. As the tongue is rolled forward from the back to the front of the mouth the separation between the two main formant frequencies increases. Thus the tongue towards the back of the mouth gives a posterior frequency of around 750 Hz and an anterior frequency of around 1850 Hz to produce a short 'a' sound, whilst with the tongue further forward a posterior frequency of around 400 Hz and an anterior of 2300 Hz produce a short 'i' sound. The size of the slit between tongue and palate gives differing qualities to the vowels: they are described as closed when the slit is narrow, and open when the slit is wide. Addition of the vestibular chamber to the anterior oral chamber lowers the anterior oral frequency and introduces a further possibility of variation.

Clicks and consonants

The second means by which sound is converted into speech is by controlling the release of the vibrating air column. Bringing together oral structures and then separating them can produce sounds without obvious phonation: the

Table 13.1
Formant frequencies (in Hz) of some vowel sounds in which anterior and posterior oral chambers are varied by moving the tongue progressively back in the mouth

	Heed	Hid	Head	Had	Hod
Anterior chamber frequency					
in males	2290	1990	1840	1720	1090
in females	2790	2480	2330	2050	1220
Prosterior chamber frequency					
in males	270	390	530	660	730
in females	310	430	610	860	850

Table 13.2
Classification of consonants by site of articulation and manner of air release

	Complete followed by release impedance	Partial stoppage in mouth, escape through nose	Partial release of airflow			
	Plosive	Nasal	Lateral	Trill/roll	Fricative	Affricative
Bilabial	p b	m			w	
Labiodental					v f	
Interdental					that thin	
Alveolar	d t	n			z s	
Prepalatal				r	v sh	j ch
Palatal			l		y	
Velar	g k	ng				
Glottal					h (aspirate)	

These sounds are indicated by the letters normally used in British or American words: the international phonetic symbols are broadly similar to these, but the letter–sound combinations are different in some other European languages – a written 's', for example, is often equivalent to the British 'sh' sound.

Consonants are produced by stopping airflow; the site and manner of stoppage give the characteristics of the sound. Thus consonants can be classified either according to the structures involved in the airflow stoppage or according to the completeness of the stoppage

action known as lip-smacking and the sound of a kiss are obvious examples involving the lips. The tongue can be used to produce clicks; these sounds, which are a non-verbal form of communication in Britain, constitute part of the speech pattern in many African countries. This kind of sound results when the articulating structures are held together and then separated over a small area to create a low pressure in that zone; the airflow into that zone when the structures are separated gives the click. However, the initiation, ending and separation of vowel sounds by stopping airflow constitute the sounds described as consonants. The consonants can be classified in two ways: by the anatomical position at which airflow is impeded, and by the degree of impedance – complete or partial. These two classifications are set out in Table 13.2. The anatomical classification is the easier to appreciate: clearly a bilabial consonant is produced by the bringing together of upper and lower lip, and labiodental, linguodental and linguopalatal are self-explanatory. However, the linguopalatal group can be further subdivided by defining the specific area of the palate involved and so the terms alveolar, prepalatal, (medio)palatal, velar and glottal are used to indicate progressively, the posterior position of the tongue stop. Although only the aspirate 'h' has been included as a glottal sound, there is also the glottal stop which substitutes for a 't' or even a 'd' in some regional speech forms and in much careless rapid speech: the northern part of the British mainland is frequently referred to as Sco'land and its inhabitants as Sco'ish.

When airflow is stopped completely and then released, with the nasal cavity sealed, a plosive sound results. Oral stoppage without the sealing of the nasal cavity results in the air leaving through the latter as a nasal sound. Thus 'b' and 'm' are both bilabials, but one is plosive and the other nasal. Both these sounds begin with the jaws slightly separated in the rest position of the mandible and are sometimes used by the dental prosthetist to estimate the rest position. The terms rolled and lateral indicate incomplete stoppage of airflow, the former by vibration of the tongue against the palate and the latter by holding the tongue towards the midline and allowing air to escape on either side. Incomplete closure, leaving a slit or rounded opening, gives the type of sound termed fricative, and the combination of this with a sudden release like that in a plosive gives an affricative sound.

Variation in the volume of airflow gives different consonantal sounds: less airflow gives a softer sound as in 'd' as opposed to 't', and 'b' as opposed to 'p'. This distinction is sometimes referred to as the difference between voiced and unvoiced consonants because the strong sounds can be produced in the absence of vocal cord vibration (unvoiced) whilst the weaker sounds are always associated with vibration of the vocal cords (voiced). The difference between the two forms of 'th' in Table 13.2 is easy to appreciate from the example words, but the 'wh' sound in English has now almost completely fallen out of use. Most people now would not distinguish between 'weather' and 'whether', although the latter should be pronounced more like 'hwether'.

Influence of malocclusion and dental procedures on speech sounds

Variations in oral structures or the position of the teeth will result in characteristic and predictable differences in speech sounds

Speech changes as a result of malocclusions or dental procedures. Any alteration in the volume of the oral and nasal resonators, or in the position or size of structures involved in impeding airflow during articulation, will affect the quality of speech. Thus, characteristic differences in timbre will be associated with high and low palatal vaults and with tongues which are large or small in relation to the size of the oral cavity. Similarly a cleft palate alters the size and shape of the oral resonator, whilst obstruction of the nasal airway by hypertrophy of the lymphoid tissues at the entrance to the pharynx reduces the size of the posterior oral resonator and reduces airflow in the nasal sounds. The reverse effect is produced when there is a deficiency in the palatal musculature or when it is functionally abnormal as in the neurotransmission defect of myaesthenia gravis. All these factors which affect the size and shape of resonating chambers may affect vowel sounds as well as the overall frequency spectrum which identifies a particular person's voice. Specific changes in consonantal sounds will be produced when the upper lip is short or a lip seal cannot be achieved, when the upper incisors are missing, malpositioned or in an abnormal occlusal relationship with the lower incisors (i.e. in other than an Angle class 1 relationship), or when tongue-to-palate contact is difficult to achieve. Thus the letters most consistently abnormal will be the bilabials, the labiodentals and the linguo-alveolar or linguo-prepalatal. Lisps may arise from almost any condition where the upper incisors are displaced or absent and where the tongue–palate relationships are changed or abnormal. An Angle's class 2 relationship, commonly inherited in the English aristocracy, is a good example of a condition predisposing to a lisp. The fitting of a denture or an orthodontic appliance often results in changes in 's' and both the 'th' sounds. Indeed, some upper dentures induce a whistle every time

Dentures and orthodontic appliances can affect the sound of speech

the wearer speaks. Adjusting the thickness of the baseplate or slightly moving the incisors may eliminate this.

Further reading

Phonetics for Speech Pathology, 2nd edition. Ball, M.J. Whurr Publishers, London, 1993

14 The ageing mouth

The general concept of ageing

If the term ageing is interpreted strictly it should refer to all the changes which occur in the body at least between birth and death and possibly from conception onwards. However, it is usual to consider age changes as those which are evident in later life, although whether that means after age 50 years, or 60 years, or 70 years, is not always defined. It is clear that most of the changes considered as age changes are slow and progressive and may be initiated relatively early in life. It is salutary to realise that the earliest signs of atherosclerosis of blood vessels – a condition usually associated with ageing – has been observed in blood vessels of the tongue in subjects below the age of 10 years.

Many of the biochemical and tissue morphology changes are observed in normal healthy individuals, but as people age they accumulate a history of past disease and most older people are receiving some kind of medication on an intermittent or continuing basis. It may be difficult to dissociate the changes due to ageing per se and the changes due to disease or pharmacological intervention. This is particularly true of changes in function as opposed to changes in tissue morphology. There are a number of studies of small groups of healthy subjects in older age groups which are attempting to look at what might be defined as normal age changes and some linear studies which are following healthy individuals over a continuing period of years. Both of the main American studies include oral and dental observations.

The study of ageing includes not only the observation of changes in healthy subjects as they grow older, but also investigations as to the mechanisms or causes of ageing. There are currently several theories to explain the phenomenon. It is possible that the genetic programme is one of ageing as well as growth. In crudely evolutionary terms the biological aim of an individual is to pass on genetic material to continue the survival of the species and there is no further need for that individual beyond the peak reproductive years or after reproduction has taken place and the offspring reared.

A less teleological view is that the genetic material suffers a continuing slight degradation. Up to a point the genes can be repaired and transcription

Ageing may be due to degradation of genetic material or accumulation of superoxide damage

errors corrected, but as errors accumulate this becomes progressively more difficult. The causes of deterioration of the genetic material may be the continuing bombardment of the body with radiation of different kinds or the accumulation in the body of free radicals (superoxides) with their powerful oxidative effects.

The age changes in the mouth and the dental tissues will mirror those in the body as a whole and so it is appropriate to summarise what is known of whole body changes before considering specifically the oral and dental tissues and functions.

Ageing changes in the body as a whole

Genetic material may deteriorate with ageing

At a molecular level there is a slowing of the rate of protein synthesis and the appearance of structurally altered proteins. Changes in the rate of protein synthesis appear to be due to changes in gene regulation and/or in the nucleoproteins rather than changes in the genes themselves as far as transcription is concerned, and changes in tRNA and mRNA as far as translation is concerned. Alterations to proteins seem to occur posttranslationally by modifications of size, charge, or conformation to correctly synthesised proteins. It is also possible that proteins may survive longer and undergo modification with time when the rate of replacement is reduced.

Collagen is an important protein whose ageing has effects on a number of tissues. This is particularly important in blood vessels because this affects the blood supply to tissues

Collagen, the main component of connective tissues, provides a specific example of a protein which changes during ageing. The turnover of collagen is slow in comparison with that of many other proteins. As it matures the degree of cross-linking increases and the tensile strength of the molecule improves. There is, however, an associated increase in stiffness. Oxidation of epsilon amino groups of lysyl and hydroxylysyl residues yields aldimine and keto cross-links near the ends of the collagen molecules. As the molecules mature these are replaced by more stable links such as pyridinoline. The amount of this cross-link increases up the end of puberty. Later other cross-links are formed more slowly by non-enzymatic reactions. One of these has been identified as histidinoalanine, formed between histidine in one peptide chain and serine or cysteine residues in a neighbouring chain.

Hormone secretion is reduced and immunological reactions are slower and less effective

At a tissue level other changes may occur. Calcified tissues which undergo turnover or apposition throughout life show varying reactions: tending to accumulate calcium and become thicker or more brittle in some areas whilst losing calcium in others and developing porosity. Although it is said that hormone secretion is reduced as subjects age, there is little evidence for this except in the special case of the sex hormones. Immunological reactions are slower and less effective in older persons and wound healing is often delayed. There is increased deposition of lipid material in the walls of blood vessels and this may calcify as time progresses. How far this should be regarded as pathological before it significantly affects the blood supply to tissues is debatable. At a tissue and organ level, the above changes will produce consequential changes in function.

Effects of ageing in relation to the mouth

Hard tissues

Enamel

Enamel is worn down with use

Enamel does not undergo any further deposition after it has been laid down by the ameloblasts. Its surface can, however, be modified grossly by abrasion, attrition, erosion or dental caries, and at a crystal level by ion exchange, demineralisation and remineralisation. Attrition – the normal wear of the tooth surface occurring during mastication of hard foods – causes loss of enamel from the occluding surfaces of teeth to produce polished facets of enamel, and then, when enamel is worn through, exposure of dentine. It is usual for the deposition of dentine to keep pace with the occlusal wear but pulpal exposure can occur if this fails. Assessment of occlusal wear is an important measure of age in forensic odontology. Lateral movement of the teeth may also cause production of facets in the interdental areas. The chemical composition of the surface enamel in the worn areas remains similar to that of the deeper layer which it originally was: its fluoride content, for example, is less than that of surface enamel. If no further wear occurs the new surface of enamel is subject to ionic exchange with its environment in the same way as the original surface. When a tooth erupts into the mouth it has a surface layer which is higher in fluoride concentration than are deeper layers. As the tooth ages it takes up fluoride from saliva or ingested water and foodstuffs so that the surface layer should steadily increase in fluoride concentration. However, surface enamel is lost by erosion, attrition and abrasion so that the actual enamel surface in an older individual may no longer be high in fluoride concentration. Other ions exchange with the surface apatite so that concentration gradients are produced through the enamel. In older people enamel becomes darker in colour and may become more liable to cracking. The colour changes may be due to progressive staining (although no obvious chemical differences have been detected which might explain the colour), or to some physical change in enamel rendering the underlying dentine more visible. One explanation of the tendency to crack has been that the outer layers of dentine may lose some water and shrink away from the enamel so that it loses its support. The most significant experimental observation on older enamel is that it is less permeable to dyes and radioactive isotopes than at an earlier stage. This suggests changes in composition in both the mineral and organic components of enamel. It is possible that some small increase in calcification occurs during ageing; this would explain the loss of permeability, and possibly make the enamel more translucent and also more brittle. Small increases in the degree of calcification would be difficult to detect in such a highly calcified tissue.

Dentine

Dentine differs from enamel in that it is can be formed continuously throughout life. As it is penetrated by the dentinal tubules which may contain cell processes or dentinal fluid, the whole thickness of dentine is in communication with fluids within the body until such time as those tubules may be obliterated.

Dentine can increase in thickness and in its degree of calcification as it ages

In the circumpulpar dentine the collagen fibres of the matrix are arranged in layers which are at right-angles to the odontoblast layer which has laid them down. This contrasts with the thin layer of mantle dentine immediately next to enamel where the fibre directions are parallel with the tubules, and with the hyaline layer next to the cementum where a similar situation exists. Regular secondary dentine is a continuation of the circumpulpar dentine which is laid down throughout life. It is usually demarcated from the circumpulpar dentine by an accentuated incremental line where a change in direction of the dentinal tubules occurs. With attrition the appearance of dentine becomes modified. Stimulation of the odontoblasts results in the rapid laying down of a layer of dentine in which the matrix fibres are much more randomly oriented and the arrangement of the tubules is disturbed. Such dentine is termed irregular secondary dentine. A second reaction, again probably mediated through stimulation of the odontoblasts, is the formation of sclerotic dentine in tubules exposed in the area of attrition. As dentine ages there is deposition of a layer of more highly calcified material on walls of the tubules. This material appears finely granular, contains collagen fibrils only as inclusions, and may be amorphous calcium phosphate rather than apatite. It is known as peritubular dentine. In sclerotic dentine the tubules are completely occluded by the further deposition of calcified material, similar in appearance to the peritubular, although it has been identified as mainly apatite. Sclerotic dentine appears translucent when viewed in ground sections in water.

The appearance of sclerotic dentine is related to attrition (or may result from dental caries) but another type of translucent dentine is produced in the normal course of ageing of dentine (Fig. 14.1). It is again produced by the deposition of apatite into the dentinal tubules, the process in this instance beginning in the root and progressing coronally. The extent of the translucent area is directly related to the age of the tooth and hence can be used as a guide to age in forensic dentistry.

The slower formation of dentine throughout life allows it to incorporate fluoride from the plasma via the pulpal tissue fluid to a greater extent. Hence the pulpal surface of dentine shows the highest concentrations of fluoride and these usually exceed those in surface enamel in older subjects (Fig. 10.4).

Cementum

Cementum is laid down throughout life. As it ages it becomes less permeable

Cementum is laid down throughout life and shows incremental growth lines which can help in determining the age of the individual from whom the tooth was removed. With age the tissue becomes less permeable to dye molecules and ions. This may explain why the deeper layers of cementum do not have viable cementocytes in them: nutritive molecules may not be able to reach them. Like dentine, cementum continues to take up fluoride where its thickness increases slowly throughout life, and relatively high concentrations may therefore be present at the surface adjacent to the periodontal ligament (Fig. 10.4).

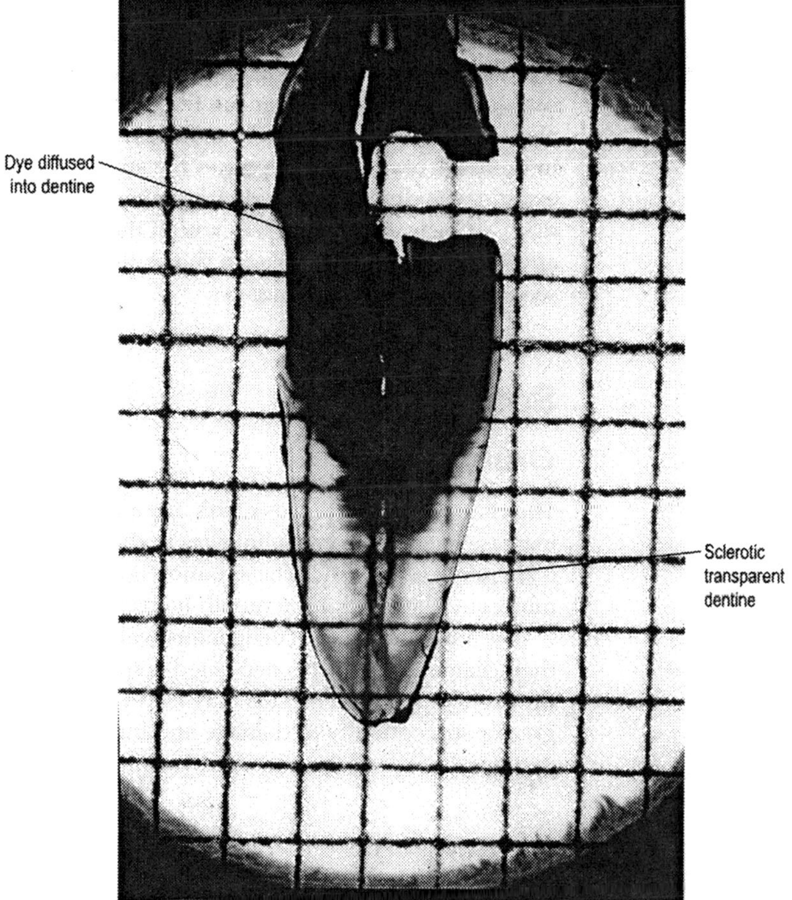

Fig. 14.1
Ground section of a tooth from an old individual. In the more coronal part dye placed in the pulp chamber has penetrated into dentine, but in the root the dentine is hypercalcified and the dye cannot penetrate. The hypercalcification or sclerosis renders the root transparent and the grid on the paper behind the tooth can be seen through the dentine.

The bone of the jaws

Loss of bone mineral – osteoporosis – is commonly associated with ageing. This occurs in the bone of the jaws

Changes of bone in ageing have been studied very extensively in women. Postmenopausal women frequently develop excessive loss of mineral from bone which manifests as osteoporosis. Between the ages of 45 and 90 years in both men and women the density of mandibular bone decreases from around 1.9 to around 1.5, but throughout these age ranges the density is some 8% less in women. These changes are parallel to those occurring in other bones such as the radius. The bone appears to be more brittle despite its lower overall density. The lamina dura is often lost and the cortical bone at the angle of the mandible becomes thinner. Histologically the mandibular bone is more *as well as elsewhere. Loss of the teeth will cause resorption of alveolar bone*

porous, principally due to an increase in the vascular spaces. The lacunae are decreased in number but occupy a greater total volume. The glycoprotein material in the lacunae is altered in its staining properties and the number of osteocytes is reduced. There are fewer but larger canaliculi in the bone. The walls of small blood vessels are thicker, and this, together with the reduction in numbers of canaliculi, reduces the supply of nutrients to the osteocytes and explains the diminution in their numbers. There is diffuse calcification in many of the canals of all sizes within the bone. The matrix of the bone is also affected by ageing: its collagen shows the typical increases in cross-linking seen in collagen in other tissues.

Soft tissues

Oral mucosa

The changes in oral mucosa with age are similar to those in skin. There is an increase in collagen cross-linkages in the dermis and a loss of elastin: the tissue is therefore less elastic. The situation is less acute than in skin because the moist environment of the mouth helps to maintain the turgor of the tissues.

The most marked changes in the oral mucosa with ageing are due to the ageing of collagen fibres

The stiffening of the collagenous walls of blood vessels and the decrease in their diameter as lipid is deposited combine to decrease the effective blood flow to the oral tissues. This may lead to a thinning of the mucosal layer and a greater susceptibility to damage and infection, a tendency enhanced by the poorer response of the immune system to new challenges.

Dental pulp

Changes in dental pulp are related to collagen fibre ageing, both directly and indirectly by its effects on the blood supply

Changes in the dental pulp in older individuals result from the progressive reduction in pulp size as secondary dentine advances into the pulp space, from changes in the fibres of its connective tissue, and from changes in blood supply and innervation (Fig. 14.2).

Change in size is also associated with a decrease in blood supply as the apical foramen is almost obliterated by secondary dentine and cementum. However, the age changes observed in the blood vessels themselves contribute to the poorer supply to the pulp. Indeed, there are reports of arteriosclerosis being observed in pulp blood vessels themselves. The number of blood vessels is reduced.

The number of cells in the pulp decreases with age in terms both of fibroblasts and of odontoblasts. The odontoblasts develop the so-called wheatsheaf appearance as intercellular and intracellular vacuoles appear. Calcified masses known as pulp stones are observed more frequently with age. They arise by calcification of collagen fibres, although some have a more dentine-like morphology with irregular tubules. It has been suggested that calcification is more likely where collagen fibres have a greater extent of cross-linking such as occurs in ageing.

The pulp decreases in size as more dentine is laid down

Despite reports that there is an increased amount of collagen in the aged dental pulp, the actual numbers of fibres is decreased. The aggregation of small fibrils into larger coarse fibrils in the smaller volume gives a false

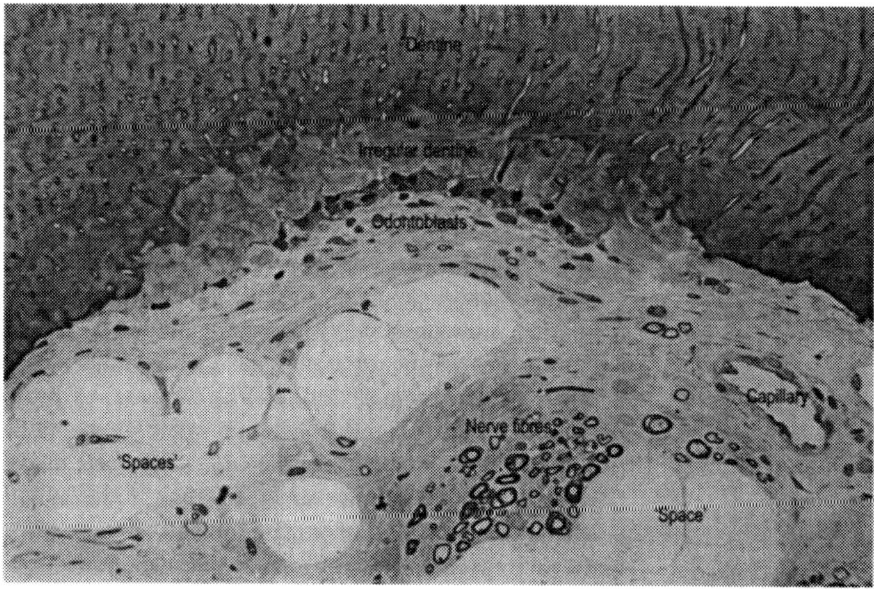

Fig. 14.2
Section through the dental pulp and dentine from an older individual. Compare this appearance with the young pulp shown in Fig. 4.1. There is loss of odontoblasts at the pulp/dentine interface, but where they remain there is irregular dentine formation. The pulp appears to have lost both fibres and cells. Blood vessels and nerves have thickened walls and the nerve sheaths in this section are showing signs of calcification. Eventually this will lead to irregular calcified deposits in the pulp.

impression of a relative increase in collagen. The rate of synthesis of collagen decreases and the existing fibres become more cross-linked. The major cross-link in human pulp collagen is dihydroxylysinonorleucine, one of the keto links referred to earlier. The amount of this cross-link increases up to the age of 40 years but decreases thereafter as other links are formed. The main collagen types in the dental pulp are types II and III; in animal observations the proportion of type III increases with age.

The number of nerve fibres decreases in the dental pulp as it ages and those which remain have thickened perineural sheaths.

Periodontal ligament

The width of the periodontal ligament decreases with age

The width of the periodontal ligament normally varies between 0.15 and 0.35 mm: this width is maintained in response to masticatory stresses. Thus, the width increases under greater masticatory loads and is less around teeth which are out of occlusal function. As cementum is laid down continuously throughout life the periodontal ligament should get narrower unless there is also resorption of an amount of alveolar bone equivalent to the amount of new cementum. This appears to be the case. However, the periodontal ligament is narrower in older individuals; this may be explained as being due to the operation of smaller masticatory forces in such individuals – but see later comments on this.

Oral functions

Salivary glands and salivary secretion

It has been known since the middle of the century that there are changes in salivary glands in older subjects. The histological changes described in the parotid, submandibular, sublingual and minor salivary glands vary slightly but the overall picture is similar. Ageing glands appear less compact with a relative loss of acinar tissue and an increase in fibrous and adipose tissue (Fig. 14.3). The relative volume occupied by ductal tissue is greater than in young glands. Some of these changes may be a result of the decreased blood supply consequent upon atherosclerosis in the salivary blood vessels, but changes still occur in glands with relatively non-affected vessels. Some ductal cells, and probably acinar cells also, transform into apparently non-functional cells termed oncocytes. They have a swollen appearance, eosinophilic staining and a central pyknotic nucleus. Mitochondria are extensive but few other organelles are present. Fat accumulation is observed in the acinar and ductal cells as well as in an infiltration of actual adipocytes.

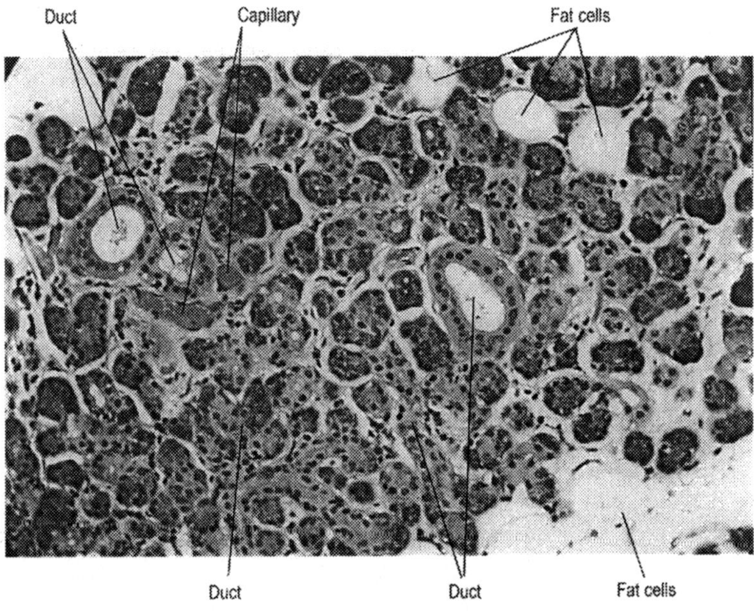

Section through a salivary gland from an older individual. The gland shows more connective tissue between the acini, the ducts are more prominent than in a younger gland and there appears to be loss of acinar tissue (compare Fig. 6.4).

In animals, focal collections of lymph cells accumulate with ageing, but in human glands lymphocytic cells are seen as single cells and as aggregations at all ages. Small plugs of protein material are found progressively more frequently in the ducts of the salivary glands. Sometimes these may calcify. They do not usually cause any problem and are lost in the normal process of salivary flow.

Saliva secretion by the parotid glands is little affected by age, although both resting and stimulated secretion by the other major glands is reduced

It is widely believed that salivary flow rates decrease with age. The evidence for this derives largely from estimates on large groups of subjects whose health and possible medication was not taken into account. More recent data from the ageing studies carried out on healthy non-medicated subjects suggest that there is little difference between stimulated whole saliva flow rates in subjects of widely differing ages. When flow from the individual salivary glands, however, is analysed the parotid glands behave differently from the other salivary glands. There is no change in salivary flow rates from the parotid glands in either the resting or the stimulated state, but both resting and stimulated flow from the other glands is reduced in older subjects. Despite this general observation the percentage increase between resting and stimulated flow rates in the older glands was greater than that in the younger. The increased incidence of xerostomia (dry mouth syndrome) in older patients probably relates, therefore, to disease or pharmacological causes, although it is possible that the slightly lower resting rate of flow of whole saliva may also give rise to a perception of dry mouth.

Changes in salivary composition are minor

There are minor changes in salivary composition with age (Table 14.1). In human stimulated parotid saliva there is a decrease in sodium concentration but no change in potassium concentration. Chloride and protein concentrations tend to be lower but the individual proteins which have been assayed separately – amylase and the acidic proline-rich proteins – show no change in concentration. This information comes from observations on groups of subjects carefully selected as being healthy and not receiving any medication. There are no data to suggest that the types of protein secreted in human saliva change as a result of ageing. However, in observations on less carefully selected, or at least less carefully defined, groups of subjects, there are reports of decreases in the absolute amounts of amylase and of acid DNase, and of changes in the proportions of different isozymes of amylase in older subjects. Animal experiments have shown a decreased uptake of

Table 14.1
Composition of stimulated parotid saliva from younger and older individuals

	Na	K	Protein (amylase)	Acidic proline-rich proteins
Males aged 40 years	30	16	3.22	0.43
Females aged 40 years	34	18	3.03	0.49
Males aged >60 years	20	18	2.67	0.41
Females aged >60 years	30	19	3.07	0.50

Concentrations of sodium and potassium are given in mmol/l, concentrations of amylase and acidic proline-rich proteins in g/l.

radioactive amino acids and a decreased rate of synthesis of exportable protein in older salivary glands.

Taste

Taste thresholds for salt and bitter are higher in older subjects, but those for sweet and acid are unaffected

Subjects frequently complain of a loss of taste sensation as they grow older. It has been known for many years that the number of taste buds declines with age. There is evidence that taste sensation is modified by nutritional state; this may account for some of the variations observed in elderly people. There is agreement, however, that the basic taste modalities of salt and bitter have increased thresholds in older subjects whilst the thresholds for sweet and acid remain very similar to those of younger subjects.

A related question is that of taste preferences; data suggest that older people find higher concentrations of salt and sugar more pleasant than do younger subjects.

Mastication and deglutition

The expected reduction in motor control in older subjects does not affect masticatory efficiency. This depends upon the maintenance of the dentition

In general, motor activity and motor control might be expected to be reduced in the elderly. This appears to be the case for the maintenance of lip seal and for swallowing, in that swallowing times are 25–50% longer in subjects over age 55 years. Masticatory efficiency as assessed by measuring the comminution of raw carrot after a fixed number of strokes and by the swallowing threshold performance index (the length of time a test food was chewed before swallowing) depends only upon the state of the dentition and there is very little difference between comparable older and younger subjects. There is an old report that biting force decreased to as little as 16% of its original value in older subjects, but no details of the experiment were given and this does not appear to have been further investigated.

Speech

Speech articulation is not affected by age, but the lower frequencies may be lost as tissue elasticity decreases

Although speech may be affected by changes in respiration and in the tissues of the mouth and larynx as people age, the process of articulation seems to be little affected. The main identifying feature of older speech is an increase in the fundamental frequencies. There is no obvious explanation of this unless it results from loss of elasticity in the tissues involved in phonation and articulation.

Further reading

The Aging Mouth. Ferguson, D.B. (editor). Karger, Basel, 1987

Index

Numbers in bold type indicate principal references where several are given; italic letters *f* and *t* refer to Figures and Tables respectively.

A

B

C

D

E

F

I

R

S

U

V

W

X

Y

Z

Printed in the United Kingdom
by Lightning Source UK Ltd.
127235UK00001B/133-140/A